Integrative Machine Learning and Optimization Algorithms for Disease Prediction

Anandhavalli Muniasamy
Department of Informatics and Computer Systems, College of Computer Science, King Khalid University, Saudi Arabia

IGI Global
Scientific Publishing
Publishing Tomorrow's Research Today

Vice President of Editorial Melissa Wagner
Director of Acquisitions Mikaela Felty
Director of Book Development Jocelynn Hessler
Production Manager Mike Brehm
Cover Design Jose Rosado

Published in the United States of America by
IGI Global Scientific Publishing
701 East Chocolate Avenue
Hershey, PA, 17033, USA
Tel: 717-533-8845
Fax: 717-533-7115
Website: https://www.igi-global.com E-mail: cust@igi-global.com

Library of Congress Cataloging-in-Publication Data

Names: Muniasamy, M. Anandhavalli editor
Title: Integrative machine learning and optimization algorithms for disease prediction / edited by Anandhavalli Muniasamy.
Description: Hershey, PA : IGI Global Scientific Publishing, 2026. | Includes bibliographical references and index. | Summary: "The integration of machine learning (ML) and optimization algorithms is revolutionizing healthcare, particularly in disease prediction, by enabling the development of predictive models that are both highly accurate and interpretable. As chronic and complex illnesses become more prevalent, these integrative approaches provide transformative solutions, leveraging large-scale biomedical data to uncover subtle patterns and relationships that traditional methods often miss"-- Provided by publisher.
Identifiers: LCCN 2024061592 (print) | LCCN 2024061593 (ebook) | ISBN 9798337310879 hardcover | ISBN 9798337310886 paperback | ISBN 9798337310893 ebook
Subjects: LCSH: Diagnosis--Data processing | Artificial intelligence--Medical applications | Machine learning
Classification: LCC RC78.7.D35 I5155 2025 (print) | LCC RC78.7.D35 (ebook) | DDC 616.07/50285--dc23/eng/20250423
LC record available at https://lccn.loc.gov/2024061592
LC ebook record available at https://lccn.loc.gov/2024061593

British Cataloguing in Publication Data
A Cataloguing in Publication record for this book is available from the British Library.

Table of Contents

Preface vii

Acknowledgment xi

Chapter 1
Introduction to Machine Learning and Optimization in Healthcare 1
Shruthi A. Gauthaman, Faculty of Medicine, Mahsa University, Malaysia
Anandhavalli Muniasamy, Department of Informatics and Computer Systems, College of Computer Science, King Khalid University, Saudi Arabia
Riyazdeen Kamaldheen, Faculty of Medicine, Mahsa University, Malaysia
Sakthynathan S. Magesh Kumar, Faculty of Medicine, Mahsa University, Malaysia
Kaurish Murugesan, Faculty of Medicine, Mahsa University, Malaysia
Mukesh Kumar Viswanathan, Faculty of Medicine, Mahsa University, Malaysia
Harini Devendran, Faculty of Medicine, Mahsa University, Malaysia

Chapter 2
Foundations of Integrative Machine Learning and Optimization for Disease Prediction 35
V. Dankan Gowda, Department of Electronics and Communication Engineering,BMS Institute of Technology and Management, Bangalore, India
B. N. Purushothamma, Faculty of Engineering, Management, and Technology (BGSIT), India
I. Nandhini, Department of Information Technology, V.S.B. Engineering College, Karur, India
Kottala Sri Yogi, Department of Operations, Symbiosis Institute of Business Management Hyderabad, India & Symbiosis International University, Pune, India
Venkatesan Hariram, Vinayaka Mission's Homoeopathic Medical College and Hospital, A Constituent College of Vinayaka Mission's Research Foundation University, Salem, India

Chapter 3
Overview of ML and Optimization Algorithms in Disease Prediction and a Comprehensive Review 63
J. Vijaya, International Institute of Information Technology, Naya Raipur, India
Pankaj Kumar Verma, International Institute of Information Technology, Naya Raipur, India
Rishi Thakur, International Institute of Information Technology, Naya Raipur, India
Shruti Soni, International Institute of Information Technology, Naya Raipur, India
Tripti Sharma, International Institute of Information Technology, Naya Raipur, India
Bhavya Chauhan, International Institute of Information Technology, Naya Raipur, India

Chapter 4
Optimization Methods in Healthcare Machine Learning: From Algorithms to Clinical Implementation........ 99
Jaswanth Sunkara, SRM Institute of Science and Technology, India
Anitha D., SRM Institute of Science and Techonology, India

Chapter 5
Optimization Algorithms for Feature Selection and Disease Prediction With Machine Learning 137
Pınar Özen Kavas, Kutahya Dumlupinar University, Turkey
Evin Şahin Şahin Sadık, Kutahya Dumlupinar University, Turkey

Chapter 6
Chronic Kidney Disease Prediction Using Machine Learning 169
G. Manodeepak, Hindusthan College of Arts and Science, India
A. V. Senthil Kumar, Hindusthan College of Arts and Science, India
Shanmugasundaram Hariharan, Vardhaman College of Engineering, India
Ismail Bin Musirin, Universiti Teknologi MARA, Malaysia
Shadi R. Masadeh, Isra University, Jordan
Rohaya Binti Latip, Universiti Putra Malaysia, Malaysia
Kyla Latrice Tennin, United Nations Peace Ambassador Foundation, USA & College of Doctoral Studies, University of Phoenix, USA & LMG, USA
Adnan Ibrahim Alrabea, Al-Balqa Applied University, Al-Salt, Jordan

Chapter 7
Acute Lymphoblastic Leukemia Classification With Deep Learning: Models Comparison 199
Prema Ganesan, Mepco Schlenk Engineering College, India
N. S. Hari Krishnaa, Mepco Schlenk Engineering College, India
S. Suraj Narayan, Mepco Schlenk Engineering College, India

Chapter 8
Harnessing Recurrent Neural Networks for Early Melanoma Diagnosis and Prevention 229
Sachin Sharma, Amity University, Mohali, India

Chapter 9
Revolutionizing Brain Tumor Diagnosis With Adaptive CNN Models 257
R. Kishore Kanna, Vel Tech Rangarajan Dr. Sagunthala R&D Institute of Science and Technology, Chennai, India
Priyanka Singh, Amity University, Noida, India
S. Raju, KPR Institute of Engineering and Technology, India
Ayodeji Olalekan Salau, Afe Babalola University, Nigeria & Saveetha Institute of Medical and Technical Sciences, Nigeria
Archibald Danquah Danquah-Amoah, Accra Technical University, Ghana
R. Gomalavalli, Sri Sai Ram institute of Technology, India
Sathea Sree, Vels Institute of Science, Technology, and Advanced Studies, India

Chapter 10
Improved Brain Tumor Segmentation Using Min-Max Normalization in a U-Net Architecture 287
K. Ramalakshmi, P.S.R. Engineering College, India
S. P. Santhoshkumar, VelTech Dr. Rengarajan Sagunthala R&D Institute of Science and Technology, India
L. Krishna Kumari, Ramco Institute of Technology, India
B. Mohan, P.S.R. Engineering College, India
S. P. Velmurugan, Kalasalingam Academy of Research and Education, India
Sravan Kumar Gunturi, Koneru Lakshmaiah Education Foundation, India
R. Subitha, AAA College of Engineering and Technology, India

Chapter 11
Advancing Mental Health Insights Through Machine Learning on EEG Data 315
Neepa Biswas, Department of Information Technology, Narula Institute of Technology, Kolkata, India
Suchismita Maiti, Department of Information Technology, Narula Institute of Technology, Kolkata, India
Sujata Kundu, Department of Information Technology, Narula Institute of Technology, Kolkata, India
Sudarsan Biswas, Department of Information Technology, RCC Institute of Information Technology, Kolkata, India

Chapter 12
Challenges and Future Directions: Emerging Trends and Limitations in ML and Optimization for Healthcare 339
Anandhavalli Muniasamy, College of Computer Science, King Khalid University, Saudi Arabia
Gauthaman Karunakaran, Government Pharmacy College, Sajong, India

Compilation of References 369

About The Contributors 407

Index 417

Preface

In recent years, the convergence of machine learning and optimization techniques has catalyzed unprecedented advances in healthcare, enabling more accurate, timely, and personalized disease prediction. As patient populations grow and clinical data proliferate in complexity and volume, innovative computational approaches are essential to extract actionable insights and to support clinicians in making data-driven decisions. **Integrative Machine Learning and Optimization Algorithms for Disease Prediction** seeks to chart this emerging landscape by presenting state-of-the-art methods, foundational principles, and real-world applications that span a broad spectrum of diseases and diagnostic challenges.

This book starts with an **Introduction to Machine Learning and Optimization in Healthcare**, setting the stage by elucidating the fundamental concepts, terminologies, and motivations that drive research at the intersection of data science and medicine. This chapter explores the integration of machine learning and optimization techniques for disease prediction in healthcare, highlighting key algorithms like SVMs, decision trees, and CNNs. It features a case study using a Kaggle dataset, where SVM achieved the highest accuracy, and discusses advanced topics such as explainable AI, federated learning, and ethical considerations in telemedicine applications.

Building upon these fundamentals, the chapter **Foundations of Integrative Machine Learning and Optimization for Disease Prediction** offers a rigorous exploration of the theoretical underpinnings that unify diverse algorithmic paradigms under a common framework for clinical inference. This chapter highlights the integration of machine learning and optimization techniques to improve disease prediction by enhancing model accuracy, efficiency, and interpretability. It reviews recent advances in feature selection and hyperparameter tuning using methods like genetic algorithms, PSO, and simulated annealing, and discusses their effectiveness in handling large medical datasets and improving prognosis for chronic and infectious diseases.

Having established this conceptual grounding, **Overview of ML and Optimization Algorithms in Disease Prediction: A Comprehensive Review** surveys the landscape of supervised, unsupervised, and hybrid learning models, alongside classical and evolutionary optimization strategies. Readers will gain an appreciation for how these algorithms are tailored to the unique statistical and regulatory demands of healthcare data. This chapter reviews the use of machine learning and optimization techniques to improve early disease diagnosis, focusing on the complexity of diseases, types of algorithms, medical data, and evaluation metrics. It highlights how these methods enhance timely and accurate detection, ultimately improving patient outcomes.

The next section—**Optimization Methods in Healthcare Machine Learning: From Algorithms to Clinical Implementation**—delves into practical considerations, from hyperparameter tuning and model calibration to resource-efficient deployment in clinical settings. This chapter explores various optimization techniques in healthcare machine learning, highlighting their applications in diagnosis, treatment, imaging, and resource management. It also addresses important implementation issues like privacy, fairness, and stakeholder involvement, and reviews emerging technologies and regulatory challenges, providing a holistic view of optimization's role in improving healthcare delivery.

In **Optimization Algorithms for Feature Selection and Disease Prediction with Machine Learning**, the focus shifts to high-dimensional data, exploring how feature selection and dimensionality-reduction techniques not only improve predictive performance but also enhance interpretability and trust in automated systems. This chapter highlights the importance of feature selection in healthcare machine learning, comparing filtering and wrapper methods and presenting a hybrid approach combining ReliefF and Genetic Algorithm. This method improves accuracy and efficiency in handling high-dimensional medical data, addressing challenges like overfitting and nonlinear relationships.

Building on these cross-cutting methods, the book then presents a series of disease-specific case studies. **Chronic Kidney Disease Prediction Using Machine Learning** examines risk stratification and early detection models. This chapter develops and evaluates a chronic kidney disease prediction model using Random Forest combined with a perceptron to handle missing clinical data. It compares this approach to other machine learning methods, demonstrating improved accuracy and robustness for early CKD detection. The chapter **Acute Lymphoblastic Leukemia Classification with Deep Learning: Models Comparison** highlights the comparative strengths of convolutional and hybrid architectures in hematologic oncology. This chapter investigates the application of deep learning models—VGG16, VGG19, InceptionV3, and MobileNetV2—for the classification and staging of Acute Lymphoblastic Leukemia (ALL) using a specialized image dataset. The study focuses on a two-step approach: first distinguishing benign from malignant cases, and then further classifying malignant samples into three stages—Early, Pre, and Pro. Performance is rigorously evaluated through metrics including accuracy, precision, recall, and confusion matrices, providing insights into the effectiveness of these models for improving ALL diagnosis and staging.

Harnessing Recurrent Neural Networks for Early Melanoma Diagnosis and Prevention demonstrates how sequence modeling can capture temporal patterns in patient history and imaging data. This chapter introduces an RNN-based framework for early melanoma detection, demonstrating high accuracy, sensitivity, and specificity. Designed to support clinicians and individuals, the system offers real-time detection with a user-friendly interface, enhancing timely diagnosis and treatment of this deadly skin cancer. **Revolutionizing Brain Tumor Diagnosis with Adaptive CNN Models** showcases adaptive learning strategies for radiographic interpretation, and presents an AI-based system for brain tumor detection using transfer learning with ResNet-152, DenseNet-121, and MobileNet models. ResNet-152 achieved the highest accuracy and reliability, while even the smaller MobileNet proved effective for resource-limited healthcare settings, demonstrating AI's potential to improve early brain tumor diagnosis.

Deepening the discussion of neuro-oncology, **Improved Brain Tumor Segmentation Using Min-Max Normalization in a U-Net Architecture** describes the integration of pre-processing techniques and specialized convolutional networks to achieve finer delineation of tumor boundaries. This chapter presents an improved UNet-based deep learning model for accurate brain tumor segmentation from MRI scans, achieving high performance with an 88.7% dice coefficient and 98.7% accuracy, offering a reliable tool to support early detection and treatment planning. **Advancing Mental Health Insights Through Machine Learning on EEG Data** ventures into neurophysiology and affective computing, illustrating how machine-learning pipelines can decode complex neural signals to inform psychiatric assessment. This chapter explores the application of machine learning techniques for classifying mental states using electroencephalography (EEG) data, highlighting its significance in neuroscience, cognitive psychology, and human-computer interaction. Seven algorithms—including decision tree, random forest, AdaBoost, K Nearest Neighbour, Naïve Bayes, Support Vector Machine, and Artificial Neural Network—were evaluated on a public EEG dataset. Among these, the random forest algorithm achieved the highest accuracy of 96%, demonstrating strong potential for advancing mental health diagnosis, treatment, and overall well-being.

Finally, **Challenges and Future Directions: Emerging Trends and Limitations in ML and Optimization for Healthcare** reflects on the ethical, technical, and regulatory hurdles that remain, and posits a roadmap for future inquiry. This chapter examines the key challenges limiting the widespread adoption of machine learning and optimization in healthcare, including issues related to data quality, model generalization, and computational constraints. It emphasizes the complexities of integrating diverse data sources such as electronic health records, wearable devices, and medical imaging, alongside the critical need for interpretable models that clinicians can trust. Addressing ethical, social, and equity considerations, the chapter explores emerging solutions like multimodal data integration, explainable AI, federated learning, hybrid models, and real-time edge computing. It concludes by highlighting future directions involving advanced model architectures, quantum computing, and interdisciplinary collaboration to foster responsible and effective healthcare innovations.

This book is intended for researchers, clinicians, data scientists, and graduate-level students who seek both foundational knowledge and applied insights into the integrative use of machine learning and optimization for disease prediction. We trust that the diverse perspectives and in-depth examples presented here will inspire new innovations and foster the responsible deployment of computational methods in healthcare.

Anandhavalli Muniasamy
Department of Informatics and Computer Systems, College of Computer Science, King Khalid University, Saudi Arabia

Acknowledgment

With heartfelt thanks, we give all praise to God. We express our deepest gratitude to the researchers, data scientists, and healthcare experts whose dedicated contributions form the foundation of this book. Special thanks to our peer reviewers, who provided critical insights and helped refine each chapter to ensure its academic rigor and practical relevance.

We gratefully acknowledge the invaluable support from various organizations and sources that provided data, tools, and case studies essential to the development of this compilation. Our sincere thanks also go to our publishers for their unwavering encouragement and guidance throughout the publishing process.

Last but not least, we extend heartfelt appreciation to our families and colleagues whose unwavering patience and support made the completion of this book possible.

Chapter 1

Introduction to Machine Learning and Optimization in Healthcare

Shruthi A. Gauthaman
https://orcid.org/0009-0007-5483-4683
Faculty of Medicine, Mahsa University, Malaysia

Anandhavalli Muniasamy
https://orcid.org/0000-0001-8940-3954
Department of Informatics and Computer Systems, College of Computer Science, King Khalid University, Saudi Arabia

Riyazdeen Kamaldheen
Faculty of Medicine, Mahsa University, Malaysia

Sakthynathan S. Magesh Kumar
Faculty of Medicine, Mahsa University, Malaysia

Kaurish Murugesan
https://orcid.org/0009-0003-3572-9205
Faculty of Medicine, Mahsa University, Malaysia

Mukesh Kumar Viswanathan
https://orcid.org/0009-0004-6483-8934
Faculty of Medicine, Mahsa University, Malaysia

Harini Devendran
https://orcid.org/0009-0007-7867-176X
Faculty of Medicine, Mahsa University, Malaysia

ABSTRACT

Machine learning (ML) and optimization techniques are revolutionizing healthcare by improving prediction accuracy and treatment efficiency. This chapter examines the evolution, integration, and application of ML algorithms—such as decision trees, SVMs, and neural networks—alongside optimization methods like linear program-

DOI: 10.4018/979-8-3373-1087-9.ch001

ming and genetic algorithms in healthcare settings. A case study using a Kaggle dataset highlights ML's role in disease prediction, utilizing data preprocessing, PCA for dimensionality reduction, and a CNN for feature extraction. CART, SVM, and Logistic Regression models were tested, with SVM achieving the highest accuracy (99.63% training, 97.62% testing). The chapter also explores explainable AI, federated learning, and real-time optimization in telemedicine, while addressing ethical issues, regulatory compliance, and equitable access—emphasizing their collective impact on the future of healthcare.

INTRODUCTION

Machine learning, a powerful branch of artificial intelligence, uses algorithms to analyze data, learn from it, and make predictions. Along with optimization techniques, it's driving significant advancements in healthcare. ML refers to the use of algorithms and statistical models to enable systems to perform tasks without explicit instructions, relying instead on patterns and inference from data. Optimization, on the other hand, involves finding the best solution to a problem from a set of feasible options, often by minimizing or maximizing an objective function. Optimization involves finding the best solution by minimizing or maximizing an objective function while satisfying given constraints. The solution space represents the set of all possible solutions that meet these requirements.

In healthcare, these technologies are applied to improve patient outcomes, streamline operations, and reduce costs. The scope of ML and optimization in healthcare spans diagnostics, treatment planning, drug discovery, resource allocation, and personalized medicine, among others. For instance, ML algorithms can analyze medical images to detect diseases like cancer, while optimization techniques can help hospitals allocate resources such as beds and staff more efficiently (Topol, 2019). Figure 1 illustrates the broad applications of ML and optimization in healthcare, highlighting their interdisciplinary nature.

Figure 1. A diagram showing the interdisciplinary applications of ML and optimization in healthcare.

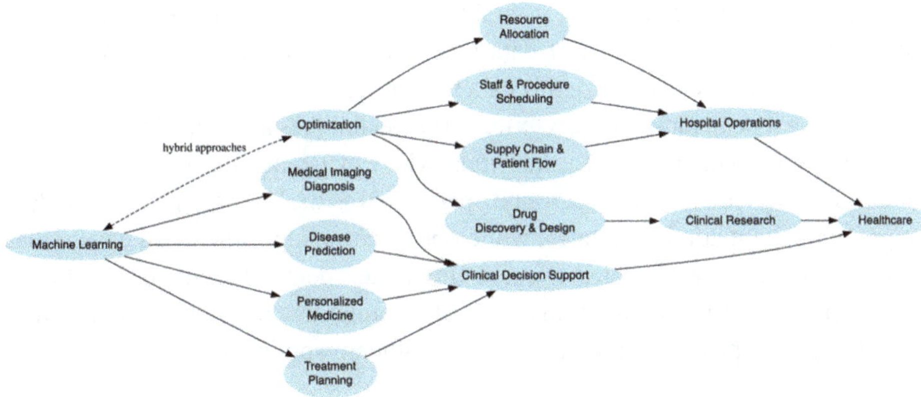

Machine learning offers various approaches to learn from data. One common method, supervised learning, involves training models on data with known labels. For example, a model could learn to diagnose diseases by analyzing medical records with confirmed diagnoses. Unsupervised learning identifies patterns in unlabeled data, useful for clustering patient populations based on similar characteristics. Reinforcement learning, which involves training models through trial and error, is increasingly used in robotic surgery and treatment optimization. Optimization techniques, such as linear programming, integer programming, and evolutionary algorithms, are used to solve complex decision-making problems. For example, linear programming can optimize the scheduling of surgeries to minimize waiting times, while evolutionary algorithms can design personalized treatment plans by exploring a vast space of possible solutions (Bishop, 2006).

The diagram illustrates the key components of machine learning and optimization and their relationships. The Machine Learning Components include data collection and preprocessing, feature engineering and selection, ML model training and evaluation, and hyperparameter tuning. The Optimization Components consist of optimization objective formulation, optimization algorithms such as gradient descent, constraints and regularization, and solution evaluation and selection. The Key Interactions between these components highlight that loss functions and performance metrics serve as the central bridge between machine learning and optimization. The optimization process plays a crucial role in hyperparameter tuning, while constraints and regularization guide the search process. Additionally, feedback loops exist between solution evaluation and model training, ensuring continuous improvement in model performance.

The relevance of ML and optimization in healthcare lies in their ability to handle large volumes of data and complex decision-making processes. With the advent of electronic health records (EHRs), wearable devices, and genomic data, healthcare systems generate vast amounts of data that can be leveraged to improve patient care. ML algorithms can analyze this data to identify trends, predict outcomes, and support clinical decision-making. Optimization techniques are crucial for resource-constrained environments, such as hospitals, where efficient allocation of resources can significantly impact patient care and operational costs. For example, ML models can predict patient admission rates, while optimization algorithms can ensure that hospital resources are allocated to meet anticipated demand (Jiang et al., 2017). Figure 2 presents a conceptual framework illustrating how machine learning (ML) and optimization processes interact within healthcare applications.

Figure 2. Conceptual framework of how ML and optimization process in healthcare

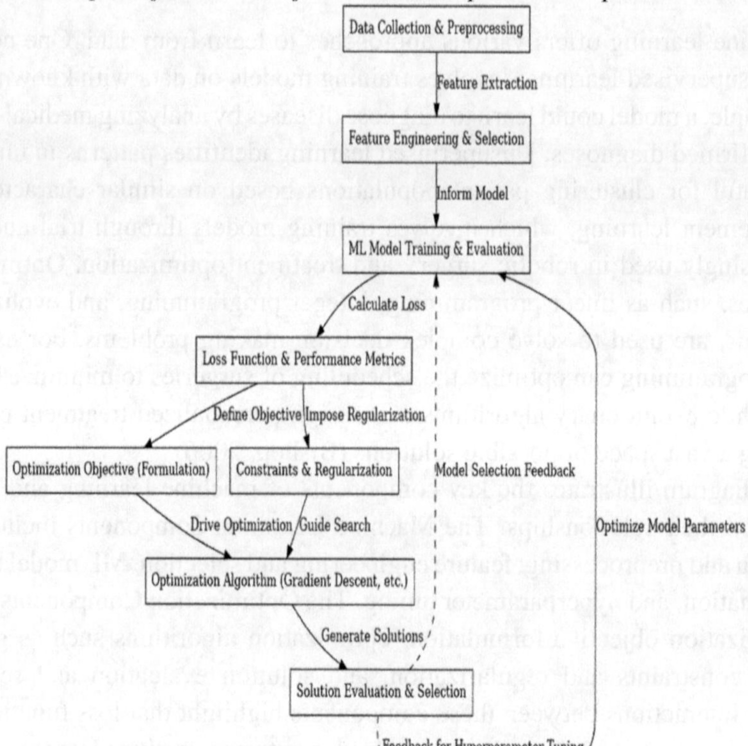

Unique Challenges in Healthcare: Despite their potential, the application of ML and optimization in healthcare faces unique challenges. One major challenge is the quality and availability of data. Healthcare data is often incomplete, inconsistent, or fragmented across different systems, making it difficult to train reliable ML models. Privacy and ethical concerns also arise, as patient data is highly sensitive and subject to strict regulations like HIPAA and GDPR. Additionally, the interpretability of ML models is a significant issue in healthcare, where decisions can have life-or-death consequences. Clinicians are often reluctant to trust "black-box" models that cannot explain their predictions. Optimization in healthcare also faces challenges due to the dynamic and uncertain nature of medical environments, where patient conditions and resource availability can change rapidly (Obermeyer & Emanuel, 2016). Figure 3 highlights the challenges of data quality and model interpretability in healthcare applications.

Figure 3. Challenges of data quality and model interpretability in healthcare applications.

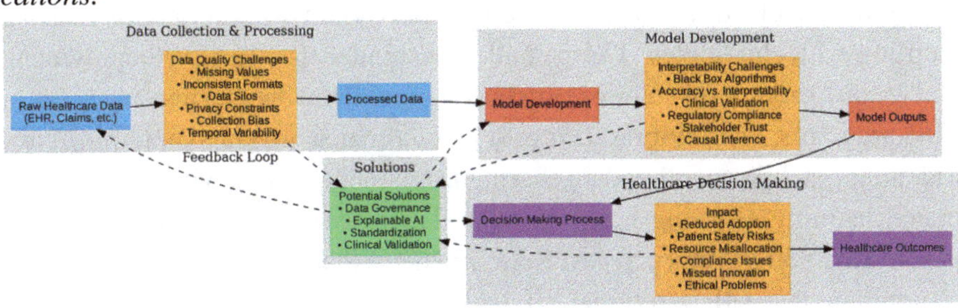

The flow from raw healthcare data through various challenges to healthcare outcomes, organized in four main clusters. The dashed lines represent how solutions can address challenges at various points in the process and create feedback loops for continuous improvement.

The integration of machine learning (ML) and optimization in healthcare begins with data collection and processing, where raw healthcare data, such as electronic health records (EHR) and insurance claims, is gathered. However, this data often flows through significant quality challenges, including missing values, inconsistent formats, and fragmentation across systems. These issues must be addressed through preprocessing steps like data cleaning, normalization, and integration, ultimately resulting in processed data that is suitable for analysis. Once the data is prepared, the next stage is model development, where the processed data is used to train ML algorithms. This phase faces its own set of challenges, particularly around interpretability.

Many advanced ML models, such as deep neural networks, operate as "black boxes," making it difficult for clinicians to understand how predictions are made. This creates a trade-off between model accuracy and interpretability, which can hinder trust and adoption. Despite these challenges, the model development process produces outputs that are intended to inform decision-making. In the healthcare decision-making stage, these model outputs are integrated into clinical and operational processes. However, the lack of interpretability and potential inaccuracies can lead to reduced adoption by healthcare providers and even pose risks to patient safety. These factors ultimately affect healthcare outcomes, potentially limiting the effectiveness of ML-driven interventions.

Bias in ML models remains a significant challenge in healthcare, where biased training data can lead to skewed outcomes, particularly for minority groups. Real-world examples, such as AI-driven skin cancer detection models underperforming for Black patients, highlight the urgent need for bias mitigation strategies like balanced datasets and fairness-aware algorithms. Real-world implementation of ML in healthcare faces barriers such as data interoperability, where hospitals struggle to integrate diverse electronic health record (EHR) systems, and clinician resistance to adopting AI technologies. These challenges hinder the effective deployment of AI and require thoughtful solutions such as standardized data formats and clinician training programs. Privacy-preserving AI plays a critical role in maintaining patient confidentiality while enabling data sharing for model training, with techniques like federated learning allowing hospitals to collaborate on AI development without compromising patient data privacy. Reinforcement learning (RL) and hybrid models, combining RL with traditional ML techniques, offer promising applications in areas like treatment optimization, robotic surgery, and decision-making systems that dynamically adapt to patient needs and improve healthcare delivery. These advanced models represent the future of personalized and efficient healthcare solutions.

The case study on AI bias highlights real-world examples, such as diagnostic models that underperformed for minority populations, leading to health disparities. Bias mitigation strategies like balanced datasets and fairness-aware algorithms are essential in ensuring equitable healthcare outcomes. AI model integration faces challenges in achieving interoperability, with standards like FHIR aiming to address data compatibility, but numerous deployment failures still occur due to inadequate system integration and clinician resistance. Regulatory challenges, including varying frameworks across regions, create complexities in AI adoption, with the FDA playing a crucial role in approving AI models for clinical use, ensuring safety and efficacy. Federated learning enables collaborative AI model development without sharing sensitive patient data, offering a privacy-preserving solution for healthcare AI. Explainable AI (XAI) provides transparency, helping clinicians trust AI-driven decisions, while emerging trends like AI in telemedicine and generative AI are revolutionizing remote healthcare (Muniasamy & Asiri, 2025) and creating synthetic data to overcome data limitations in rare diseases.

To address these challenges, potential solutions can be implemented at each stage. For example, robust data governance frameworks can improve data quality during collection and processing, while explainable AI (XAI) techniques can enhance model interpretability during development. Additionally, feedback loops can be established to ensure that insights from decision-making and outcomes inform earlier stages, such as refining data collection practices or improving model training processes. This iterative approach ensures that solutions are continuously refined, creating a more effective and trustworthy integration of ML and optimization in healthcare.

The key Objectives of the Chapter are as follows:

- Explain the concepts of machine learning (ML) and optimization, outlining their significance, applications, and challenges in the healthcare sector.
- Provide an overview of commonly used ML algorithms (e.g., decision trees, support vector machines, neural networks) and optimization techniques (e.g., linear programming, genetic algorithms, gradient descent) with their healthcare-specific applications.
- Highlight the synergy between ML and optimization in solving complex healthcare challenges such as predicting patient outcomes and optimizing treatment plans.
- Demonstrate the application of ML models with optimized feature extraction using convolutional neural network (CNN) in disease prediction to determine the most effective predictive model.
- Explore recent advancements in ML and optimization, such as explainable AI, real-time optimization in telemedicine and remote monitoring.
- Discuss ethical considerations, regulatory compliance, and the necessity of equitable access to ML and optimization technologies in healthcare.

BACKGROUND

The historical development of machine learning (ML) and optimization in healthcare is rooted in the broader evolution of computational technologies and data science. Early applications of optimization in healthcare date back to the mid-20th century, with operations research techniques being used to solve logistical problems such as hospital resource allocation and scheduling. The advent of electronic health records (EHRs) in the 1960s and 1970s marked a significant milestone, providing a structured digital format for patient data that could be analyzed computationally. The rise of ML in the 1980s and 1990s, fueled by advancements in algorithms and computing power, enabled more sophisticated data analysis, particularly in areas like medical imaging and diagnostics. The 2000s saw the integration of ML with big data, as the proliferation of wearable devices, genomic data, and telemedicine generated vast amounts of health-related information. This era also witnessed the emergence of deep learning, which revolutionized tasks such as image recognition and natural language processing, further expanding ML's role in healthcare. Today, ML and optimization are integral to modern healthcare, driving innovations in predictive analytics, personalized medicine, and operational efficiency, while continuing to evolve with advancements in artificial intelligence and data-driven technologies (Topol, 2019; Jiang et al., 2017).

Progression of Machine Learning Techniques in Healthcare: From Rule-Based Systems to Deep Learning. It could include the following stages:

1. Rule-Based Systems (1960s–1980s):
   - o It depicts a simple decision tree or flowchart representing rule-based logic.
   - o Example: "If symptom X and Y are present, diagnose condition Z."
2. Statistical Learning Models (1980s–2000s):
   - o It represents algorithms like logistic regression, support vector machines (SVM), and k-nearest neighbors (KNN).
   - o Example: "Logistic regression for predicting disease risk based on patient data."
3. Modern Machine Learning (2000s–2010s):
   - o It includes representations of ensemble methods like random forests and gradient boosting.
   - o Example: "Random forests for analyzing electronic health records (EHRs)."
4. Deep Learning (2010s–Present):
   - o It illustrate a neural network with multiple layers, highlighting its complexity.
   - o Example: "Convolutional neural networks (CNNs) for medical image analysis."
5. Applications in Healthcare:
   - o Real-world applications, such as medical imaging, natural language processing (NLP), and genomics.
   - o Example: "Deep learning for tumor detection in MRI scans."

Milestones in Integrating ML and Optimization in Healthcare:

The integration of Machine Learning (ML) and optimization algorithms in healthcare has led to significant breakthroughs in diagnostics, personalized medicine, and operational efficiency. Over the past few decades, these technologies have evolved to transform patient care, improve decision-making, and enhance resource utilization.

One of the earliest milestones in ML-driven healthcare was the use of decision trees and support vector machines for medical diagnosis in the late 20th century. These techniques laid the groundwork for modern deep learning approaches used in image-based diagnostics. For instance, convolutional neural networks (CNNs) now achieve dermatologist-level accuracy in detecting skin cancer from medical images (Esteva et al., 2017). Similarly, ML models have been instrumental in detecting diabetic retinopathy and lung cancer, improving early diagnosis rates (Ardila et al., 2019).

Personalized medicine has seen remarkable progress due to ML and optimization techniques. The development of predictive models using genomic and clinical data enables tailored treatments based on an individual's genetic profile. Advances such as IBM Watson's AI-powered oncology solutions have demonstrated the potential of ML in recommending cancer treatment plans by analyzing vast datasets of medical literature and patient records (Kourou et al., 2015). Optimization algorithms further refine drug dosage calculations and treatment scheduling, ensuring maximum efficacy with minimal side effects.

Operational efficiency in healthcare has also benefited from ML and optimization. Hospitals utilize predictive analytics to forecast patient admissions and optimize staff scheduling, reducing overcrowding and enhancing service delivery. Optimization algorithms assist in resource allocation, such as optimizing emergency room workflows and streamlining supply chain management for pharmaceuticals (Topaloglu & Powell, 2006). AI-powered robotic systems now aid in minimally invasive surgeries, increasing precision and reducing recovery times (Rajeswaran et al., 2017).

Despite these milestones, challenges remain in integrating ML and optimization in healthcare, including data privacy concerns, model interpretability, and ethical considerations. As research progresses, future advancements will likely focus on enhancing transparency, improving interoperability between AI systems and medical professionals, and ensuring equitable access to AI-driven healthcare solutions. Figures illustrating ML applications in disease diagnostics, personalized treatment models, and hospital resource optimization can provide deeper insights into these advancements.

Commonly Used Machine Learning Algorithms in Healthcare:

Several ML algorithms play a crucial role in disease prediction and medical decision-making. Some of the most commonly used techniques include:

- Decision Trees: These hierarchical models classify data based on a sequence of decision rules. They are widely used in diagnosing diseases such as heart conditions and diabetes due to their interpretability (Quinlan, 1996).
- Support Vector Machines (SVMs): These algorithms identify optimal hyperplanes for classifying medical data, making them effective in detecting cancers and neurological disorders (Cortes & Vapnik, 1995).
- Neural Networks: Deep learning models, such as convolutional and recurrent neural networks, process complex medical images and sequential data, improving accuracy in radiology and genomics (LeCun et al., 2015).
- Random Forests: A collection of decision trees that enhance prediction stability and accuracy, frequently applied in medical risk assessment (Breiman, 2001).
- K-Nearest Neighbors (KNN): This algorithm classifies data based on similarity, commonly used in medical image retrieval and pattern recognition (Cover & Hart, 1967).

Optimization Techniques and Their Healthcare Adaptations:

Optimization techniques ensure efficient resource allocation, scheduling, and treatment planning in healthcare. Some widely used methods include:

- Linear Programming: A mathematical approach to optimizing hospital resource management, such as staffing and supply chain logistics (Dantzig, 1963).
- Genetic Algorithms: Inspired by evolutionary principles, these algorithms optimize treatment protocols and medical imaging enhancements by evolving the best solutions (Holland, 1975).
- Gradient Descent: A fundamental optimization technique in deep learning, enabling neural networks to learn from medical data and refine diagnostic accuracy (Rumelhart et al., 1986).
- Integer Programming: Used in radiation therapy planning to optimize dosage schedules while minimizing adverse effects (Lv et al., 2017).
- Simulated Annealing: Applied in medical image registration and surgery planning, finding optimal solutions by mimicking physical annealing processes (Kirkpatrick et al., 1983).

These ML and optimization algorithms continue to shape healthcare advancements, ensuring precise diagnostics, efficient treatment plans, and enhanced operational performance. Future research should focus on hybrid approaches that combine ML's predictive power with optimization's efficiency for better healthcare delivery.

Commonly used deep learning algorithms in healthcare

Deep learning algorithms have gained prominence in healthcare applications due to their ability to process vast amounts of unstructured data and identify complex patterns. Some of the widely used deep learning algorithms include:

- Convolutional Neural Networks (CNNs): Primarily used for medical image analysis, CNNs have shown exceptional performance in detecting diseases such as diabetic retinopathy, pneumonia, and skin cancer by analyzing radiological scans and dermatological images (Krizhevsky et al., 2012).
- Recurrent Neural Networks (RNNs) and Long Short-Term Memory (LSTM) Networks: These models are effective in analyzing sequential medical data such as electrocardiograms (ECGs) and electronic health records (EHRs) for predictive analytics and anomaly detection (Hochreiter & Schmidhuber, 1997).
- Autoencoders: Used for unsupervised learning, autoencoders help in feature extraction and anomaly detection in medical imaging and genomics (Hinton & Salakhutdinov, 2006).
- Transformers: These models, including BERT and GPT, have been applied in medical natural language processing (NLP) tasks such as clinical text summarization, medical chatbot development, and automated diagnosis reports (Vaswani et al., 2017).
- Generative Adversarial Networks (GANs): GANs generate synthetic medical images for training deep learning models, helping overcome data scarcity issues in medical imaging applications (Goodfellow et al., 2014).

Optimization techniques and their healthcare adaptations:

Optimization techniques are essential for enhancing the efficiency and effectiveness of deep learning models in healthcare. Some commonly used optimization methods include:

- Gradient Descent and Its Variants: Stochastic gradient descent (SGD), Adam, and RMSprop optimize deep learning models by adjusting weights to minimize loss functions. These techniques are crucial in training CNNs and RNNs for disease diagnosis and prognosis (Kingma & Ba, 2014).

- Bayesian Optimization: Applied in hyperparameter tuning for deep learning models, Bayesian optimization improves the accuracy of medical predictive models by selecting optimal hyperparameter configurations (Snoek et al., 2012).
- Genetic Algorithms: Inspired by natural evolution, genetic algorithms are used in optimizing treatment plans, feature selection for medical diagnosis, and neural architecture search (Holland, 1975).
- Particle Swarm Optimization (PSO): A bio-inspired algorithm that fine-tunes deep learning model parameters, PSO has applications in optimizing radiotherapy treatment planning and medical signal processing (Kennedy & Eberhart, 1995).
- Simulated Annealing: Employed in scheduling and resource allocation problems, this technique ensures efficient hospital management and treatment scheduling (Kirkpatrick et al., 1983).

These deep learning algorithms and optimization techniques continue to drive innovation in healthcare, enhancing diagnostic accuracy, improving patient outcomes, and optimizing hospital resource management. The future of AI-driven healthcare will likely focus on integrating interpretable and ethical AI models to ensure trust and reliability in clinical decision-making.

Examples of ML and Optimization in Healthcare:

- **Predicting Patient Outcomes:** Predicting patient outcomes, such as the likelihood of recovery, disease progression, or risk of complications, is one of the primary applications of ML. For example, ML models can analyze patient data to predict the probability of a patient developing diabetic retinopathy based on features like glucose levels, age, and blood pressure (Kumari & Upadhayay, 2025). Once these models provide predictions, optimization methods can be used to tailor individual patient care plans. For instance, Bayesian Optimization can be employed to find the optimal parameters for a treatment regimen that maximizes the chance of recovery based on predicted patient outcomes (Jones et al., 1998).
- **Optimizing Treatment Plans:** Personalized treatment plans are another area where the synergy between ML and optimization can have a significant impact. ML algorithms can process patient data to predict how a patient will respond to different treatments based on factors such as genetics, past treatments, and comorbidities. For example, in cancer treatment, deep learning models can

predict which chemotherapy regimen would be most effective for a specific patient by analyzing genomic data and other clinical variables (Vamathevan et al., 2019). After predicting the likely outcomes, optimization techniques can be used to fine-tune the treatment strategy. Linear Programming can help optimize schedules for chemotherapy sessions, ensuring that resources are used effectively, minimizing wait times for patients, and avoiding overuse or underuse of treatment protocols (Kolasa et al., 2023). By combining ML for prediction and optimization for decision-making, healthcare providers can offer treatments that are not only tailored to the individual patient but also efficiently managed at the healthcare system level.

- **Optimizing Healthcare Resource Allocation:** Another critical application of ML and optimization synergy is in the allocation of healthcare resources. ML can predict patient demand for services based on historical data, seasonal trends, and demographics, while optimization techniques can determine the best allocation of resources, such as staff, hospital beds, and medical equipment, to meet that demand efficiently. For example, ML models can predict the number of patients likely to require intensive care at any given time, and optimization models can be used to allocate ICU beds, ventilators, and medical staff to maximize patient throughput and minimize resource wastage (Rajagopal, et al., 2024).
- **Surgical Scheduling Optimization:** Surgical scheduling is a complex task involving various constraints, including surgeon availability, operating room time, patient urgency, and the complexity of procedures. Machine learning models can predict surgery durations and recovery times based on patient history and the type of surgery. Using this data, optimization algorithms, such as constraint programming or mixed-integer linear programming, can schedule surgeries to minimize delays, reduce operating room idle time, and ensure timely interventions for critical cases (Al Amin et al., 2024).

The synergy between machine learning and optimization provides a powerful framework for addressing complex healthcare challenges. While machine learning excels at predicting patient outcomes and uncovering hidden patterns in data, optimization techniques fine-tune those predictions and ensure the best decision-making processes, from personalized treatment planning to efficient resource allocation. This integration can significantly enhance patient care, improve operational efficiency, and reduce healthcare costs. As healthcare continues to evolve, the collaboration between ML and optimization will play an increasingly vital role in transforming clinical practices and healthcare delivery systems.

Federated learning offers a robust solution for secure data-sharing in healthcare by enabling collaborative model training without centralizing sensitive patient data, ensuring compliance with regulations like GDPR and HIPAA. This approach allows hospitals and healthcare institutions to work together on AI development while maintaining patient confidentiality. Real-world examples of AI bias in healthcare, such as diagnostic models underperforming for specific demographic groups, emphasize the need for explainable AI techniques like SHAP and LIME, which provide transparency and accountability in AI-driven decisions. A hybrid ML-optimization case study, combining machine learning with optimization techniques, demonstrates practical applications in resource allocation and patient treatment planning, offering more efficient and personalized healthcare solutions. Emerging trends in healthcare AI, such as reinforcement learning, federated learning, and generative AI, are revolutionizing areas like autonomous treatment optimization, secure data-sharing, and synthetic data generation for rare disease research. AI's increasing role in telemedicine is enhancing remote healthcare by enabling virtual diagnoses, continuous patient monitoring, and improving access to healthcare in underserved regions.

CASE STUDY

This study focuses on developing a model to accurately predict 40 different diseases. The model analyzes relevant features to determine the presence or absence of these diseases. The primary objective is to develop a model that can accurately classify and identify various medical conditions based on patient data. Figure 4 illustrates the workflow, encompassing data processing, feature selection, model training, and prediction. This approach aims to improve diagnostic accuracy and assist healthcare professionals.

Figure 4. Proposed human disease prediction system.

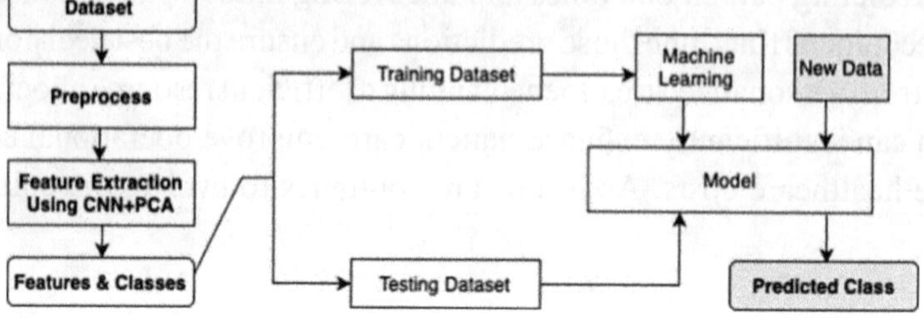

- **Dataset**

The study utilizes a human disease dataset (Dataset, 2025) containing 4,920 patient records, each with 132 features representing various symptoms, and a final column indicating one of 40 possible diagnoses. This dataset enables the model to learn relationships between symptoms and diseases for accurate prediction.

- **Data Preprocessing**

The data preprocessing steps encompassed handling missing values, dimensionality reduction, encoding categorical data, standardizing data, and splitting it into training and testing sets. Additionally, feature selection was performed to identify the most relevant variables for disease prediction before training machine learning models. During the data cleaning phase, the dataset was thoroughly examined for incomplete entries to ensure data integrity, which was essential given its size. Notably, the dataset contained no missing values, allowing for a more reliable analysis and model training.

- **Data Normalization**

It was applied using the formula $z = (x - \mu) / \sigma$, where μμ represents the mean of the training samples and σσ is the standard deviation, ensuring consistent scaling of features.

- **Dimensionality Reduction**

It was achieved through Principal Component Analysis (PCA) (Jolliffe, 2002), which projects high-dimensional data into a lower-dimensional space while preserving most of the original variance. PCA identifies principal components (PCs) that maximize variance, with the first PC capturing the highest variance and subsequent PCs remaining orthogonal to maximize data representation. This approach helps generate more independent feature sets, reducing the risk of high correlation among variables.

- **Labeling Disease Classes**

It was accomplished using one-hot encoding, a technique that converts categorical values into binary columns, where 1 indicates the presence of a category and 0 signifies its absence. This method eliminates any implied ordinal relationships between categorical values, allowing machine learning models to correctly interpret and learn from the data without assuming hierarchical associations among variables.

- **Optimize Feature Extraction using CNN**

The basic convolution neural network (CNN) architecture which involves feature extraction and classification is illustrated in Figure 5. For this study, CNN with 1D (one dimension) has been used to work various symptom variables of the dataset for feature extraction. The proposed CNN architecture which consists of 2 convolution layers, followed by MaxPooling and Flatten layers. The principal component analysis (PCA) feature selection generated 1D numerical array each features that is used as an input for the CNN model and move with Flatten layer to shape up how the input variables are going to be represented through the Dense layer using 16 filters of 'relu' activation function. For the multi-class classification, fully connected 'Dense' sequents followed by 'Softmax' layer funtion. In “Dense” layer, for each neuron, outputs weighted sum of all input symptom variables resulting in the Disease prognosis types mixed on an equal proportion.

Figure 5. Basic CNN architecture.

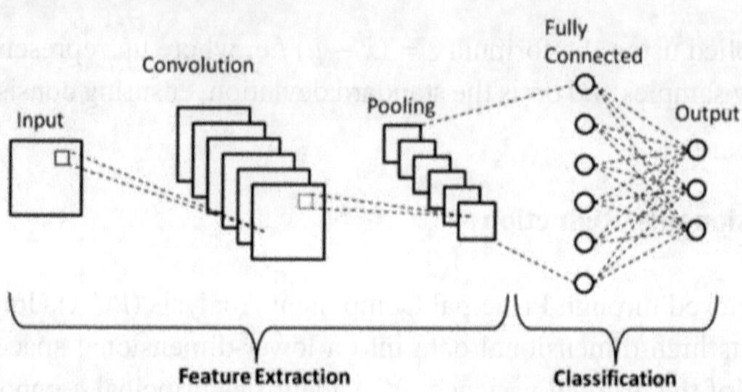

Table 1 shows the hyperparameters used for the proposed CNN model, which provides the insights into the configuration and tuning of the network for optimal performance.

Table 1. Hyperparameter Values of the Proposed CNN model

Parameter	Values
Epochs	10
Pooling	MaxPooling with size 2
Convolution layer activation	Relu
Dropout	0.3
Filters	32
Dense layer activation	SoftMax
Compiler optimizer	Adam
Compiler loss	Categorical cross entropy

- **Machine Learning Models**

Three models classes have been trained on the dataset; these three models are CART, SVM and Logistic Regression. The models were done in python 3, using the sklearn modules which provide a powerful set of tools for machine learning. The SVM model, recognized for its capacity to manage high-dimensional data, identifies an appropriate hyperplane to distinguish the classes. Logistic Regression, a commonly used approach for binary classification, was utilized to forecast the probability of disease. Each of these models was trained and evaluated to identify the most accurate and efficient approach for disease prediction.

Classification and Regression Trees (CART): CART is a unique machine learning algorithm which can be applied for regression as-well classification models. CART assigns a class label to each leaf node based on majority classes of the observations falling into that leaf node. For regression tasks, the outcomes in the leaf nodes are averaged and return. CART model has broad usefulness across various domains such as healthcare or finance because it still retains simplicity with respect to both the calculation and representation of results (Davis & Hoh, 2020).

Logistic Regression (LR): Logistic Regression is a linear model predicts for the values of categorical response variables, that is a disease exists or not. It estimates the probability of the symptom variable taking a particular value. The output probability final value could be used to get the conclusion once for each input it is calculated after the logistic regression probability. This shows which category is more probable, 0 or 1 (Alquhtani & Muniasamy, 2022).

Support Vector Machines (SVM): SVM is the efficient technique to solve prediction of disease because it can work well with high dimensional data and nonlinear relationships. It utilizes the 'kernel trick', a method to solve non-linear separation problems by transforming the initial non-linearly separable points into a higher-dimensional space. Then, this modified feature space was classified using a linear classifier (Alquhtani & Muniasamy, 2022). It performs quite well when the classes are well separated in a feature space thus making it applicable to disease cases that show appropriate symptoms.

- **Performance Evaluation**

Table 2 recapitulates the evaluation metrics applied for the proposed ML models, which are crucial to understand and evaluate the predictive capabilities of trained ML models. As for evaluation, key metrics like Accuracy, Precision, Recall and F1-score are must when evaluating the model performance (Buckland & Gey, 1994). These metrics define the tradeoff between precision and recall as a background, hence it provides us to derive relevant formulas over this table. True negatives (TN) and true positives (TP) are those that were correctly classified, while false negatives (FN) and false positives (FP) represent samples that are incorrectly classified. In combination, the metrics represent a broad scope to assess the ubiquity of making exact predictions on trained models using execution time(ET).

Table 2. Performance Metrics Illustration

Name of the Metrics	Formula
Classification Accuracy	(TP+TN) / Total Records
Precision (PR)	TP / (TP + FP)
Recall (RE)	TP / (TP + FN)
F1-Score	2* [(PR*RE) / (PR + PE)]

- **Results and Analysis**

Table 3 presents the results of evaluating training and testing accuracy of all models. As the result states that 97.60% for testing accuracy and >99% for the training accuracy has achieved to predict the disease class correctly all. Precision score is high in the achieved result rate of false positive is less in the evaluation of the models, which means that misclassifying a negative disease case as positive (FP) costs less than misclassifying a positive case as negative (FN). Embracing a specific threshold of false positives can motivate individuals to get medical care promptly by notifying them about possible disease instances. Recall, which is critical for minimizing false negatives, was consistently high across all models, with a score of 97.62%. The F1-Score, a balanced metric that takes both precision and recall into account, was also considered, especially important for achieving a trade-off between false positives and false negatives. Our objective focused on accurately identifying positive disease cases, aiming to enhance recall while minimizing the impact on precision.

Table 3. Summary of Performance Metrics for ML classifiers

Model	Train_ accuracy	Test_ accuracy	AUC	ET	PR	RE	F1
SVM	0.997	0.976	0.999	0.42	98.80	97.62	97.62
CART	1.0	0.976	0.994	0.013	98.81	97.62	97.62
LR	1.0	0.976	1.0	2.31	98.80	97.62	97.62

The results indicate no major differences in the overall performance of the models regarding accuracy, precision, recall, and F1-Score. Our key objective is to precisely identify true disease cases while reducing false positives. An ideal model would exhibit a significantly high area under the curve (AUC) alongside high values in the other metrics. In this study, the LR model achieved the highest AUC of 100%, followed closely by the SVM at 99.9%. To determine the best classifier among the three, we also measured the elapsed time for the classification process. Notably, SVM consumed the least execution time. Consequently, we consider SVM to be the best classifier in this study, as it balances both high predictive performance and efficiency in execution.

The case study now focuses on deployment challenges, highlighting real-world difficulties such as data interoperability, integration with existing IT systems, and clinician resistance to adopting AI technologies. Privacy concerns are addressed, emphasizing the importance of secure data-sharing mechanisms like federated learning to maintain patient confidentiality while enabling AI advancements. Regulatory compliance is also explored, examining the role of frameworks like HIPAA and GDPR in shaping AI adoption in healthcare, ensuring that AI models meet stringent privacy and ethical standards.

SOLUTIONS AND RECOMMENDATIONS

Machine learning and deep learning are transforming healthcare by improving how clinicians make decisions and streamlining healthcare operations. These technologies address a broad range of challenges, from enhancing diagnostic accuracy and treatment planning to streamlining administrative tasks and improving patient outcomes. Below, we explore how ML and DL algorithms tackle these diverse challenges.

Improving Clinical Decision-Making

- Enhanced Diagnostic Accuracy: ML and DL algorithms can analyze vast amounts of medical data, including patient records, medical imaging, and laboratory results, to identify patterns that may be difficult for human clinicians to detect. Deep learning, specifically Convolutional Neural Networks (CNNs), excels at analyzing medical images like X-rays, MRIs, and CT scans, achieving highly accurate results. These algorithms can automatically detect abnormalities like tumors, fractures, and other pathologies, often outperforming human radiologists in accuracy and speed.
- Predictive Analytics for Early Diagnosis: ML models can predict the onset of diseases based on historical data. For example, predictive models for diabetes or cardiovascular diseases leverage patient data such as age, lifestyle factors, and genetic predispositions to identify high-risk individuals early. By providing early alerts, these algorithms enable timely intervention, potentially preventing disease progression and improving patient outcomes.
- Personalized Treatment Plans: ML and DL can help personalize treatment plans by analyzing individual patient data to recommend tailored therapies. In oncology, for example, algorithms can analyze genomic data to recommend the most effective treatment for specific cancer types, considering the patient's genetic makeup and the tumor's characteristics. This level of personalization improves treatment efficacy and reduces adverse reactions.
- Decision Support Systems: ML-powered decision support systems assist clinicians by suggesting potential diagnoses, treatment options, or drug prescriptions based on a patient's symptoms, medical history, and other relevant factors. These systems can also flag inconsistencies or errors in clinical decision-making, ensuring that the chosen course of action aligns with best practices and guidelines.

Synergy Between Machine Learning (ML) and Optimization in Healthcare

Machine learning (ML) and optimization techniques are increasingly being combined to address complex healthcare problems, demonstrating a powerful synergy in various domains. Both ML and optimization are fundamental to advancing healthcare technologies, but they serve different yet complementary roles. Machine learning focuses on learning from data to make predictions or classifications, while optimization seeks to fine-tune models and decisions to achieve the best possible outcomes. By combining these two approaches, healthcare systems can achieve more accurate predictions, personalized treatments, and optimized resource management, leading to better patient outcomes and reduced costs.

ML and Optimization Complement each other in the following ways

- ML in Predictive Analytics and Data Modeling: Machine learning algorithms excel in learning patterns from large datasets and can handle complex, high-dimensional information that is often encountered in healthcare. These models are capable of identifying relationships between patient characteristics (such as age, gender, genetic factors, and lifestyle habits) and disease outcomes. For instance, ML algorithms such as Random Forest, Support Vector Machines (SVM), and Neural Networks have been successfully used in predicting patient outcomes, such as predicting the onset of chronic diseases, post-surgical complications, or the progression of diseases like cancer or diabetes (Kolasa et al., 2023).
- Optimization in Model Calibration and Decision-Making: While ML models provide predictions, optimization techniques are used to fine-tune parameters, optimize model performance, and select the best course of action. In healthcare, optimization is often applied to adjust the hyperparameters of ML models or optimize decision-making processes, such as resource allocation or treatment planning. For example, optimization methods like Genetic Algorithms (GA), Particle Swarm Optimization (PSO), and Bayesian Optimization can help to adjust the parameters of ML models, such as the regularization term in SVMs or the learning rate in deep learning models, to enhance accuracy and generalization (Hastie et al., 2009).
- Integrating ML with Optimization to Solve Complex Healthcare Problems: The combination of ML and optimization enables solving multi-faceted problems in healthcare, such as predicting patient outcomes, optimizing treatment regimens, and managing healthcare resources. ML provides the predictive capabilities needed to model complex relationships between variables, while optimization refines the decision-making process to ensure the best possible results. A key example of this synergy can be seen in predicting patient outcomes and optimizing treatment plans. For instance, ML can be used to predict the likelihood of a patient developing a particular disease or experiencing a complication, while optimization techniques can help devise personalized treatment plans that take into account the patient's unique risk profile and maximize the chances of a favorable outcome.

Impact and Current Trends in Machine Learning, Optimization, and Healthcare Technologies

The integration of machine learning (ML) and optimization with healthcare systems is rapidly transforming clinical decision-making, patient care, and healthcare logistics. Recent advancements in technologies such as Explainable AI (XAI), Federated Learning, and Real-Time Optimization are driving improvements in telemedicine, remote monitoring, and various clinical applications. These innovations offer enhanced accuracy, transparency, and scalability while addressing pressing challenges in healthcare, including ethical considerations, regulatory compliance, and equitable access to technology.

Current Trends in Machine Learning, Optimization, and Healthcare Technologies

In recent years, the convergence of machine learning (ML), optimization algorithms, and healthcare technologies has significantly transformed the healthcare industry. These interdisciplinary advancements are driving innovations in diagnosis, treatment planning, operational efficiency, and patient care, marking a paradigm shift in how healthcare systems operate and deliver services. This article explores current trends in machine learning, optimization strategies, and healthcare technologies, emphasizing their integration and impact on modern medicine.

- **Machine Learning in Healthcare**

Machine learning, a subset of artificial intelligence (AI), plays a crucial role in extracting patterns from complex datasets and making data-driven predictions. In healthcare, ML is increasingly employed in diagnostic imaging, genomics, personalized medicine, drug discovery, and predictive analytics.

One of the most impactful applications is diagnostic imaging, where ML models—especially convolutional neural networks (CNNs)—achieve expert-level performance in interpreting radiographs, MRIs, and CT scans. These models are used for early detection of conditions such as cancer, neurological disorders, and cardiovascular diseases.

Natural language processing (NLP) is another key area, facilitating the extraction of meaningful insights from unstructured clinical notes, electronic health records (EHRs), and medical literature. Tools like BERT-based models and GPT variants are used to automate clinical documentation and decision support.

Moreover, ML is instrumental in predictive analytics, helping clinicians anticipate patient deterioration, readmission risks, or disease progression. These models improve care by enabling timely interventions, particularly in chronic disease management.

- **Optimization Techniques in Healthcare**

Optimization algorithms are essential in solving complex healthcare challenges where resources are limited and outcomes are critical. Recent trends highlight the use of both classical and evolutionary optimization techniques, such as linear programming, genetic algorithms, particle swarm optimization, and reinforcement learning.

Resource allocation and scheduling represent key application domains. Hospitals use optimization models to streamline staff scheduling, allocate operating rooms efficiently, and manage ICU bed utilization. These efforts reduce costs, minimize patient wait times, and improve care delivery.

In treatment planning, especially in radiation therapy and chemotherapy, optimization algorithms help personalize dosages and schedules to maximize efficacy while minimizing adverse effects. Multi-objective optimization techniques are particularly valuable in balancing conflicting goals, such as treatment intensity versus patient comfort.

Supply chain and logistics optimization has gained momentum, especially post-COVID-19, ensuring the timely delivery of medical supplies, vaccines, and equipment through smart inventory control and transportation planning.

- **Emerging Healthcare Technologies**

Recent advances in healthcare technologies are characterized by the integration of AI, the Internet of Medical Things (IoMT), wearable devices, robotics, and blockchain.

Wearable health technologies, such as smartwatches, fitness trackers, and biosensors, continuously collect physiological data including heart rate, blood pressure, glucose levels, and oxygen saturation. This data is fed into ML models to monitor patient health in real time, detect anomalies, and provide personalized health recommendations.

IoMT connects medical devices and systems to facilitate real-time data sharing between patients and providers. It improves chronic disease monitoring, remote diagnostics, and telemedicine—expanding access to care, especially in rural or underserved regions.

Robotic-assisted surgery is another rapidly evolving area. Surgical robots enhance precision, reduce complications, and shorten recovery times. These systems often use real-time imaging and ML algorithms to guide procedures.

Blockchain technology is being explored to secure and streamline health data exchange. It enables tamper-proof, decentralized storage of medical records while preserving patient privacy and enhancing interoperability across institutions.

- **Integration and Interoperability**

One of the central trends is the push toward integrated health ecosystems, where ML, optimization, and healthcare technologies work synergistically. Electronic health records are becoming more interoperable, enabling AI tools to access comprehensive data for robust predictive analytics. Platforms that combine ML with optimization models can dynamically adjust treatment plans or resource allocation based on real-time data inputs.

Federated learning is emerging as a solution to the challenge of data privacy. It allows ML models to be trained across decentralized data sources without transferring sensitive patient data, maintaining compliance with regulations like HIPAA and GDPR.

Recent Advancements in Healthcare Technologies

- Explainable AI (XAI) in Healthcare: One of the most significant challenges of deploying machine learning in healthcare has been the "black-box" nature of many deep learning models. These models, while highly accurate, often fail to provide insights into how predictions or decisions are made. Explainable AI (XAI) is a response to this issue, aiming to make AI models more interpretable and understandable for healthcare professionals (Miller, 2019). In healthcare, XAI is particularly crucial, as clinicians need to trust the system's decision-making process, especially when it involves high-stakes decisions like diagnoses or treatment plans.
- Recent advancements in XAI have enabled models to not only predict outcomes but also provide explanations that can help clinicians understand why a particular decision was made. For instance, algorithms used in predicting cardiovascular diseases or cancer outcomes can now offer interpretable visualizations that highlight which features (e.g., age, cholesterol levels, or genetic markers) influenced the model's decision, thus improving the decision-making process (Gilpin et al., 2018). The ability to explain model outputs is especially valuable in improving trust and ensuring that AI-based tools align with clinical standards and regulations.
- Federated Learning: Federated learning (Li et al., 2020) allows multiple institutions to collaboratively train machine learning models without directly sharing sensitive patient data. Instead of pooling data in a central location,

the data remains on local devices or within individual organizations, and only model updates are exchanged. This approach enhances privacy and security in healthcare applications. (McMahan et al., 2017). This approach tackles the vital issue of keeping patient data private and secure, which is especially important in healthcare. Since medical information is very sensitive and protected by laws like HIPAA, this technique offers a way to analyze data while maintaining confidentiality.

- Real-Time Optimization in Telemedicine and Remote Monitoring: The integration of real-time optimizationwith telemedicine and remote monitoring technologies is revolutionizing healthcare delivery, particularly for chronic disease management and post-operative care. Wearable sensors and mobile health apps allow for continuous tracking of patient data, including vital signs, activity levels, and other important health indicators. This remote monitoring provides valuable insights into a patient's health status outside of traditional clinical settings.. Machine learning models can then analyze this data in real-time, offering timely insights into a patient's health status. Real-time optimization techniques are being used to adapt treatment plans based on this ongoing data collection. For example, in managing diabetes, real-time optimization algorithms can adjust insulin dosage by processing glucose level data from continuous glucose monitors (CGMs) and predicting future trends. This ensures patients receive the correct dosage at the right time, preventing complications and improving outcomes (Wang et al., 2020). Similarly, in telemedicine, real-time optimization can optimize resource allocation by predicting patient demand for virtual consultations, helping healthcare providers schedule appointments efficiently, thus minimizing wait times and maximizing healthcare delivery efficiency.

High-quality data is essential for effective machine learning models. However, healthcare data is often fragmented and inconsistent. Additionally, patient privacy must be safeguarded, requiring strict adherence to regulations like HIPAA. Machine learning models, especially deep learning models, can be complex and difficult to interpret. This lack of transparency can be a barrier to their adoption in clinical settings where understanding the reasoning behind a decision is crucial. Integrating ML and optimization solutions with existing healthcare IT systems can be challenging. Interoperability standards and a clear implementation strategy are necessary for seamless integration.

ETHICAL CONSIDERATIONS AND REGULATORY COMPLIANCE

- Ethical Challenges in AI and ML in Healthcare: The deployment of AI and ML in healthcare raises several ethical concerns. One of the primary issues is bias in AI models, which can lead to inequitable healthcare outcomes. If the training data used for ML models is not representative of diverse populations, models may perpetuate health disparities, particularly for minority groups. For example, a model trained primarily on data from one demographic (e.g., Caucasian populations) might perform poorly for other racial or ethnic groups, leading to misdiagnoses or suboptimal care (Obermeyer et al., 2019). To ensure fairness and avoid bias in healthcare AI, it's crucial to use diverse and high-quality data when training these systems. Additionally, ongoing evaluation is essential to confirm that the AI is providing equitable care to all patients.
- As machine learning, optimization, and advanced healthcare technologies become deeply integrated into modern medicine, ethical considerations are paramount. A key concern is patient privacy and data security, as vast amounts of sensitive health information are used to train algorithms. Ensuring compliance with regulations like HIPAA and GDPR is essential to protect patient rights. Another pressing issue is algorithmic bias. If models are trained on unrepresentative or biased datasets, they may produce inaccurate or discriminatory outcomes, especially for minority or underserved populations. Fairness and inclusivity must be embedded in model design and validation. Transparency and explainability are also critical. Many machine learning models, especially deep learning systems, operate as "black boxes," making it difficult for clinicians to understand or trust their outputs. Developing explainable AI (XAI) is essential to support informed clinical decision-making. Furthermore, accountability and liability in AI-driven decisions remain unclear. Determining who is responsible when a machine learning model makes an incorrect prediction is a legal and ethical challenge.
- Another ethical concern is informed consent when using AI tools in healthcare. Patients must be fully aware of how their data is being used, and they must have the right to refuse participation in AI-driven healthcare processes. This is especially relevant for AI tools that analyze sensitive medical data, such as genomics or mental health data. Ensuring transparency in how AI models make decisions and how data is handled is essential to maintaining patient trust (Boppana, 2020). Lastly, informed consent must be updated to reflect AI usage, ensuring that patients understand how their data will be used and how AI may influence their care. Ethical oversight, continuous evalua-

tion, and interdisciplinary collaboration are essential to responsibly advance these technologies in healthcare.

- Regulatory Compliance: The use of AI and ML in healthcare must comply with various regulatory frameworks to ensure patient safety and privacy. In the US, AI tools used in healthcare must follow regulations set by the Food and Drug Administration (FDA). This includes software that assists with diagnosis or treatment, ensuring these tools meet safety and effectiveness standards. The FDA's recent efforts to establish clear guidelines for AI and machine learning-based medical devices (FDA, 2025) are important steps in ensuring that these tools are safe, effective, and reliable.
- AI tools used in healthcare must follow strict data protection rules. In the US, this means complying with HIPAA, which safeguards patient privacy. In Europe, GDPR(General Data Protection Regulation) sets a high standard for data protection and requires patient consent for data use. These regulations ensure responsible and ethical development of AI in healthcare. As healthcare systems become more reliant on AI and machine learning, ensuring compliance with these regulations is essential to prevent misuse of sensitive patient data and to protect patients' rights.
- Equitable Access to Healthcare Technologies: While AI and ML have the potential to revolutionize healthcare, there is an urgent need to ensure equitable access to these technologies. In many parts of the world, especially in low-resource settings, access to AI-driven healthcare tools may be limited due to factors such as infrastructure challenges, cost, and a lack of digital literacy. To prevent the widening of health inequalities, efforts must be made to make these technologies accessible to all populations, including marginalized and underserved communities.
- Telemedicine and remote monitoring offer opportunities to bridge the gap in healthcare access, particularly in rural or remote areas. By leveraging mobile health technologies and low-cost sensors, it is possible to provide remote monitoring of chronic diseases, reducing the need for frequent hospital visits. However, challenges such as internet connectivity, affordability, and lack of proper training for both patients and healthcare providers must be addressed to ensure that these technologies benefit everyone (Nallamothu & Cuthrell, 2023).

The advancements in explainable AI, federated learning, and real-time optimization are reshaping healthcare by improving clinical decision-making, patient care, and healthcare logistics. While these technologies hold immense potential, ethical considerations, regulatory compliance, and equitable access must be prioritized to ensure their responsible and inclusive use. By addressing issues such as data privacy, bias, and accessibility, healthcare systems can ensure that AI and optimization tools improve patient outcomes while remaining fair, transparent, and compliant with global regulations.

FUTURE RESEARCH DIRECTIONS

The future of machine learning and optimization in healthcare is bright. With ongoing improvements in algorithms, growing amounts of health data, and increasingly powerful computers, we can expect exciting new developments in this field. Collaborative efforts between data scientists, healthcare professionals, and policymakers will be essential in realizing the full potential of these technologies.

While ML and DL offer tremendous potential, their implementation in healthcare is not without challenges. Data privacy and security remain a significant concern, as medical data is highly sensitive. It's essential to make sure that algorithms used in healthcare follow important data protection laws like HIPAA in the US and GDPR in Europe. This ensures that patient privacy is protected.

Additionally, there is a need for transparent and interpretable models. It can be difficult for healthcare professionals to understand how some deep learning models make their predictions, because these models can be like "black boxes" where the internal workings are hidden. This lack of transparency can make it harder for clinicians to trust and use these models in real-world medical settings. Efforts to develop explainable AI (XAI) models are underway to address these concerns.

Another challenge is the integration of ML and DL algorithms into existing healthcare infrastructure. Many hospitals still rely on legacy systems, making it difficult to adopt advanced technologies without significant investment in IT infrastructure. It's important to provide ongoing training for healthcare professionals so they can confidently and effectively use AI tools in their daily work.

The application of machine learning (ML) in healthcare is revolutionizing clinical practices through several key avenues. Real-time analytics enables clinicians to leverage up-to-the-minute data for immediate decision-making, significantly enhancing patient care. Furthermore, telemedicine and remote monitoring utilize ML to analyze data collected from wearable devices, providing actionable insights that facilitate proactive and personalized healthcare. Finally, genomic medicine harnesses the power of ML to analyze complex genomic data, driving the discovery of novel treatments and deepening our understanding of disease mechanisms, ultimately paving the way for more targeted and effective therapies.

CONCLUSION

Machine learning and deep learning have the potential to revolutionize healthcare. By improving diagnoses, personalizing treatments, and making operations more efficient, these technologies can lead to better results for patients, lower costs, and a more effective healthcare system overall. However, hurdles like data privacy, model interpretability, and integration with current systems must be addressed. As these technologies progress, they are set to play a pivotal role in shaping the future of healthcare. Timely and accurate medical diagnoses are crucial, as early disease detection significantly improves treatment success and can save lives. However, diagnosis is often complex and demanding, requiring both precision and speed. The proposed study explored the use of machine learning plus feature extration optimization to predict diseases, comparing three different models. The Support Vector Machine (SVM) emerged as the most effective in providing accurate predictions. This success highlights the importance of careful data preparation and model optimization, including fine-tuning model parameters, to achieve the best results in disease forecasting. Combining machine learning with optimization methods offers a particularly exciting avenue for disease prediction, allowing us to convert massive datasets into practical solutions. This innovative approach could revolutionize healthcare by enhancing accuracy, lowering expenses, and fueling research into novel prediction techniques. The potential benefits for society are vast, emphasizing the need for ongoing development and broad implementation. While challenges remain, the continued evolution and integration of these technologies hold the key to a more effective and efficient healthcare system.

REFERENCES

Al Amin, M., Baldacci, R., & Kayvanfar, V. (2024). A comprehensive review on operating room scheduling and optimization. *Operations Research*, •••, 25.

Alquhtani, S. A., & Muniasamy, A. (2022). Analytics in support of e-commerce systems using machine learning. In *2022 International Conference on Electrical, Computer and Energy Technologies (ICECET)* (pp. 1–5). Prague, Czech Republic. DOI: 10.1109/ICECET55527.2022.9872592

Ardila, D., Kiraly, A. P., Bharadwaj, S., Choi, B., Reicher, J. J., Peng, L., & Corrado, G. (2019). End-to-end lung cancer screening with three-dimensional deep learning on low-dose chest computed tomography. *Nature Medicine*, *25*(6), 954–961. DOI: 10.1038/s41591-019-0447-x PMID: 31110349

Bishop, C. M. (2006). *Pattern Recognition and Machine Learning*. Springer.

Boppana, V. R. (2020). Ethical implications of big data in healthcare decision making. *SSRN*.

Buckland, M., & Gey, F. (1994). The relationship between recall and precision. *Journal of the American Society for Information Science*, *45*(1), 12–19. DOI: 10.1002/(SICI)1097-4571(199401)45:1<12::AID-ASI2>3.0.CO;2-L

Cortes, C., & Vapnik, V. (1995). Support-vector networks. *Machine Learning*, *20*(3), 273–297. DOI: 10.1007/BF00994018

Cover, T., & Hart, P. (1967). Nearest neighbor pattern classification. *IEEE Transactions on Information Theory*, *13*(1), 21–27. DOI: 10.1109/TIT.1967.1053964

Dantzig, G. B. (1963). Linear programming and extensions. Princeton University Press., Dataset https://www.kaggle.com/datasets/kaushil268/disease-prediction-using-machine-learning, Retrieved March 21, 2025, from.

Davis, D., & Hoh, S. (2020). Application of decision trees in predicting heart disease. *International Journal of Medical Informatics*, *142*, 104205.

Esteva, A., Kuprel, B., Novoa, R. A., Ko, J., Swetter, S. M., Blau, H. M., & Thrun, S. (2017). Dermatologist-level classification of skin cancer with deep neural networks. *Nature*, *542*(7639), 115–118. DOI: 10.1038/nature21056 PMID: 28117445

FDA. (2025). *Artificial Intelligence and Machine Learning in Software as a Medical Device*. U.S. Food and Drug Administration.

Gilpin, L. H.. (2018). *Explaining explanations: An overview of interpretability of machine learning. Proceedings of the 2018 CHI Conference on Human Factors in Computing Systems.* DOI: 10.1109/DSAA.2018.00018

Goodfellow, I., Pouget-Abadie, J., Mirza, M., Xu, B., Warde-Farley, D., Ozair, S., & Bengio, Y. (2014). Generative adversarial nets. *Advances in Neural Information Processing Systems*, •••, 27.

Hastie, T., Friedman, J. H., & Tibshirani, R. (2009). *The elements of statistical learning: Data mining, inference, and prediction.* Springer Science & Business Media. DOI: 10.1007/978-0-387-84858-7

Hochreiter, S., & Schmidhuber, J. (1997). Long short-term memory. *Neural Computation, 9*(8), 1735–1780. DOI: 10.1162/neco.1997.9.8.1735 PMID: 9377276

Holland, J. H. (1975). *Adaptation in natural and artificial systems.* University of Michigan Press.

Jiang, F., Jiang, Y., Zhi, H., Dong, Y., Li, H., Ma, S., Wang, Y., Dong, Q., Shen, H., & Wang, Y. (2017). Artificial intelligence in healthcare: Past, present, and future. *Stroke and Vascular Neurology, 2*(4), 230–243. DOI: 10.1136/svn-2017-000101 PMID: 29507784

Jolliffe, I. T. (2002). *Principal component analysis* (2nd ed.). Springer.

Jones, D. R., Schonlau, M., & Welch, W. J. (1998). Efficient global optimization of expensive black-box functions. *Journal of Global Optimization, 13*(4), 455–492. DOI: 10.1023/A:1008306431147

Kennedy, J., & Eberhart, R. (1995). Particle swarm optimization. *Proceedings of ICNN'95 - International Conference on Neural Networks*, 4, 1942-1948. DOI: 10.1109/ICNN.1995.488968

Kingma, D. P., & Ba, J. (2014). Adam: A method for stochastic optimization. *arXiv preprint arXiv:1412.6980.*

Kirkpatrick, S., Gelatt, C. D.Jr, & Vecchi, M. P. (1983). Optimization by simulated annealing. *Science, 220*(4598), 671–680. DOI: 10.1126/science.220.4598.671 PMID: 17813860

Kolasa, K., Admassu, B. Y., Holownia, M., & Kędzior, K. J. (2023). *Systematic reviews of machine learning in healthcare: A literature review* (Version 1). Research Square. DOI: 10.21203/rs.3.rs-3035548/v1

Kourou, K., Exarchos, T. P., Exarchos, K. P., Karamouzis, M. V., & Fotiadis, D. I. (2015). Machine learning applications in cancer prognosis and prediction. *Computational and Structural Biotechnology Journal*, *13*, 8–17. DOI: 10.1016/j.csbj.2014.11.005 PMID: 25750696

Krizhevsky, A., Sutskever, I., & Hinton, G. E. (2012). ImageNet classification with deep convolutional neural networks. *Advances in Neural Information Processing Systems*, •••, 25.

Kumari, S., & Upadhayay, A. (2025). Diabetic retinopathy prediction using machine learning. *Journal of Neonatal Surgery*, *14*(18S), 767–781.

LeCun, Y., Bengio, Y., & Hinton, G. (2015). Deep learning. *Nature*, *521*(7553), 436–444. DOI: 10.1038/nature14539 PMID: 26017442

Li, T., Sahu, A. K., Talwalkar, A., & Smith, V. (2020). Federated learning: Challenges, methods, and future directions. *IEEE Signal Processing Magazine*, *37*(3), 50–60. DOI: 10.1109/MSP.2020.2975749

Lv, M., Li, Y., Kou, B., & Zhou, Z. (2017). Integer programming for improving radiotherapy treatment efficiency. *PLoS ONE, 12*(7), e0180564.Breiman, L. (2001). Random forests. *Machine Learning*, *45*(1), 5–32.

McMahan, B.. (2017). *Communication-efficient learning of deep networks from decentralized data. Proceedings of the 20th International Conference on Artificial Intelligence and Statistics.*

Miller, T. (2019). Explanation in artificial intelligence: Insights from the social sciences. *Artificial Intelligence*, *267*, 1–38. DOI: 10.1016/j.artint.2018.07.007

Muniasamy, A., & Asiri, F. (2025). Advanced human activity recognition on wearables with multi-scale sparse attention. *Multimedia Tools and Applications*. Advance online publication. DOI: 10.1007/s11042-024-20475-6

Nallamothu, P. T., & Cuthrell, K. M. (2023). Artificial intelligence in health sector: Current status and future perspectives. *Asian Journal of Research in Computer Science*, *15*(4), 1–14. DOI: 10.9734/ajrcos/2023/v15i4325

Obermeyer, Z., & Emanuel, E. J. (2016). Predicting the future—Big data, machine learning, and clinical medicine. *The New England Journal of Medicine*, *375*(13), 1216–1219. DOI: 10.1056/NEJMp1606181 PMID: 27682033

Obermeyer, Z., Powers, B. W., Vogeli, C., & Mullainathan, S. (2019). Dissecting racial bias in an algorithm used to manage the health of populations. *Science*, *366*(6464), 447–453. DOI: 10.1126/science.aax2342 PMID: 31649194

Quinlan, J. R. (1996). Improved use of continuous attributes in C4.5. *Journal of Artificial Intelligence Research*, *4*, 77–90. DOI: 10.1613/jair.279

Rajagopal, A., Ayanian, S., Ryu, A. J., Qian, R., Legler, S. R., Peeler, E. A., Issa, M., Coons, T. J., & Kawamoto, K. (2024). Machine learning operations in health care: A scoping review. *Mayo Clinic Proceedings. Digital Health*, *2*(3), 421–437. DOI: 10.1016/j.mcpdig.2024.06.009 PMID: 40206123

Rajeswaran, A., Kumar, V., Gupta, A., Schulman, J., Todorov, E., & Levine, S. (2017). Learning complex dexterous manipulation with deep reinforcement learning and demonstrations. *arXiv preprint arXiv:1709.10087.*

Rumelhart, D. E., Hinton, G. E., & Williams, R. J. (1986). Learning representations by backpropagating errors. *Nature*, *323*(6088), 533–536. DOI: 10.1038/323533a0

Snoek, J., Larochelle, H., & Adams, R. P. (2012). Practical Bayesian optimization of machine learning algorithms. *Advances in Neural Information Processing Systems*, •••, 25.

Topaloglu, H., & Powell, W. B. (2006). Dynamic-programming approximations for stochastic, time-staged integer multicommodity flow problems. *INFORMS Journal on Computing*, *18*(1), 31–42. DOI: 10.1287/ijoc.1040.0079

Topol, E. J. (2019). *Deep Medicine: How Artificial Intelligence Can Make Healthcare Human Again.* Basic Books.

Vamathevan, J., Clark, D., Czodrowski, P., Dunham, I., Ferran, E., Lee, G., Li, B., Madabhushi, A., Shah, P., Spitzer, M., & Zhao, S. (2019). Applications of machine learning in drug discovery and development. *Nature Reviews. Drug Discovery*, *18*(6), 463–477. DOI: 10.1038/s41573-019-0024-5 PMID: 30976107

Vaswani, A., Shazeer, N., Parmar, N., Uszkoreit, J., Jones, L., Gomez, A. N., & Polosukhin, I. (2017). Attention is all you need. *Advances in Neural Information Processing Systems*, •••, 30.

ADDITIONAL READING

Dhiman, P., Bonkra, A., Kaur, A., Gulzar, Y., Hamid, Y., Mir, M. S., Soomro, A. B., & Elwasila, O. (2023). Healthcare Trust Evolution with Explainable Artificial Intelligence: Bibliometric Analysis. *Information (Basel)*, *14*(10), 541. DOI: 10.3390/info14100541

Ingole, P. (2024). Optimizing resource allocation in hospitals using predictive analytics and information systems. *Journal of Information Systems Engineering & Management, 10*(1s), 400–415. DOI: 10.52783/jisem.v10i1s.224

Mittermaier, M., Raza, M. M., & Kvedar, J. C. (2023). Bias in AI-based models for medical applications: Challenges and mitigation strategies. *npj. Digital Medicine, 6*, 113. PMID: 37311802

Pati, S., Kumar, S., Varma, A., Edwards, B., Lu, C., Qu, L., Wang, J. J., Lakshminarayanan, A., Wang, S., Sheller, M. J., Chang, K., Singh, P., Rubin, D. L., Kalpathy-Cramer, J., & Bakas, S. (2024). Privacy preservation for federated learning in health care. *Patterns (New York, N.Y.), 5*(7), 100974. DOI: 10.1016/j.patter.2024.100974 PMID: 39081567

Showrov, A. A., Aziz, M. T., Nabil, H. R., & Jim, J. R. (2024). Generative adversarial networks (GANs) in medical imaging: Advancements, applications, and challenges. *IEEE Access, PP*, (99), 1–1.

KEY TERMS AND DEFINITIONS

Machine Learning (ML): A branch of AI that uses algorithms to analyze data, learn patterns, and make predictions without explicit programming.

Optimization: The process of finding the best solution to a problem by minimizing or maximizing an objective function while adhering to constraints.

Supervised Learning: A type of ML where models are trained on labeled data to make predictions or classify new data.

Reinforcement Learning: A method of ML where models learn through trial and error, improving based on feedback from the environment.

Explainable AI (XAI): Techniques in AI that aim to make machine learning models more interpretable and understandable to human users.

Chapter 2
Foundations of Integrative Machine Learning and Optimization for Disease Prediction

V. Dankan Gowda
https://orcid.org/0000-0003-0724-0333
Department of Electronics and Communication Engineering, BMS Institute of Technology and Management, Bangalore, India

B. N. Purushothamma
https://orcid.org/0000-0002-3919-2703
Faculty of Engineering, Management, and Technology (BGSIT), India

I. Nandhini
Department of Information Technology, V.S.B. Engineering College, Karur, India

Kottala Sri Yogi
https://orcid.org/0000-0002-3671-7420
Department of Operations, Symbiosis Institute of Business Management Hyderabad, India & Symbiosis International University, Pune, India

Venkatesan Hariram
https://orcid.org/0000-0003-2237-7071
Vinayaka Mission's Homoeopathic Medical College and Hospital, A Constituent College of Vinayaka Mission's Research Foundation University, Salem, India

DOI: 10.4018/979-8-3373-1087-9.ch002

ABSTRACT

Integrative Machine Learning (ML) and optimization have risen to the challenges associated with disease prediction through improvement of accuracy, efficiency, and decision-making in health. This chapter focuses on the integration of the feature selection and hyperparameter tuning with predictive improvement of an ML algorithm through the help of some optimization techniques. While a literature review presents novel developments in the use of ML for the prognosis of chronic and infectious diseases and optimization techniques as genetic algorithms, PSO, SA. Additionally, the chapter analyzes the tendencies in the integrative approaches' effectiveness compared to the standard methods for knowledge discovery; how it may address big quantities of medical data; and how enhancing the interpretability of results is achieved. This work underlines the relevance and potential of integrative ML and optimization in improving the health care results.

INTRODUCTION

Modern health care system can not imagine its functioning without disease prediction as a part of successful and timely treatment providing and efficient resources utilization. As chronic and infectious diseases become a growing problem, successful prediction models have emerged as vital tools in assessing and preventing health risks, optimizing patients' recovery, and minimizing health care expenditures. Statistical methodologies have had successes in certain cases but are unable to efficiently deal with the rising complexity and dimensionality of the medical data (Asha, et al., 2024). This has created the ground for the implementation of Machine Learning (ML), which is numerically superior in detection of patterns, associations and tendencies in the huge amount of data.

Some other Machine Learning techniques like Decision Trees, Support Vector Machines (SVM), Artificial Neural Networks (ANN) and Convolutional Neural Networks (CNN) performed really well in predicting the diseases. For example, ML models can employ and interpret disparate types of medical data, clinical documentation, patient's genomic data, or imaging data and can diagnose or predict a variety of diseases that include diabetes, cardiovascular diseases, or cancers (Pankajavalli, et al., 2021). On top of increasing predictiveness of the model, when using advanced feature selection and deep learning in the design of ML models, interpretability of the outcomes is equally boosted. Still, these models highly rely on selecting the correct hyperparameters such as the features to use and the setting up the learning process (Balafas et al., 2023).

This is where optimization techniques bear an important role in calculations. Several advanced models like Genetic Algorithm (GA), Particle Swarm Optimization (PSO) and Simulated Annealing (SA) are used to improve the relevant ML models and some of the important parameters and features are optimized from them.For example, from a dataset with n features DDD, an optimization procedure aims at selecting the subset F⊆DF that best approximates the performance measure M(F) which can be accuracy or AUC or similar performance measure.sed to enhance ML models by identifying optimal parameters and features (Divya, et al., 2024). For example, given a dataset DDD with n features, an optimization algorithm can identify the subset F⊆DF that maximizes the performance metric M(F), such as accuracy or area under the curve (AUC). Such methods also help in achieving faster convergence, and avoids over training that a common problem in ML, which hinders generalization of models to unseen data (Abdellatif, et al., 2022). Furthermore, other integration of ML with optimization is being developed more widely, in which, optimization techniques improve feature selection and the learning process toward building efficient, accurate and comprehensible models.

The combination of Machine Learning and optimization in the current work to predict disease is proposed to counter some of the biggest issues that arise in the advancement of Healthcare analytics namely; dealing with imbalanced data, missing data and the rising concern of fairness and explainability in the decision-making process (Agarwal et al., 2024). In addition, the above integrative approaches also facilitate the prediction in real time, especially in intensive care as well as epidemic monitoring.

The objectives of this chapter are threefold: Thus, this paper aims to: (1) Provide an introduction to basic concepts of Machine Learning, especially when applied to disease prediction and using optimization; (2) Discuss prior studies to conceptualize major advancements and issues related to integrative methods; (3) Include case studies and real-life applications to show the potential combination of Machine Learning and optimization for healthcare improvement (Abdulmalek et al. 2022). This chapter therefore presents a general understanding of these ideas with the hope of enabling both researchers and practitioners, as well as healthcare providers to build new solutions to disease risk prediction.

Altogether, the conjunction of Machine Learning and optimization heuristics is a change of healthcare analytics paradigm. By integrating the two techniques, the high level of accuracy, optimization and ethical approaches of the ML with problem solving techniques few as optimization to accurately predict the disease outcome in future, gives healthcare modern face.

BACKGROUND

Foundations Of Integrative Machine Learning And Optimization

Many diseases have been predicted with the aid of Machine Learning (ML), which gives the potential to handle and analyze large amounts of di- and multi-dimensional medical data to discover relationships and make predictions. ML techniques are broadly categorized into three paradigms: of which are classification learning, clustering learning, and the reward-based learning (Gowda et al., 2024). The most used class in disease prediction is supervised learning because labeled data is utilized to train models to categorize outcomes or values. Algorithms which are frequently used in this area are Decision Trees, Support Vector Machines SVM and Neural Networks (Patil et al., 2024). For instance, Design Tree for example, can diagnose a patient as being a high risk or a low risk based on features such as age, blood pressure and cholesterol, whereas SVM can identify non-linear patterns reducing diagnostic error (Gowda eta al., 2024). Neural Networks are particularly Convolutional Neural Networks (CNN) have played a major role in diagnosing medical image such as the case of tumors detected in radiology images (Prasad et al., 2024). In contrast, the methods of unsupervised learning, including clustering and decreasing dimensionality, are employed for exploring the concealed structures in the data that are not labelled, for example, subgroups of patients with similar signs of the disease. Reinforcement learning while is less frequently employed, is steadily being incorporated into improvement of treatment plans and precision medicine.

Like in case of disease prediction, optimization techniques are as important a tool that helps to fine tune the ML models. Optimization means the use of methods for selecting the best possible solution from a particular set of solutions having certain constraints (Vasanthakumar and Singh, 2024). Applicable machine learning algorithms in this area comprise of Genetic Algorithms (GA), Particle Swarm Optimization (PSO) and Simulated Annealing (SA). Genetic algorithms mimic the basic natural selection for generation of better solutions with the help of which, feasible features can be selected dynamically in high dimensionality along with tuning of hyperparameters (Arora et al., 2023). For instance, let a given data set have n features; this is where a GA is capable of detecting the F that is a subset of DF such that M(F) is the best achievable performance. PSO, a simulation of bird flocking, is used for fine-tuning model parameters by adjusting solutions through social and cognitive components of particles (Mallikarjun & Kawale, 2023). The probabilistic technique used is Simulated Annealing to click through solution space to avoid solution space of false local minimum to reach a globally ideal configuration.

The combination of both MH and optimization presents a formidable union that partially offsets some of the major problems of disease prediction. Enhancement in this regard thus optimizes the process by reducing the number of predictors to only those that are most relevant to perform computations at reduced complexity and the level of overfitting is also brought under control. It also is important for choosing between different parameters for a given ML algorithm such as a learning rate, number of layers in a neural net, kernel type for SVM and so on. For instance, an integrated approach we may be to use PSO to identify the kernel parameter of an SVM which would yield the maximum classification accuracy in case of heart disease. Thirdly, optimization make decisions easier to make as the outputs are easy to interpret and act on such as risky patient groups or interventions to take.

In conclusion, the use of ML Hand the integration of productive optimization methods offer a stable environment for disease prediction. Whereas, the standard ML gives a model-based computational vision for managing the large amount of medical data, the optimization helps to fine-tune that model, to be more effective and correct for handling the healthcare data analysis. Combined, they create the foundation that leads to a progression in existing predictive models that can impact the management of care for patients.

Applications In Disease Prediction

Artificial intelligence (AI) and optimization in general have been key in reshaping the area of disease prediction in a myriad of ailments. Such integrative approaches deliver increased accuracy, speed and capacity for scalability that benefits health-care systems in risk factor profiling, disease prognosis and patient customisation. It ranges from chronic diseases, infectious diseases, and single disease conditions, clearly showing the areas that have the potential for being used by, and for the advancement of, modern ML-aided optimization in healthcare.

In the context of chronic diseases, they utilize the ML models needed to detect the diseases and the risk segregation as well. For instance, in diabetes prediction, the supervised learning contains decision trees, support vector machine etc. and clinical features like glucose level, age, and BMI to predict about chance of getting diabetes. Feature selection and hyperparameter tuning are glorified here as valuable optimization methods enable the improvement of the performance of ML models (Gowda et al., 2023). For instance, a genetic algorithm will be useful in developing an efficient method to search through a population of predictive features that require packaging into a box of limited space, to maximize model efficiency and minimize required computational resources. Similarly in predicting cardiovascular diseases, enhanced risk scores have been developed with the help of Machine Learning assisted by optimization techniques such as Particle Swarm Optimization (PSO).

Combining these approaches, practitioners can better determine those for whom the most dangerous treatment is possible and take necessary precautions.

However, in infectious diseases rapid and accurate predictions have become important especially with the COVID-19 pandemic. Many cases of employing ML algorithms include the analysis of epidemiological data as well as the prognosis of disease rates and results of the patients' treatment. Some common approaches like Convolutional Neural Network's or CNNs have been applied in radiography image diagnostics for instance in diagnosing COVID-19 from chest x-rays or CT scans. Various optimization algorithms take these models to the next level by, featuring the main discriminating features and increasing classification's accuracy (Jadhav and Kaur, 2023). For instance, Simulated Annealing has been employed to review CNN architectures, to guarantee that the identified models connect high performance with efficiency. In addition to COVID-19, ML and optimization have been used globally on cases of tuberculosis through integrating genomic information and public health data to predict the distribution rate and effects in order to inform policy on where to allocate limited resources and efforts.

It has applied even to rare diseases, which normally do not have enough labeled data needed for raw analysis and/or optimization. This aspect of unsupervised learning methods and in particular, clustering is exceptionally useful in diagnosing rare genetic disorders given that their patterns in high dimensions are rare. In the literature, reinforcement has been used to model treatment paths for patients and proactively predict their 'hard to maneuver' results (Kalpana, and Hariram, 2023). Techniques such as Bayesian optimization are utilized to further refine the models optimality so as to perform well even when confronted with a small number of data inputs. To illustrate, Bayesian optimization can be employed for the hyperparameters selection in applied neural networks trained with genomics data to enhance diagnostic performance and reveal new diagnostics' features.

ML and optimization integration is most useful in feature extraction and optimizing the model is an emerging trend in feature extraction and in the enhancement of the models. For example, when anticipating the onset of diabetes, inputs diminished from original large data sets utilizing Principal Component Analysis (PCA) to streamline higher formative factors. This also means that a model is correct not only numerically but also semantically thereby making it easy for clinicians to make right decisions on the results they find most applicable since the results will be as expected.

Thus, the use of ML and optimization in the prediction of diseases has made remarkable progress for different diseases, both ordinary and unusual. These techniques serve as the groundwork for building descriptive models that are elaborate, precise, and can therefore be used to build an effective analytic model of personalized medicine.

Literature Survey

The combination of Machine Learning (ML) and optimization in disease prediction has been assessed and revealed satisfactory outcomes within different areas of medicine. Earlier literature has shown that diagnostic accuracy and predictive capacities have been enriched by the use of ML. Convolutional Neural Networks (CNNs) are widely used in healthcare related roles, including tumour detection, classification of Diabetic Retinopathy, and diagnosis of pneumonia (Pandidurai & Senthil Kamalesh, 2023). For instance, CNN models have achieved high performance on images of lungs and chest X-ray and CT scans in detecting lung cancer and COVID-19. These models take advantage of the substructure extraction capacity of CNNs to distinguish patterns that might not be discerned by human beings. In the same regard, other supervised learning algorithms have been used in risk stratification of chronic diseases including predicting probability of cardiovascular disease from clinical features.

Several optimization methods have been used in future enhancement of the performance of ML models in diseases prediction (Ramesha et al., 2022). For example, Genetic Algorithms (GA) have been employed in feature selection, a process of feature subset counseling in big data to have only relevant features. Through optimum selection of features, GA raises the efficiency and reliability of the resultant ML models. Particle Swarm Optimization (PSO) has also been used for hyperparameter optimization to guarantee optimal performance of ML telmodels with low costs on resources. For instance, in a diabetes prediction model, the parameters of the neural networks have been optimized thru PSO resulting to high degree of accuracy of prediction. Optimization problems that can lead to local minimum issues in an algorithm have been solved using Real Simulated Annealing (SA) making ML even more resilient.

Recent trends in the field emphasize privacy-preserving and scalable approaches to disease prediction. There is federated learning, which is a decentralized ML approach, that doesn't require sharing patients' data but trains models on different datasets (Tanguturi and Poornima, 2022). CV use has been most relevant in healthcare, where the issue of data protection is critical. Research shows that federated learning can be employed to forecast diseases such as diabetes and Parkinson's with very high precision while preserving patients' identities (Rashmi & Chinamuttevi, 2022). Another ongoing development is that transformer models are starting to be applied to healthcare mainly for time series data. Originally used for NLP, transformers are again proven to excel with sequential data such as patients' vitals and medical records. For example, delivery transformer models have been applied in performance of sepsis and other important states in ICU wards with enhanced interpretation capacity and accuracy compared to some normal models.

However, current research in this area is not without its weaknesses. Most of the programs investigated address the aspects of either the ML or the optimization strategies on their own (Reddy, et al., 2021). Further, issues such as data imbalance, interpretability, and scalability questions are still unanswered in many applications. Perhaps, there is lack of globe-wide effective frameworks that incorporate both ML and optimization to tackle these challenges adequately (Chauhan and Kaur, 2023). Secondly, although federated learning and transformer models appear promising, they remain largely experimental due to computations' limitations and lacking best-practice guidelines in healthcare (Chen et al., 2017).

In conclusion, literature confirms the value of bringing changes in disease predicting models through the use of ML and optimization. However, the implementation of these techniques, amongst others together with some of the recent trends like federated learning and transformers, is pivotal to fill the existing gaps and to advance the field further. To fill these research gaps, this chapter will look at more advanced integrative techniques for disease prediction.

CASE STUDY

The current research methodology depicts a conceptual framework that lays a groundwork for combining ML and optimization to improve disease prediction models. As it will be explained in the following sections, this approach arises from the fact that ML can easily handle a large amount of data and a high number of features while optimization allows refining the parameters of model and selecting the relevant ones to guarantee accuracy, feasibility, and readability. The methodology is intended to solve issues such as, imbalance of data, over fitting, and excessive computations which are frequent in the health care field. Moreover, the Figure.1. depicts an extensive and detailed glossary of an ML/optimization workflow for improving disease prediction models. The process starts with data acquisition, then data preprocessing and more specifically missing value treatment for the dataset validity. There is normalization and standardization to reduce variability and methods like SMOTE employ while handling over or undersampled class data. Genetic Algorithms are used for feature selection, as optimization algorithms which enables to find the best subsets of features. In ways of Hyper tuning of the model, optimization procedures like Particle Swarm Optimization are also employed to fine-tune the ML parameters.

Figure 1. Workflow of Integrative Machine Learning and Optimization for Disease Prediction

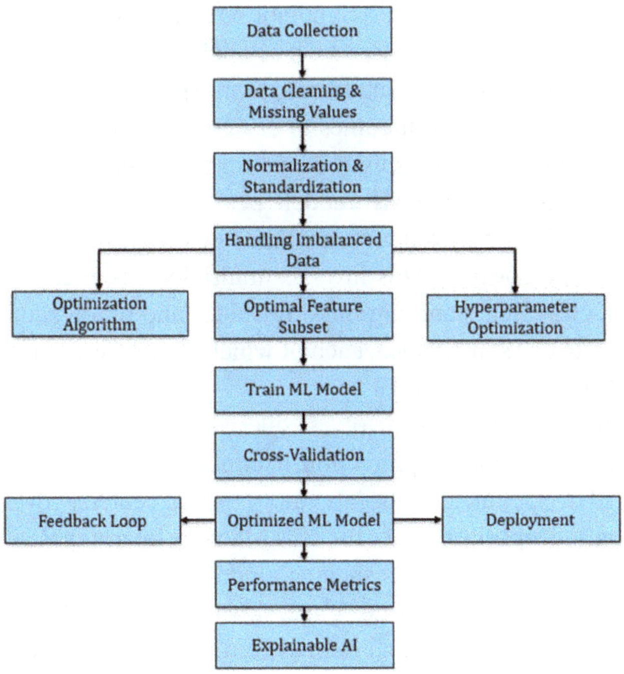

There is a progression to train the ML models, and cross-validation procedures, and construction of the best optimized model provider using performance indicators such as accuracy and precision. Others make it interpretable by simply giving detail features that need to be paid attention to in features importance. The last is the deployment phase in which the model is integrated into a clinical decision-support system. A feedback mechanism can be used to prevent feedback from forming a loop of its own back into the stages of prediction. This workflow in a nutshell illustrates that how both ML and optimization assist to overcome various aspects of healthcare and helps in the accurate disease prediction.

The conceptual framework consists of four key stages: acquisition and cleaning, transformation and feature extraction and reduction, building and training, tuning and assessing. The workflow can be applied to any disease dataset, such as a dataset for predicting diabetes or cardiovascular diseases, by following these steps:

Data Preprocessing: The first step is data acquisition and data cleansing in this process. For a diabetes data set this may include extracting simple attributes like glucose intake, body mass index, age, and their hereditary factors. The analysis for this data deals with the treatment of missing values, which are then followed by imputation process, and outliers treatment with the aim of creating accurate data set.

Features are then made logical or consistent by normalizing data or making them standard especially when features are of different scales. For imbalance of data, one can apply some of the method such as, Synthetic Minority Oversampling Technique (SMOTE) to balance the target classes such as Diabetic and Non Diabetic.

Data preprocessing is a fundamental and essential phase in any machine learning (ML) pipeline. Especially when it comes to disease prediction tasks such as diagnosing diabetes, the integrity, cleanliness, and relevance of the dataset are pivotal in ensuring that the downstream ML models perform optimally. Preprocessing is the first step in transforming raw healthcare data into meaningful inputs suitable for feeding into an ML algorithm. This involves multiple sub-processes such as data acquisition, data cleansing, handling missing values and outliers, data normalization, and addressing class imbalance, each of which significantly contributes to the performance of the predictive models.

To begin with, data acquisition involves collecting data from reliable and diverse sources. In the context of diabetes prediction, datasets may be sourced from electronic health records (EHRs), clinical trials, laboratory testing centers, government health databases, and online repositories like the UCI Machine Learning Repository. These datasets typically contain attributes such as glucose levels, insulin concentration, blood pressure, BMI (Body Mass Index), age, skin thickness, and personal or family history of diabetes. The diversity and richness of the dataset are crucial in creating a robust and generalizable model.

Following data acquisition is data cleansing, which focuses on correcting or removing erroneous, inconsistent, or incomplete data. In medical datasets, missing values are a common issue. Patients might miss appointments or certain tests may not be administered due to various constraints. If left untreated, these gaps can severely affect model performance. To handle this, various imputation techniques are applied. Basic methods include filling missing values with the mean, median, or mode of a feature, depending on its distribution. More advanced techniques include K-Nearest Neighbors (KNN) imputation, which predicts missing values based on the values of neighboring data points, or multiple imputation by chained equations (MICE), which iteratively estimates missing data using a sequence of regression models.

Handling outliers is another key step. Outliers in medical data could result from manual entry errors or rare but valid physiological measurements. Outliers can skew statistical analyses and mislead the learning process. Techniques such as Z-score, interquartile range (IQR), and visual tools like boxplots or scatter plots help detect these anomalies. Once detected, outliers can be addressed through transformation techniques such as logarithmic or square root scaling, or be capped using winsorization. In some cases, if an outlier is confirmed to be an error, it may be removed entirely.

Normalization or standardization is often necessary to bring all features to the same scale. Machine learning algorithms such as Support Vector Machines (SVM) and K-Nearest Neighbors (KNN) are sensitive to the range of input features. For example, glucose levels might range from 50 to 300, whereas age ranges from 0 to 100. If not normalized, higher magnitude features may dominate the learning process. Normalization typically scales data between 0 and 1, while standardization transforms data to have a mean of zero and a standard deviation of one.

Another major challenge in diabetes prediction datasets is class imbalance. In most real-world datasets, the number of non-diabetic patients significantly outweighs the number of diabetic patients. This skewness can lead to biased models that favor the majority class. To mitigate this, resampling techniques like Synthetic Minority Over-sampling Technique (SMOTE) are used. SMOTE works by creating synthetic instances of the minority class, thus balancing the dataset. Other techniques include Adaptive Synthetic Sampling (ADASYN), Tomek Links, and undersampling the majority class.

Feature Selection Using Optimization: Feature selection plays a primary role of dimensionality reduction and improving on the models. Genetic Algorithm (GA), for instance, is used in picking the best features out of the abundant ones. The objective function M(F) is defined to optimize a hypothetical measure such as accuracy or expect it to minimize the error rates, whereby F interprets as the chosen feature set. For example, for diabetes data set, algorithm may find out that glucose level, BMI and family history as potential important predictor variables. This step is to avoid using irrelevant features and ultimately it decreases computational analysis and increases readability.

Feature selection is the process of identifying and selecting a subset of relevant features for model construction. In the context of healthcare, this step is not only essential for improving model accuracy and efficiency but also for enhancing interpretability. Feature selection helps in eliminating redundant or irrelevant variables that may introduce noise and overfitting.

One of the most effective approaches to feature selection involves optimization algorithms. Among these, Genetic Algorithms (GA) are particularly notable for their ability to explore large search spaces efficiently. GAs are inspired by the principles of natural evolution and operate through selection, crossover, and mutation of a population of candidate feature sets. An objective function, often model accuracy or another performance metric, evaluates each candidate set. The algorithm iteratively evolves the population toward optimal solutions.

For instance, in a diabetes dataset, a GA might identify glucose level, BMI, age, and family history as the most predictive features. These features are biologically plausible and corroborated by medical literature, thus adding to the clinical credibility of the model. The feature set is represented as a binary chromosome, where each gene corresponds to a feature. A value of 1 indicates selection and 0 denotes exclusion.

Other optimization-based feature selection methods include Particle Swarm Optimization (PSO), Simulated Annealing (SA), and Ant Colony Optimization (ACO). PSO simulates the social behavior of birds or fish to iteratively improve solutions, whereas SA mimics the annealing process in metallurgy, and ACO draws inspiration from the path-finding behavior of ants.

These techniques are particularly useful when the number of features is large or when interactions between features are complex. They help in reducing computational complexity, enhancing model generalizability, and improving prediction accuracy. Importantly, by reducing dimensionality, they also make the final model more interpretable for clinicians.

Model Development Using Machine Learning: The next step in feature selection is data transformation where a Random Forest, Support Vector Machines (SVM) or Neural Networks is trained on the processed dataset. For example the Random Forest classifier can be used where the model is to predict diabetes using the features above; though not all of them. The model is then trained on portion of the data (Possessing training set) then tested on the other portion of the data (Possessing validation set). To determine the model's credibility, there is cross-validation including independent k-fold cross-validation.

After selecting the optimal features, the next step involves training machine learning models to learn patterns from the data and make predictions. Several algorithms are suitable for binary classification tasks like predicting diabetes, including Decision Trees, Random Forests (RF), Support Vector Machines (SVM), and Neural Networks.

Random Forest is an ensemble learning method that constructs multiple decision trees during training. The final prediction is made by aggregating the predictions of all trees. RF is robust to overfitting, handles high-dimensional data well, and can capture complex interactions among features. For example, an RF model trained on glucose, BMI, and age might be able to accurately classify a patient as diabetic or non-diabetic based on learned thresholds and combinations of these attributes.

Support Vector Machines are another powerful tool for classification. SVMs work by finding the optimal hyperplane that separates data points of different classes. The choice of kernel function (e.g., linear, polynomial, radial basis function) allows SVMs to model complex, non-linear relationships. The regularization parameter C controls the trade-off between achieving a low error on training data and maintaining a large margin between classes.

Neural Networks, particularly Deep Learning models, have gained traction in healthcare due to their ability to model highly non-linear and intricate patterns in data. A basic artificial neural network consists of input, hidden, and output layers.

Each layer comprises neurons that perform weighted summations of inputs followed by a non-linear activation function. The network is trained using backpropagation and gradient descent to minimize a loss function.

Model development involves splitting the dataset into training and test sets, typically using an 80/20 or 70/30 ratio. To ensure that the model generalizes well to unseen data, cross-validation techniques like k-fold cross-validation are used. This involves partitioning the data into k subsets, training the model on k-1 subsets, and validating it on the remaining one. This process is repeated k times, and the average performance is recorded.

Optimization and Evaluation: To attain the final optimization of the hyperparameters of the ML model normal optimization parameters such as Particle Swarm Optimization (PSO), or Bayesian Optimization are used. For instance, in the case of SVM model, PSO can work on kernel functions and could search for the optimum value of, C the regularization term to give the best accuracy in classification. The optimized model thus can be tested on a test set in terms of such parameters as accuracy, precision, recall and F1-score. Moreover, there is a way of including other Explainable AI (XAI) approaches after this work to explain the weights assigned to every feature.

Even with a good model and selected features, hyperparameter tuning plays a critical role in enhancing performance. Hyperparameters are parameters that define the model's structure or how it is trained (e.g., learning rate, number of trees in a forest, or kernel type in SVM). Unlike weights, they are not learned during training and must be set beforehand.

Particle Swarm Optimization and Bayesian Optimization are commonly used for this purpose. PSO optimizes hyperparameters by simulating a swarm of particles moving through the hyperparameter space. Each particle adjusts its position based on its own experience and that of its neighbors. In contrast, Bayesian Optimization uses a surrogate model to predict performance and guide the search for optimal hyperparameters.

Once optimized, models are evaluated using metrics like accuracy, precision, recall, F1-score, and the Area Under the Receiver Operating Characteristic Curve (AUC-ROC). Accuracy measures the proportion of correctly classified instances, precision quantifies how many predicted positives are true positives, and recall assesses how many actual positives are correctly identified. The F1-score balances precision and recall, and AUC-ROC evaluates the trade-off between sensitivity and specificity.

To further enhance trust in model predictions, Explainable AI (XAI) techniques like LIME (Local Interpretable Model-Agnostic Explanations) and SHAP (SHapley Additive exPlanations) can be applied. These methods provide insight into how each feature influences a prediction, thus making the model more transparent and acceptable to clinicians.

Deployment and Feedback: The last is the application or deployment of the model that is the best in the clinical environment or basically in any decision-making system. To evolve the model furthermore feedback from healthcare professionals can be given continuously for the better usage of the model.

This integrated method is driven from the prediction capacity of ML and the ability of optimization to fine tune it, this makes the disease prediction to be robust. In this way, the described methodology helps to create realistic, reliable and intelligible models that can be useful for early diagnosis as well as for choosing the proper treatment for patients. After successful training and evaluation, the final step is model deployment. In a clinical setting, the deployed model should integrate seamlessly with existing hospital information systems. This might involve developing a user-friendly interface where healthcare professionals can input patient data and receive diagnostic predictions in real-time.

Deployment can be done via APIs, web-based platforms, or mobile applications. The model should be continuously monitored for performance degradation, which can occur due to changes in patient demographics, disease profiles, or treatment practices over time. Incorporating a feedback loop where healthcare professionals can validate and comment on predictions is essential for maintaining and improving model performance. Furthermore, retraining the model periodically with new data ensures its relevance and accuracy. This adaptive learning capability is vital in dynamic environments like healthcare.

In conclusion, the process of developing a robust, reliable, and interpretable diabetes prediction model using machine learning and optimization techniques involves several critical steps. Beginning with thorough data preprocessing, followed by strategic feature selection, model development, hyperparameter tuning, and culminating in thoughtful deployment, each phase plays a vital role in ensuring the model's success. The synergy of machine learning's predictive power with optimization techniques' fine-tuning capabilities offers a comprehensive solution to early disease diagnosis, ultimately improving patient outcomes and aiding healthcare professionals in clinical decision-making.

SOLUTIONS AND RECOMMENDATIONS

The improvement returns acquired by combining ML and optimization approaches show better efficiency than conventional approaches to disease prediction. To measure how effective the integrated models are, or are not, accuracy and precision and recall and AUC-ROC are used as measures to weigh the integrative models with non-optimized models. The effect of applying type of oversampling known as Synthetic Minority Oversampling Technique (SMOTE) when handling class imbalance in the dataset is shown in Figure 2. First, this dataset was imbalanced, containing 70% of samples in Class 1 and 30% in Class 0. When we performed SMOTE, the number of instances in each class was equal to 70 percent as evident from bar plot. This step enhanced the model's sensitivity by avoiding the over-representation of the dominant class which normally occurs with the other probability estimation techniques.

The GA based optimized fatures set importance score is presented in Figure 3. The data depicted in this bar chart also shows that some features have much higher importance scores than others, for example, Feature 4 and Feature 1, with scores of 0.9 and 0.8 respectively. By choosing these high importance features, the integrative approach dimensionality of the dataset significantly decreased, but its predictive ability remained intact. The training and validation accuracy of the ML model can be observed in Figure 4. below, after 20 iterations through the data. The graph demonstrates the general increase in the training accuracy and validation accuracy; although for the training accuracy is 98% for the epoch 4, while the validation accurate is 95% for the epoch 4.; The convergence trend proves that tuning of hyperparameters reduces overfitting and improves the generality of the model.

Figure 5 shows the model performance using the confusion matrix. Looking at the matrix below it can be seen that the model achieved 85 true positives and 90 true negatives with acceptable levels of errors, 15 false positives and 10 false negatives. Consequently, it was determined that the specificity is 92.5%, sensitivity is 85%, and the measure of precision is 89%. It is clear from the value add balanced performance metrics that the integrative model is quite solid. Concerning the quantitative criteria, the Receiver Operating Characteristic (ROC) curve is portrayed in Figure 6 which signifies the vice versa relationship of TPR & FPR. They can reach partly to 0.94 of Area Under the curve (AUC) to demonstrate the excellent discrimination of the model. This result reinstated the applicability of the integrative approach as a means of demarcating between positive and negative cases.

Figure 2. Data Preprocessing - Class Imbalance Handling Using SMOTE

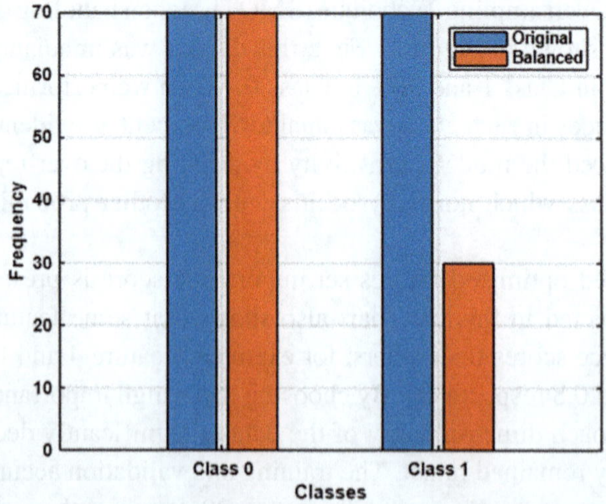

Figure 3. Feature Importance Using Optimization Algorithms

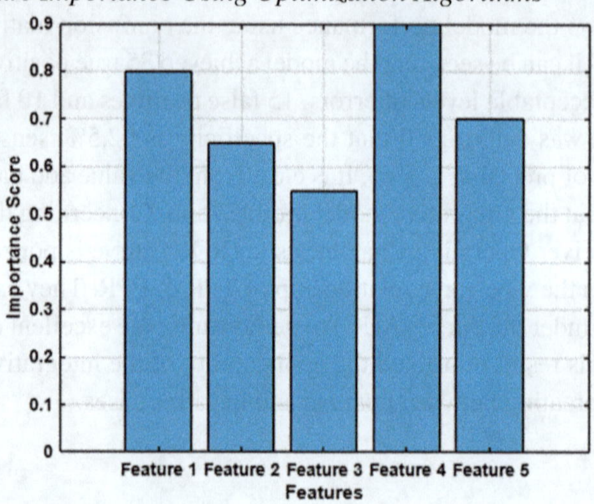

Figure 4. Model Training Accuracy vs. Epochs

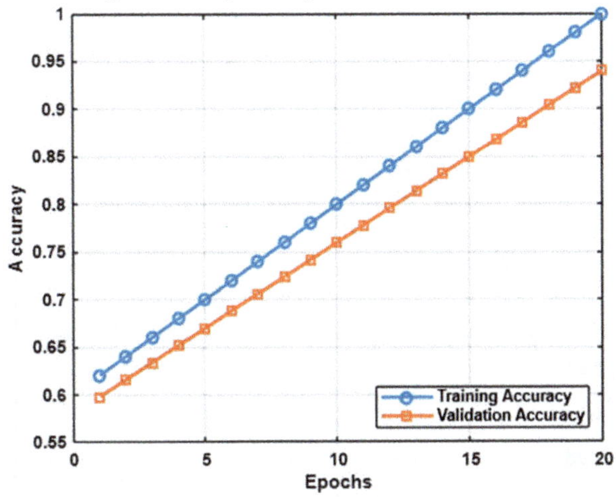

Figure 5. Confusion Matrix for Model Performance

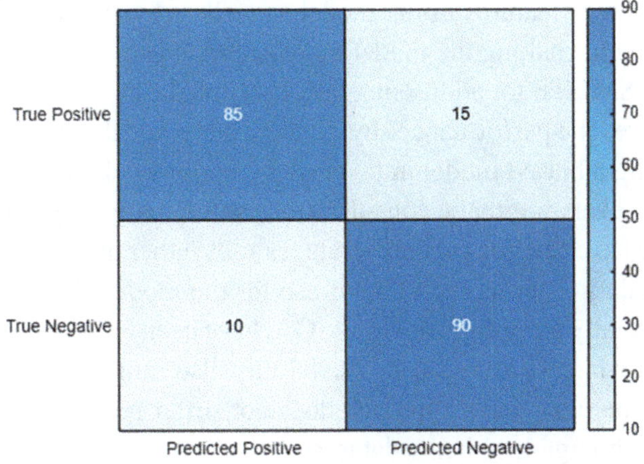

Figure 6. ROC Curve

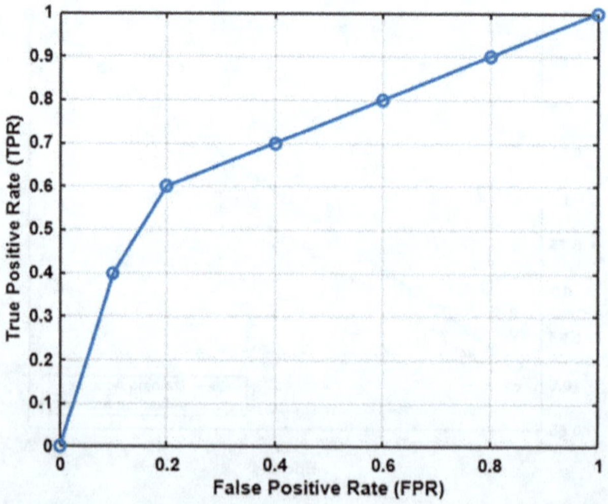

The results obtained clearly indicate that incorporation of ML and optimization significantly improves the quality of the models. The use of optimization algorithms enhances selection of features in the model as well as hyperparameters displayed in figures 3 & 4 thus making the model more accurate and easier to interpret. Furthermore, using SMOTE for addressing the class imbalance in our study (Figure 2) generally improves the performances by giving a better recall rate and reducing the chances of having a biased model in favor of the majority class.

That said however, pragmatic considerations still remain a mystery. This is why it is important to have categorical or discrete features rather than continuous metrics – otherwise the data is too noisy to be of use for the model. Another issue is that techniques, especially for optimization like GA, have been found to be computationally expensive for large-featured data. Scalability also remains a concern in order to confirm that the integrative approach does not suffer performance degradation when dealing with large healthcare datasets.

Finally, the presented framework of the combined ML and optimization process can be deemed as a highly reliable approach to disease prediction applied in healthcare analytics as a continuation of the existing models' development. The findings indicate the possibility of utilizing this approach and outline they way for further studies and practical work.

IMPACT AND CURRENT TRENDS IN MACHINE LEARNING, OPTIMIZATION, AND DISEASE PREDICTION

- **The Transformative Impact of Machine Learning and Optimization in Disease Prediction**

The integration of machine learning (ML) and optimization algorithms into disease prediction has ushered in a new era in healthcare, marked by data-driven decision-making, proactive patient management, and personalized medicine. Traditional diagnostic methods, often reliant on subjective clinical judgment and limited datasets, are increasingly being supplemented—or even replaced—by AI systems capable of processing vast and diverse datasets with remarkable accuracy. ML models, particularly deep learning networks, are trained on electronic health records (EHRs), genetic information, imaging data, and real-time physiological signals to detect complex patterns and forecast disease onset long before clinical symptoms become apparent. This predictive capability has proven invaluable in chronic conditions such as diabetes, cardiovascular diseases, and various cancers, where early intervention significantly improves patient outcomes. Additionally, time-series models like LSTM (Long Short-Term Memory) and transformer-based architectures have demonstrated their effectiveness in forecasting disease trajectories, enabling dynamic treatment planning. Optimization plays a critical role in refining these predictive models by tuning hyperparameters, selecting relevant features, and minimizing error functions, thereby enhancing model precision and reliability. Furthermore, optimization techniques are central to clinical decision support systems (CDSS), where they help prioritize interventions, allocate resources, and design individualized treatment plans based on predicted risks. For example, genetic algorithms and swarm intelligence methods are increasingly used to determine the optimal combination of biomarkers or symptoms for accurate disease classification. These developments collectively empower clinicians with predictive insights that were previously unattainable, fostering a shift from reactive to preventive healthcare models.

- **Current Trends in Machine Learning and Optimization for Disease Prediction**

Recent advancements in machine learning and optimization are setting transformative trends in disease prediction, driven by innovations in algorithm design, data accessibility, and computing power. One of the most prominent trends is the rise of multi-modal learning, where algorithms integrate diverse data types—such as genomic sequences, radiological images, wearable sensor data, and patient histories—to form a holistic view of patient health. This fusion significantly improves diagnostic precision, especially in complex and multifactorial diseases like Alzheimer's, where single-source data is insufficient. Another trend is the increasing use of federated learning models, which enable training ML algorithms across decentralized healthcare systems without compromising patient privacy. This approach is especially useful in scenarios where patient data cannot be centrally pooled due to regulatory or ethical concerns, yet collective intelligence is required for robust disease prediction. Additionally, reinforcement learning is gaining traction in sequential decision-making tasks, such as drug dosage optimization and treatment path recommendations, where the model learns optimal strategies over time based on simulated or real clinical outcomes. In parallel, explainable AI (XAI) is becoming a standard requirement rather than an optional feature. With healthcare decisions having direct implications on human lives, black-box models are increasingly being replaced or augmented with interpretable models like decision trees, SHAP (SHapley Additive exPlanations), and LIME (Local Interpretable Model-agnostic Explanations), which provide transparency and build clinician trust. Furthermore, optimization algorithms are evolving beyond classical approaches; hybrid and metaheuristic techniques are now being employed to solve high-dimensional, nonlinear problems typical in genomics and epidemiological modeling. These trends reflect a broader shift toward precision health, where predictive analytics is not just a tool but a foundational pillar of modern clinical practice.

- **Real-World Applications, Challenges, and the Road Ahead**

The application of machine learning and optimization in disease prediction is no longer confined to theoretical research—it is actively transforming clinical workflows, public health initiatives, and pharmaceutical research. In clinical settings, predictive algorithms are embedded in EHR systems to flag patients at risk of sepsis, cardiac arrest, or mental health crises, allowing for timely interventions. Startups and healthcare institutions are deploying AI-powered platforms for cancer detection using histopathological images and radiographic data, with some models achieving diagnostic accuracies on par with, or surpassing, trained pathologists. In the context of public health, machine learning models are being used to track and predict the spread of infectious diseases, such as influenza and COVID-19, by analyzing mobility data, social media trends, and environmental factors. Optimization algorithms support these efforts by enhancing model efficiency and enabling real-time response planning. Despite these successes, several challenges persist. Data quality and interoperability remain significant barriers, as healthcare data is often noisy, fragmented, and siloed. Ethical concerns regarding bias, patient consent, and algorithmic accountability further complicate widespread adoption. There is also a critical need for standardized benchmarks and validation frameworks to assess model performance across diverse populations and clinical settings. Moving forward, the convergence of cloud computing, quantum algorithms, and edge AI is expected to further accelerate disease prediction capabilities. Integrating AI into medical curricula and clinical training will also be essential to ensure that healthcare professionals can effectively utilize these tools. In summary, while the journey toward fully AI-integrated disease prediction is complex and multifaceted, the combined power of machine learning and optimization holds unparalleled potential to transform global healthcare delivery and outcomes.

FUTURE DIRECTIONS

Disease prediction with the help of machine learning (ML) and optimization techniques have huge scope for more developments. However, as the progress in the field continues on, few promising areas stand out that may greatly improve the effectiveness, explainability, and versatility of predictive models in the field of healthcare. The six directions are using quantum computation, adopting XAI, and using IoT and Wearable Technology data in real-time.

It is also, one of the most promising areas where quantum computing may be utilized to optimize for the ML models. Optimization is a much simpler task in which complex computations can be achieved via quantum computing at far higher speeds. Future developments such as Quantum Approximate Optimization Algorithm (QAOA) could be used for feature selection and hyperparameters optimization problems. For example, in high-dimensional medical datasets, quantum computing could efficiently find set-features that would give maximal results for improved model accuracy with minimal Resource consumption. Besides, with sufficient quantum advancements, the analysis of the extensive medical databases like genomics, or even imaging databases could be performed in real time, opening new horizons in disease diagnosis.

One important areais the existing and potential function of Explainable AI (XAI) in enhancing model interpretability. Indeed, even if the deep learning technique allows finding good predictions, it often lacks interpretability, which hinders its use in clinical practice. XAI solves this problem by helping the HE professionals understand how those models arrive at certain decisions. For instance, methods such as SHAP and LIME can draw attention to the critical features affecting the prediction of diseases. For instance when a patient is diagnosed with cancer, XAI could assist the doctor in understanding why a particular biomarker is ranked highly by a particular model. Moreover, the coupling of XAI with optimization can ascertain that interpretability does not suffer, even when achieving high levels of accuracy is the goal.

There is another significant possibility for increasing the rate of illness prediction and that is using IoT devices and wearable technology data in near-real-time. Smartwatches and fitness trackers consume health information that is produced in real-time, including heart rate, blood pressure, and motion. When integrated with ML models, this real-time data can help in prompt diagnosis of various ailments such as arrhythmias, hypertension, or even manifestations-of mental health ailments. For instance, when developing an application that uses wearables, optimization methods can be used to choose the data streams for these wearables, and make models logical and economical. However, real time data integration can indeed enhance personalized health care as prediction and recommendations can be adjusted according to the changing status of the health status.

Nevertheless, there are some issues which are still open, for example, the high price of quantum devices, the lack of suitable methods for XAI, and the question of how to protect real-time health information. Such challenges can only be solved by professionals including computer science, health care practitioner and policy maker.

Altogether, the future perspectives of the integrative use of machine learning and optimization in diseases' prediction can be bright with the accounted influences of prospective quantum computing, the further development of XAI, and the increased usage of IoT for continuous data streaming. All these gains are predesigned not only to increase the performance of the model, its predictive abilities, and the wholesale interpretation of the results but also to strengthen the Patient's outcomes and thus, move the health sector from a purely reactive one to a proactive one.

CONCLUSION

The coupling of ML and solution methods as a revolutionary model has clearly emerged as the best approach in the domain of disease prediction. This chapter demonstrates how integrative models outperform conventional models using accuracy, precision, recall, and improved interpretability. Utilization of feature selection using Genetic Algorithm, hyper parameter tuning using Particle Swarm Optimization, and managing class imbalance using SMOTE have shown to be useful in handling of various challenges facing health data analytics. Besides, it is evident that the models used produce dependable results through the application of enhanced visualizations such as confusion matrices and ROC curves.

This integrative system has significant implications for the present and future practice and science of health care. Since these models help in identifying diseases at their early stages and with high accuracy, the clinicians can be in a better position in taking right decisions that will lead to better patient care as well as reducing diagnostic errors. It is evidenced that when models are both accurate and interpretable, they are trustful, thanks to the use of Explainable AI. Further, the applicability of wearable and IoT data for real-time information integration may bring drastic changes in the conventional health care delivery system, where care is given in advance and in accordance with the needs of the patients.

Therefore, ML combined with optimization may be considered as a new direction in disease prediction that demonstrates a significant potential to translate big data into realistic solutions. This approach will in the long run improve the healthcare delivery and reduce costs as well as open up research in prediction techniques for healthcare delivery. This potential calls for the significance of enhancing this field as a result of its potential in being taken up by the society in large scale.

REFERENCES

Abdellatif, A., Abdellatef, H., Kanesan, J., Chow, C.-O., Chuah, J. H., & Gheni, H. M. (2022). An effective heart disease detection and severity level classification model using machine learning and hyperparameter optimization methods. *IEEE Access : Practical Innovations, Open Solutions*, *10*, 79974–79985. DOI: 10.1109/ACCESS.2022.3191669

Abdulmalek, S., Nasir, A., Jabbar, W. A., Almuhaya, M. A. M., Bairagi, A. K., Khan, M. A., & Kee, S. H. (2022). IoT-based healthcare-monitoring system towards improving quality of life: A review. *Healthcare (Basel)*, *10*(10), 1993. DOI: 10.3390/healthcare10101993 PMID: 36292441

Agarwal, S., P. P. S., S. D., & Kumari, G. S. (2024). Optimizing IoT-based healthcare systems with scalable AI and machine learning using cloud platforms. In *Proceedings of the 2024 First International Conference on Innovations in Communications, Electrical and Computer Engineering (ICICEC)* (pp. 1–7).

Arora, D., Suneetha, S., & Patil, S. R. (2023). Advancements in multi-cloud applications for enhanced e-healthcare services. In *Proceedings of the 2023 International Conference on Artificial Intelligence for Innovations in Healthcare Industries (ICAIIHI)* (pp. 1–7).

Asha, A., Dhiyanesh, B., Kiruthiga, G., Shakkeera, L., Jacob, V., & Venaik, A. (2024). Efficient coronary heart disease prediction: Enhanced neural network with chaos salp decision and feature optimization. *International Journal of Intelligent Systems and Applications in Engineering*, *12*(20s), 440–450.

Balafas, V., Karantoumanis, E., Louta, M., & Ploskas, N. (2023). Machine learning and deep learning for plant disease classification and detection. *IEEE Access : Practical Innovations, Open Solutions*, *11*, 114352–114377. DOI: 10.1109/ACCESS.2023.3324722

Chauhan, N. K., & Kaur, N. (2023). Predicting cardiovascular diseases using machine learning integrated with feature selection through blue whale optimization. In *Proceedings of the 2023 10th IEEE Uttar Pradesh Section International Conference on Electrical, Electronics and Computer Engineering (UPCON)* (pp. 464–469). DOI: 10.1109/UPCON59197.2023.10434597

Chen, M., Hao, Y., Hwang, K., Wang, L., & Wang, L. (2017). Disease prediction by machine learning over big data from healthcare communities. *IEEE Access : Practical Innovations, Open Solutions*, *5*, 8869–8879. DOI: 10.1109/ACCESS.2017.2694446

Gowda, D., Shindhe, R., Simha, S. K., & Yashwanth, T. (2023, December). Healthcare Energized by Motion Harnessing Piezoelectric Energy in Conjunction with IoT for Medical Innovations. In *2023 International Conference on Artificial Intelligence for Innovations in Healthcare Industries (ICAIIHI)* (Vol. 1, pp. 1-7). IEEE.

Gowda, D. V., Sharma, A., Mukherjee, S., & Rahman, M. (2024). Optimizing resource allocation in healthcare facilities through IoT and machine learning predictive analysis. In *Universal threats in expert applications and solutions* (pp. 177–187).

Jadhav, M. R., & Kaur, M. (2023). Predictive modeling of dental health outcomes based on fluoride concentrations using AI. In *Proceedings of the 2023 3rd International Conference on Smart Generation Computing, Communication and Networking (SMART GENCON)* (pp. 1–7).

Kalpana, V., & Hariram, V. (2023). Artificial intelligence-based health monitoring system on IoT platform. In *Proceedings of the 2023 Second International Conference on Augmented Intelligence and Sustainable Systems (ICAISS)* (pp. 1458–1463).

Mallikarjun, S. S. D., & Kawale, S. R. (2023). Cloud-based multi-layer security framework for protecting e-health records. In *Proceedings of the 2023 International Conference on Artificial Intelligence for Innovations in Healthcare Industries (ICAIIHI)* (pp. 1–7).

Ramesha, M., Anughna, N., Nareshkumar, A., Gowda, D., & Gururaj, B. (2022, November). An integrated IoT technology for health and traffic monitoring system with smart ambulance. In *2022 IEEE North Karnataka Subsection Flagship International Conference (NKCon)* (pp. 1-6). IEEE.

Pandidurai, M., & Senthil Kamalesh, M. S. C. (2023). Design of IoT-based rural health helper using natural language processing. In *Proceedings of the 2023 4th International Conference on Electronics and Sustainable Communication Systems (ICESC)* (pp. 328–333).

Pankajavalli, P. B., Karthick, G. S., & Sakthivel, R. (2021). An efficient machine learning framework for stress prediction via sensor integrated keyboard data. *IEEE Access : Practical Innovations, Open Solutions*, *9*, 95023–95035. DOI: 10.1109/ACCESS.2021.3094334

Patil, N. J., Sharma, A., Prasad, K. D. V., & Kottala, S. (2024). IoT-enabled predictive healthcare monitoring using machine learning models. In *Universal threats in expert applications and solutions* (pp. 165–175). DOI: 10.1007/978-981-97-5146-4_15

Prasad, K., S. R., & A. K. N. (2024). Design and implementation of an AI and IoT-enabled smart safety helmet for real-time environmental and health monitoring. In *Proceedings of the 2024 IEEE International Conference on Information Technology, Electronics and Intelligent Communication Systems (ICITEICS)* (pp. 1–7).

Rashmi, G. R., & Chinamuttevi, V. S. (2022). IoT-based smart healthcare system to monitor COVID-19 patients. *International Journal of Electrical and Electronics Research, 10*(1), 36–40. DOI: 10.37391/IJEER.100105

Reddy, K. V. V., Elamvazuthi, I., Aziz, A. A., Paramasivam, S., Chua, H. N., & Pranavanand, S. (2021). Prediction of heart disease risk using machine learning with correlation-based feature selection and optimization techniques. In *Proceedings of the 2021 7th International Conference on Signal Processing and Communication (ICSC)*(pp. 228–233). DOI: 10.1109/ICSC53193.2021.9673490

Tanguturi, R. C., & Poornima, G. (2022). An intelligent system for remote monitoring of patients' health and the early detection of coronary artery disease. In *Proceedings of the 2022 International Conference on Smart Generation Computing, Communication and Networking (SMART GENCON)* (pp. 1–6).

ADDITIONAL READING

Balaji, P., Chaurasia, M. A., Bilfaqih, S. M., Muniasamy, A., & Alsid, L. E. G. (2023). Hybridized deep learning approach for detecting Alzheimer's disease. *Biomedicines, 11*(1), 149. DOI: 10.3390/biomedicines11010149 PMID: 36672656

Balaji, P., Muniasamy, V., Bilfaqih, S. M., Muniasamy, A., Tharanidharan, S., Mani, D., & Alsid, L. E. G. (2023). Chimp optimization algorithm influenced type-2 intuitionistic fuzzy C-means clustering-based breast cancer detection system. *Cancers (Basel), 15*(4), 1131. DOI: 10.3390/cancers15041131 PMID: 36831474

Muniasamy, A., Alquhtani, S. A. S., Alshehri, A. H., Begum, A., & Sabahath, A. (2025). Investigating hybrid quantum-assisted classical and deep learning model for MRI brain tumor classification. *Journal of Image and Graphics, 13*(1). Advance online publication. DOI: 10.18178/joig.13.1.123-129

Muniasamy, A., Begum, A., Sabahath, A., & Yaqub, H. (2023). Lung cancer histopathology image classification using transfer learning with convolution neural network model. *Journal Name, volume*(issue), 1–12.

Muniasamy, A., Begum, A., Sabahath, A., Yaqub, H., & Karunakaran, G. (2024). Coronary heart disease classification using deep learning approach with feature selection for improved accuracy. *Technology and Health Care*, *32*(3), 1991–2007. DOI: 10.3233/THC-231807 PMID: 38339946

Muniasamy, A., Begum, A., Sabahath, A., Yaqub, H., & Karunakaran, G. (2024). Coronary heart disease classification using deep learning approach with feature selection for improved accuracy. *Technology and Health Care*, *32*(3), 1–17. Advance online publication. DOI: 10.3233/THC-231807 PMID: 38339946

Vasanthakumar, G., & Singh, M. (2024). Quantum machine learning in healthcare: Diagnostics and drug discovery. In Raj, P., Song, H., Le, D., & Vyas, N. (Eds.), *Quantum Machine Learning: Quantum Algorithms and Neural Networks* (pp. 39–64). De Gruyter.

KEY TERMS AND DEFINITIONS

Disease Prediction: The process of using computational models and data-driven techniques to estimate the likelihood of a disease developing in an individual or population.

Feature Selection: A process in machine learning where the most relevant input variables (features) are identified and retained to improve model accuracy, reduce complexity, and enhance interpretability.

Federated Learning: A decentralized machine learning approach where models are trained across multiple devices or servers holding local data samples, without exchanging the actual data, thereby preserving privacy and data security.

Genetic Algorithms (GAs): A type of evolutionary algorithm inspired by the process of natural selection, used to find optimal or near-optimal solutions by iteratively selecting, crossing, and mutating candidate solutions.

Healthcare Analytics: The application of data analysis techniques to healthcare data in order to improve patient outcomes, optimize operations, and support clinical decision-making.

Hyperparameter Tuning: The process of selecting the optimal configuration of hyperparameters—settings that control the learning process of a machine learning model—to improve its performance.

Machine Learning (ML): A branch of artificial intelligence (AI) that enables systems to learn from data, identify patterns, and make decisions or predictions with minimal human intervention.

Optimization Techniques: Mathematical and computational strategies used to adjust model parameters or processes to achieve the best possible performance, often by maximizing accuracy or minimizing error.

Predictive Models: Statistical or machine learning models designed to predict future outcomes or trends based on historical data.

Chapter 3
Overview of ML and Optimization Algorithms in Disease Prediction and a Comprehensive Review

J. Vijaya
https://orcid.org/0000-0002-9948-8573
International Institute of Information Technology, Naya Raipur, India

Pankaj Kumar Verma
International Institute of Information Technology, Naya Raipur, India

Rishi Thakur
International Institute of Information Technology, Naya Raipur, India

Shruti Soni
International Institute of Information Technology, Naya Raipur, India

Tripti Sharma
International Institute of Information Technology, Naya Raipur, India

Bhavya Chauhan
International Institute of Information Technology, Naya Raipur, India

ABSTRACT

Globally, there is a significant unmet need for effective and timely disease diagnosis. The complexity of various disease mechanisms, along with the diverse symptoms presented by patients, creates substantial challenges in the development of early diagnosis tools and effective treatments. Machine learning (ML), a subfield of artificial intelligence (AI), and Optimization techniques has emerged as a powerful tool to address some of these challenges. By leveraging advanced algorithms and large datasets, ML enables the early identification and classification of numerous diseases, thus improving patient outcomes and facilitating timely interventions. In medical domains, Optimization techniques focus on developing algorithms and tech-

DOI: 10.4018/979-8-3373-1087-9.ch003

niques to ensure accurate disease diagnosis. The review explores recent trends and methodologies in disease prediction, focusing on critical factors such as the types of algorithms used, the diseases diagnosed, the nature of the data employed, and the various applications and evaluation metrics used to assess model performance.

INTRODUCTION

Medical diagnosis involves identifying the diseases or conditions that explain a person's symptoms and signs, typically relying on information gathered from the patient's history and physical examination. This process is often challenging because many symptoms and signs can be ambiguous, requiring expert interpretation. In countries with limited healthcare professionals, such as Bangladesh and India, providing adequate diagnostic procedures for the entire population becomes a significant issue. Additionally, diagnostic procedures often involve medical tests, which can be costly and inaccessible for low-income individuals (Mishra and Vijaya, 2024). Human errors in medical diagnoses are not uncommon, potentially leading to issues like overdiagnosis, unnecessary treatments, and subsequent impacts on health and the economy. The majority of people will make at least one diagnostic mistake in their lifetime, according to a 2015 research by the National Academies of Sciences, Engineering, and Medicine. Factors contributing to misdiagnoses include the lack of noticeable symptoms, the presence of rare diseases, or the omission of certain conditions from consideration. Machine learning (ML) has emerged as a powerful tool in healthcare, offering innovative solutions for disease diagnosis that are both cost-effective and time-efficient (Ram et al., 2024). Unlike traditional diagnostic processes, which are constrained by human limitations, ML systems can process large datasets and operate continuously without exhaustion. These systems utilize various types of healthcare data, such as medical images (e.g., X-rays, MRIs) and structured data (e.g., patient demographics and clinical metrics), to perform tasks like disease classification and regression with remarkable accuracy. ML, a subset of AI, applies mathematical functions to process data and generates outputs such as classifications or predictions. For example, ML techniques can simplify the detection of malignant cells in microscopic images, a task that is typically complex for human experts. Recent advancements in Deep Learning (DL), a specialized form of ML, have further enhanced the accuracy of disease diagnosis, often exceeding 90% in detecting conditions like Alzheimer's disease, heart failure, and breast cancer.

These developments underscore the transformative potential of ML in the medical field (Prasanna and Vijaya, 2022).

Optimization techniques provide data-driven solutions for disease diagnosis, medical imaging, personalized treatment, drug discovery, and hospital resource management. However, given the complexity, heterogeneity, and high-dimensional nature of medical data, ML models require robust optimization techniques to improve predictive accuracy, computational efficiency, and interpretability. Optimization plays a crucial role in fine-tuning hyper parameters, selecting relevant features, and enhancing the performance of deep learning models, making them more suitable for real-world healthcare applications (Vijaya et al. 2023). PSO (Particle Swarm Optimization) has been particularly effective in optimizing convolutional neural networks (CNNs) for brain tumor classification by fine-tuning learning rates, filter sizes, and network depths, thereby minimizing classification errors (Vijaya and Rao, 2022). ACO (Ant Colony Optimization) has demonstrated its efficiency in medical image segmentation by simulating the natural foraging behavior of ants to identify optimal pixel clusters, significantly improving tumor detection accuracy (Xia et al., 2024). ABC (Artificial Bee Colony) has been applied to cardiovascular disease prediction by selecting the most relevant patient features, enhancing classification accuracy while reducing computational costs (Khan et al., 2024). Despite the significant advancements achieved through ML-driven optimization techniques in healthcare, several challenges persist. Computational complexity remains a critical issue, as some optimization algorithms require extensive computational resources, making real-time healthcare applications difficult to implement. Data privacy concerns also pose challenges, as ML models rely on vast amounts of patient data, necessitating the development of privacy-preserving optimization techniques such as federated learning. Model interpretability continues to be a major concern, particularly in high-stakes clinical decision-making, requiring further research into Explainable AI (XAI) methods that provide transparent and trustworthy predictions. Selecting the most suitable optimization algorithm for a given healthcare problem remains a challenge due to the diversity of medical data, necessitating the development of adaptive and hybrid optimization techniques (Rao et al., 2024; Ramesh and Lakshmanna, 2024).

Future research directions in ML-based healthcare optimization emphasize the need for more interpretable, adaptive, and multi-objective optimization strategies. Explainable AI (XAI) ensures that clinicians can trust and understand AI-generated recommendations. Adaptive optimization techniques that dynamically adjust their strategies based on evolving patient data and real-time clinical requirements will be essential for personalized medicine (Islam, Majumder, Hussein, et al., 2024). Multi-objective optimization will be critical in balancing trade-offs between model accuracy, computational efficiency, and interpretability, leading to more robust and clinically applicable solutions. Federated learning and privacy-preserving optimization techniques will be vital for enabling decentralized AI models that protect patient confidentiality while leveraging collaborative learning across multiple healthcare institutions (Mienye and Jere, 2024). Hybrid optimization approaches that combine multiple techniques, such as swarm intelligence with evolutionary algorithms, will further improve model convergence rates and generalization capabilities. Quantum-inspired computing holds promise for tackling complex optimization problems in healthcare, leveraging quantum mechanics principles to accelerate the search for optimal solutions. Bias-aware optimization techniques will be necessary to ensure fairness in AI-driven healthcare, reducing disparities across different patient demographics. The continuous evolution of these optimization methodologies will be instrumental in advancing the field of AI-driven healthcare, ultimately improving diagnostic accuracy, treatment efficacy, and patient outcomes (Vijaya et al., 2023).

This review begins with a bibliometric analysis of 1,216 publications sourced from the Scopus and Web of Science (WOS) databases. The analysis identifies the most prolific authors, countries, organizations, and the most cited articles in the field of Machine-Learning-Based Disease Diagnosis (MLBDD). The review then explores recent trends and methodologies in MLBDD, focusing on critical factors such as the types of algorithms used, the diseases diagnosed, the nature of the data employed, and the various applications and evaluation metrics used to assess model performance. Furthermore, the review highlights the challenges and limitations faced in the application of ML in disease diagnosis, including issues related to data quality, algorithm interpretability, and model generalization. Finally, the paper provides insights into the future directions and opportunities for ML in healthcare, outlining potential breakthroughs and emphasizing the need for further research to overcome existing obstacles and enhance the adoption of ML techniques in real-world clinical settings.

BACKGROUND

Machine learning in healthcare has undergone a profound evolution since its early inception in the mid-20th century. Initial efforts in ML were characterized by rule-based systems, exemplified by MYCIN in the 1970s, which was developed for diagnosing bacterial infections. These early systems relied heavily on hand-crafted rules and logical inference, offering groundbreaking potential at the time but lacking scalability and adaptability to complex, dynamic healthcare environments (Skender and Zhang, 2024). These advancements have enabled AI applications to extend far beyond diagnostics, encompassing areas like personalized medicine, drug discovery, and robotic-assisted surgery. The integration of increasing computational power with access to large, diverse healthcare datasets has been instrumental in this transformation. This evolution highlights a shift from deterministic, rule-based approaches to probabilistic, data-intensive methodologies, underscoring the growing role of AI in enhancing healthcare delivery (Serrano et al., 2024). Traditionally, disease prediction has relied on human expertise, involving a combination of clinical observations, systematic investigations, and the application of extensive medical training. Physicians traditionally followed a linear diagnostic workflow for symptom identification, hypothesis generation, targeted testing, and data interpretation all of which depended on human cognitive processes. While laboratory tests and imaging technologies complemented clinical judgment, the process remained susceptible to inherent limitations such as cognitive biases, memory constraints, and variability in expertise. Diagnosis often hinged on a physician's experience and subjective pattern recognition, which introduced an element of inconsistency, particularly in complex cases with overlapping or subtle symptoms.

This conventional approach, while foundational to modern medicine, struggled to synthesize vast and complex data, limiting its effectiveness in addressing multifaceted diagnostic challenges (Taha et al., 2024). ML has shown significant promise in various diagnostic applications. For example, it has been utilized to enhance the accuracy of radiological assessments by analyzing imaging data alongside patient demographics and clinical histories. Hulsen et al (2023) Studies indicate that ML models (Supervised, Unsupervised, and Reinforcement Learning) can outperform traditional diagnostic methods by reducing false positive and negative rates significantly. Furthermore, ML algorithms can quickly adapt to new data, making them invaluable during emerging health crises, such as outbreaks of infectious diseases. This capability is particularly beneficial for early disease detection and personalized treatment plans.

Machine learning in healthcare encompasses a wide range of applications, including disease prediction, medical imaging analysis, personalized treatment, drug discovery, and hospital resource management. Supervised learning methods, Decision Tree, Support Vector Machine, Naïve Bayes, K Nearest Neighbor, Artificial Neural Network and Logistic Regression (DT, SVM, NB, KNN, ANN, LR), and deep learning-based convolutional neural networks (CNNs) are widely used for tasks like medical diagnosis and image classification. Unsupervised learning techniques, including clustering and dimensionality reduction, assist in patient segmentation and anomaly detection, while reinforcement learning is increasingly being explored for clinical decision support and robotic surgeries (Padmavathi et al., 2023; Arumugam et al., 2023). However, achieving high accuracy and efficiency in ML-driven healthcare applications often requires the application of advanced optimization algorithms that fine-tune models, select the most relevant features, and improve decision-making processes. Despite the remarkable success of ML in healthcare, these models require extensive fine-tuning and optimization to achieve the best performance. Factors such as selecting the right hyper parameters, feature subsets, and training strategies play a crucial role in ensuring that ML models provide reliable and interpretable results. This is where optimization algorithms become essential.

Optimization techniques possess the remarkable capability of continuous learning, where each processed disease case refines the system's diagnostic accuracy and predictive capabilities. Unlike static human knowledge, optimization enables real-time adaptation and improvement, a critical advantage in the fast-evolving medical landscape. For instance, machine learning algorithms have demonstrated the ability to detect minute textural changes in medical images, identify genetic markers with high precision, and predict disease progression through sophisticated multivariate analyses. This represents a fundamental shift from reactive to proactive diagnostics, facilitating earlier detection and personalized risk assessments (Vijaya, et al., 2023). Evolutionary algorithms, inspired by natural selection and genetic evolution, have also contributed significantly to healthcare optimization. The Genetic Algorithm (GA) has been widely applied to disease prediction strategies. GA operates by evolving candidate treatment plans over multiple generations, selecting the most effective combinations while minimizing adverse effects (Vijaya, 2023). Differential Evolution (DE) has been instrumental in drug discovery and molecular docking simulations by optimizing molecular interactions, leading to the identification of novel drug compounds for treating various diseases. Physics-based optimization techniques, inspired by natural physical phenomena, have further contributed to ML-driven healthcare solutions (Pesaramelli and Sujatha, 2024). Simulated Annealing (SA) has been successfully applied to optimize hospital resource allocation, ensuring efficient scheduling of beds, medical staff, and equipment to meet patient demand while minimizing operational costs. SA mimics the annealing process in metallurgy, exploring the search space for optimal solutions by probabilistically accepting suboptimal configurations to escape local minima. This stochastic approach has proven valuable in dynamic healthcare environments where resource constraints and demand fluctuations are common (Gangadevi et al., 2024). The Gravitational Search Algorithm (GSA) has been employed in electrocardiogram (ECG) signal classification for heart disease detection by optimizing deep learning models. GSA leverages gravitational forces to guide solutions toward optimal classifications, improving the accuracy of normal and abnormal ECG pattern detection. These physics-based techniques have demonstrated their effectiveness in optimizing complex medical systems, enhancing both predictive capabilities and resource utilization (Ezzat et al., 2021).

This literature section goes into further detail about the case study of Non-Alcoholic Fatty Liver Disease (NAFL) disease prediction systems in humans. Goldman, Orit, et al (2021) analyzed the two parameters such as fatty liver index and fibrosis 4 which are significant reasons for NAFL liver disease in humans. They used a real-time dataset from a survey named TAMCIS for validation through classification models such as the CHAID algorithm. Finally, they concluded that the identified two parameters influence non-alcoholic fatty liver disease and they suggested mechanisms for how to control or change the two parameters in the affected humans also they ranked the importance of features that are highly correlated to the disease (Goldman et al. 2021). Lee et al., (2022) studied the relationship between the two diseases gestational diabetes mellitus (GDM) and NAFL disease through real-time experimental setups. They chose around 1500 women patients have analyzed the impact of the identified disease using Machine Learning (ML) models with the predicted five most important features. A unique blended Random Forest (RF) classification with a (DT and three classification models such as the augmented LR model, SVM, and Deep Neural Network (DNN) are used to build a model for their works. They concluded that non-alcoholic fatty liver disease increases the likelihood that pregnant women may develop Gestational Diabetes Mellitus (GDM). Ke et al (2025) analyzed the performance of the ML models in the field of NAFL disease management systems realistically. They collaborated with multiple liver clinics in the United States and collected real-time data for the patients involved in liver disease in 6-month durations. In this process, they included 1370 patients' information along with 17 useful pieces of information given to the three ML models such as LR, RF, and ANN. This model is used to analyze the connections and flow between the various significant stages of this disease and the models are evaluated by the known parameters of the classification models.

Castañé et al (2021) surveyed NAFL disease from their perceptive which includes different research dimensions. They segmented 8 important features such as age, sex, body mass index, Homa Ir, T2Dm, Hta, drugs, and dyslipidemia for sample preparation. The plasma sample and lipid extraction of the identified sampled patients' data are pre-processed by univariate and multi-variant data analysis. Then the pre-processed data is given to ML models. The four factors of the steatosis fibrosis of the NAFL disease from the previous stage (Hepatokines lipid mediators) are diet lipid mediators; insulin, hypertrophy, and inflammatory cell infiltration are identified. Kumar et al (2023) studied children with NAFL disease which leads to childhood fatigue and they collected unstructured data (digital descriptions and ultrasounds). The input of the machine learning model is pixel images which are capable of categorizing the input images into normal and diseased liver tissues. They used the representative Region of Interest (ROI) methodology to identify the top features that are given to multiple machine learning models such as SVM, NN, and Extreme Gradient Boost. In their implementation, 93 non-diseased images, 39 diseased images, and 28 texture-featured images are collected from 744 images of 42 children. They performed a comparative study between them and finally concluded which performs better classification for NAFL disease in children. CA

Kezer et al. (2021) reviewed the application of ML methods, such as deep learning (DL), neural networks, supervised learning, and natural language processing in hepatology systems. They segmented the role of ML in hepatology systems into six which include diagnosing the disease, distinguishing the stages, grade severity of images, prognosticate variables, evaluating for transplant, and the outcome of the transplant. They studied the seven most widespread chronic diseases including NAFL diseases each of which ends up causing a person's death. G Feng et al (2021)) analyzed fibrosis in biopsy which affects the levels of NAFL disease and their seriousness. They proposed a solution that is based on machine learning principles such as Least Absolute Shrinkage and Selection Operator (LASSO) logistic regression algorithm for the same by real-world experiments which is funded by the China Research Foundation and concluded that the proposed system showed the highest Area-Under-Curve (AUC) value. Liu et al (2023) studied the NAFL disease of Chinese patients around 15000 with a class distribution of 2:1 through ML models. The implemented chronicle illness data varies in size and the number of individual features to test the efficiency of learning algorithms and classification methods. Finally, they concluded that XG-Boost algorithms performed better than the other models, however, the output of the prediction system is purely dependent on the historical data used in the study.

Ganiger et al. (2018) evaluated 12 distinct algorithms for classification on multiple databases, each one with 400 records and 24 features. To assess prediction performance, they evaluated it by comparing their anticipated results to real outcomes. They measured the effectiveness of the classifiers using performance measures such as accuracy and other relevant parameters and it should be noted that NAFL disease is indeed common. The varying degrees of chronic inflammation linked to several lifestyle-related illnesses, including cardiovascular disease, stroke, lung cancer, colorectal cancer, and depression are examined by Subramanian et al. (2022). They proposed a new multi-label artificial neural network technique (ML-ANN) for predicting NDFL chronic illnesses that integrates a neural network and a multi-label training technique based on a cross-entropy loss mechanism and a backward propagation method. In 5 quality metrics, the suggested technique outperformed 14 traditional multi-label learning techniques on 10 chronic conditions and 19733 patients. The findings show that the suggested technique can effectively predict chronic illnesses and help doctors identify and treat sick people. Veerankutty et al. (2021) have presented their ideas for a computerized method for diagnosing a non-alcoholic fatty liver disease that uses a convolution neural network to examine the illness's inevitability (CNN). Utilizing a CT scan, the technique has been utilized to identify non-alcoholic fatty liver disease. Disease diagnosis could be a task that is occasionally very simple and other times may be a little trickier. To prevent life-threatening side effects for the victim, elevated concentrations of care and assistance are typically needed. Diagnosis is essential and victim severity evaluation seems to be the two most visible actions during ICU admission. To identify and evaluate illnesses, an embedded disorder identification and intensity assessment model (IDDSAM) has been proposed by Kaur et al. (2022). Reddy et al. (2024) introduced machine learning models that combine neural networks to detect non-alcoholic fatty liver disease. The suggested strategy consistently outperformed 14 conventional multi-label learning techniques for Asian patients in 5 performance metrics. The outcomes show that the suggested strategy may accurately forecast non-alcoholic fatty liver and help medical professionals identify and treat individuals. The research methodology employed in this review focuses on systematically exploring and analyzing the integration of optimization and ML within Disease prediction. The methodology consists of several stages, including data collection, analysis, and evaluation of findings from both theoretical and practical.

MAIN FOCUS OF THE CHAPTER

Figure 1 provides an in-depth exploration of how ML and optimization techniques are transforming healthcare. It covers:

Figure 1. Disease prediction system using ML and Optimisation Techniques

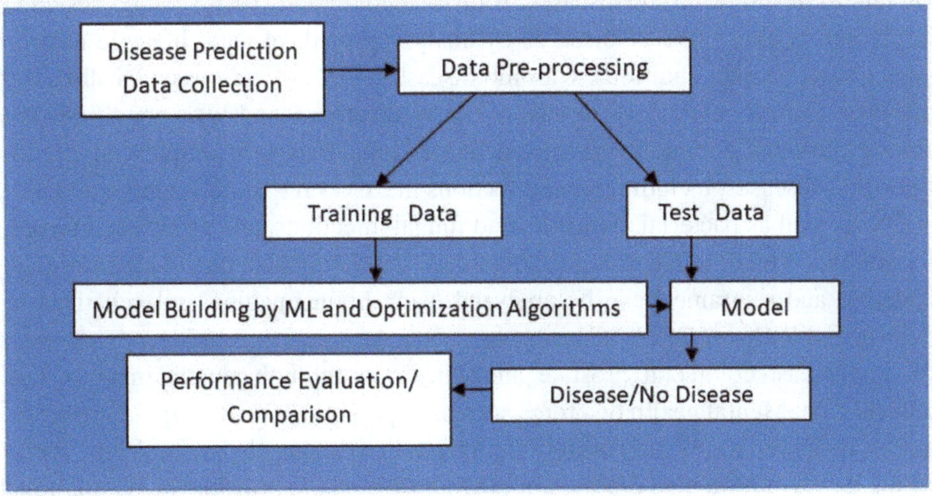

- The fundamental principles of ML in healthcare and its key applications.

- The role of optimization in enhancing ML models for disease detection, treatment planning, and medical imaging.
- A detailed review of various swarm-based, evolutionary, physics-based, and animal behavior-inspired algorithms used in healthcare AI.
- Case studies demonstrating how these algorithms improve the performance of disease prediction.

By leveraging ML and optimization together, healthcare professionals and researchers can develop more precise, interpretable, and efficient AI-driven solutions.

Type of Diseases in Disease Prediction System

Any Government must successfully implement a Health Care Management System (HMS) and it can create a long-term relationship between patients and healthcare providers. Healthcare service suppliers supply healthcare specialties to a patient through the hospital infrastructure, ambulance services, pharmacies, doctors with a variety of specialties, nurses, and other healthcare staff. A healthcare management system has various research facets, including disease diagnosis and identification, medicine production, bioinformatics issues, individualized care, patient image processing, and more.

There are two forms of disease diagnosis based on the nature of the disease including Acute and Chronic diseases. A disease prediction system can be designed to predict various types of diseases by analyzing medical data, lifestyle factors, and environmental conditions. Chronic diseases such as cardiovascular diseases, diabetes, chronic respiratory diseases, kidney disorders, and liver conditions are among the most commonly predicted due to their long-term impact on health. Infectious diseases, including viral infections like COVID-19, influenza, and HIV/AIDS, as well as bacterial, parasitic, and fungal infections, are also crucial targets for prediction models. Neurological disorders, including Alzheimer's, Parkinson's, epilepsy, and migraines, can be analyzed using brain imaging and genetic data (Vijaya and Rishabh, 2023). Cancer prediction systems focus on identifying risks for lung, breast, colorectal, prostate, and skin cancer through genetic, imaging, and clinical data. Mental health disorders such as depression, anxiety, bipolar disorder, and schizophrenia are increasingly being predicted using behavioral and social media data. Autoimmune diseases, including rheumatoid arthritis, lupus, multiple sclerosis, and Type 1 diabetes, can also be detected early using biomarkers and genetic analysis. Additionally, gastrointestinal disorders like irritable bowel syndrome (IBS), inflammatory bowel disease (IBD), and acid reflux, along with dermatological diseases such as eczema, psoriasis, and skin cancer, can be monitored for early warning signs. Genetic and hereditary conditions like cystic fibrosis, sickle cell anemia, and thalassemia are predicted using DNA sequencing and family history data. Rare and emerging diseases, such as genetic syndromes and new infectious outbreaks like Ebola or Nipah virus, can also be modeled for risk assessment. By integrating these various disease categories, prediction systems can provide early diagnosis, improve treatment strategies, and enhance preventive healthcare, ultimately reducing morbidity and mortality rates (Jha et al., 2024).

Disease Prediction Data sets

For disease prediction, various types of data are utilized to enhance accuracy and reliability. Clinical data, including electronic health records (EHRs), medical imaging, pathology reports, and doctor's notes, provide direct insights into a patient's medical history. Genomic and molecular data, such as DNA sequences, proteomics, and metabolomics, help in identifying genetic predispositions and biomarkers for diseases. Behavioral and lifestyle data, including diet, physical activity, sleep patterns, and habits like smoking or alcohol consumption, contribute to understanding risk factors. Environmental factors, such as air pollution, water quality, and climate conditions, play a crucial role in disease outbreaks and chronic illnesses. Wearable and sensor data, including heart rate, blood oxygen levels, glucose monitoring, and sleep tracking, enable continuous health monitoring. Social and epidemiological data, like demographic details, contact tracing, and disease outbreak reports, aid in tracking disease spread and risk assessment. Additionally, microbiome data particularly gut and skin micro biota, influence immunity and disease susceptibility (Ogunpola et al., 2024). Multi-omics data, integrating genomics, transcriptomics, and proteomics, provide a holistic approach to disease prediction. Drug and treatment response data, including pharmacogenomics and treatment efficacy, help in personalized medicine. Furthermore, text and natural language data from medical literature, social media, and research papers contribute to AI-driven insights and early warning systems. Integrating these diverse data sources improves disease prediction models, aiding in preventive healthcare and personalized treatment strategies (Islam & Miah et al., 2024).

Sources of Disease Prediction Data sets

Here are some publicly available datasets for disease prediction across various categories:

1. General Medical and Clinical Datasets
    a. MIMIC-III/MIMIC-IV (Medical ICU Data) – https://physionet.org/content/mimiciv

b. Electronic Health Records (EHRs) - eICU Collaborative Research Database – https://eicu-crd.mit.edu/
c. UCI Machine Learning Repository (Various Healthcare Datasets) – https://archive.ics.uci.edu/ml/index.php

2. Cardiovascular Disease Prediction
   a. Heart Disease Dataset (Cleveland, UCI) -https://archive.ics.uci.edu/ml/datasets/Heart+Disease
   b. Framingham Heart Study – https://www.framinghamheartstudy.org/
3. Diabetes Prediction
   a. Pima Indians Diabetes Dataset (UCI) – https://www.kaggle.com/datasets/uciml/pima- Indians-diabetes-database
4. Cancer Prediction
   a. Breast Cancer Wisconsin Dataset – https://archive.ics.uci.edu/ml/datasets/Breast+Cancer+Wisconsin+(Diagnostic)
   b. TCGA (The Cancer Genome Atlas) – https://portal.gdc.cancer.gov/
5. Neurological Disorders
   a. Epileptic Seizure Recognition Dataset (UCI) – https://archive.ics.uci.edu/ml/datasets/Epileptic+Seizure+Recognition
   b. Alzheimer's Disease Neuroimaging Initiative (ADNI) – https://adni.loni.usc.edu/
6. Infectious Disease and COVID-19
   a. COVID-19 Open Research Dataset (CORD-19) – https://www.kaggle.com/datasets/allen-institute-for-ai/CORD-19-research-challenge
   b. Tuberculosis Dataset – https://www.kaggle.com/datasets/raddar/tuberculosis-genomics-dataset
7. Mental Health and Depression Prediction
   a. Mental Health in Tech Industry (Kaggle) – https://www.kaggle.com/datasets/osmi/mental-health-in-tech-survey
8. Autoimmune and Chronic Diseases
   a. Chronic Kidney Disease Dataset (UCI) – https://archive.ics.uci.edu/ml/datasets/chronic_kidney_disease
9. Wearable and Sensor-Based Health Monitoring
   a. PhysioNet Wearable Sensor Data – https://physionet.org/about/database/

Data Preprocessing in Disease Prediction

Data preprocessing is a crucial step in disease prediction systems as it ensures the quality, consistency, and reliability of the data before feeding it into predictive models. The process begins with data collection from various sources such as electronic health records (EHRs), medical imaging, wearable sensors, and laboratory reports. Since raw medical data often contains missing values, inconsistencies, and noise, preprocessing techniques such as data imputation, outlier detection, and normalization are applied. Missing values can be handled using methods like mean/mode imputation, k-nearest neighbor (KNN) imputation, or advanced deep learning-based techniques. Additionally, duplicate and irrelevant features are removed to improve computational efficiency and model accuracy. Standardization or normalization of numerical features is performed to ensure uniformity across different scales, particularly for physiological parameters such as blood pressure, glucose levels, and heart rate. Categorical data, such as patient history and diagnostic codes, are encoded using one-hot encoding or label encoding, making them suitable for machine-learning models (Islam & Jannaty et al., 2024).

Feature engineering and dimensionality reduction play a significant role in optimizing disease prediction. Feature selection techniques like Principal Component Analysis (PCA), Recursive Feature Elimination (RFE), and mutual information help reduce redundant or non-informative variables while retaining essential predictors. For text-based medical records, Natural Language Processing (NLP) techniques such as tokenization, stemming, and word embeddings (e.g., Word2Vec or BERT) are used to extract meaningful insights. In medical imaging, preprocessing includes noise reduction, contrast enhancement, and image segmentation to highlight disease-related patterns. Data balancing methods like SMOTE (Synthetic Minority Over-sampling Technique) are often used to handle imbalanced datasets, ensuring that rare disease cases are not overshadowed by common conditions. Finally, data is split into training, validation, and testing sets to prevent over fitting and enhance generalizability. Proper preprocessing not only improves model performance but also ensures that predictions are clinically meaningful, aiding in early diagnosis and effective treatment planning (Dubey et al., 2024).

These techniques help in handling missing values, eliminating inconsistencies, and optimizing data for machine learning algorithms.

1. Data Cleaning

Medical datasets often contain missing values, duplicate records, noise, and inconsistencies. Several techniques are used to handle these issues:

a. Missing Value Imputation:
    i. Mean/Median/Mode Imputation: Filling missing numerical values using statistical measures.
    ii. K-Nearest Neighbours (KNN) Imputation: Predicting missing values based on the closest neighbors in the dataset.

iii. Multivariate Imputation by Chained Equations (MICE): Iterative modeling to estimate missing values.
iv. Deep Learning-Based Imputation: Autoencoders and GANs (Generative Adversarial Networks) can predict missing values.

b. Noise Removal:
i. Moving Average Smoothing: Used for time-series biomedical data such as ECG signals.
ii. Wavelet Transform: Used for denoising medical imaging and bio signals.
iii. Gaussian Filters & Median Filters: Used to remove artifacts in medical images (e.g., X-rays, MRIs).

c. Duplicate Record Removal:
i. Exact Matching: Identifying and removing duplicate rows.
ii. Fuzzy Matching (Levenshtein Distance, Jaccard Similarity): Detecting similar but non-exact duplicate records.

2. Data Transformation

Data from different sources might have varying formats, requiring standardization and encoding:

a. Standardization (Z-score normalization): Transforms numerical data to have a mean of 0 and standard deviation of 1.
b. Min-Max Normalization: Scales values between 0 and 1, often used for biometric data like glucose levels.
c. Log Transformation & Box-Cox Transformation: Helps normalize skewed distributions in lab test data.
d. One-Hot Encoding: Converts categorical variables (e.g., disease types, patient demographics) into binary vectors.
e. Label Encoding: Assigns numerical values to categorical labels (e.g., "Male" → 0, "Female" → 1).
f. Ordinal Encoding: Converts categorical variables with an inherent order (e.g., disease severity: Mild → 0, Moderate → 1, Severe → 2).

3. Feature Engineering

Feature engineering enhances disease prediction models by creating more informative input features:

a. Polynomial Features: Generates interaction terms (e.g., BMI^2) to capture non-linear relationships.
b. Binning: Converts continuous variables into categorical bins (e.g., age groups: 0-20, 21-40, 41-60).

c. Time-Series Feature Extraction:
   i. Rolling Mean & Standard Deviation: Used for ECG/EEG signals.
   ii. Fourier Transform & Wavelet Transform: Identifies periodic patterns in bio signals.
d. Feature Construction: Creating new meaningful features, e.g., "Cholesterol-to-HDL Ratio" for cardiovascular risk.
   4. Feature Selection

Selecting relevant features improves model performance and reduces overfitting:

a. Filter Methods:
   i. Correlation Analysis (Pearson, Spearman, Kendall): Removes redundant features with high correlation.
   ii. Mutual Information: Measures how much information a feature provides about the target variable.
b. Wrapper Methods:
   i. Recursive Feature Elimination (RFE): Iteratively removes the least important features.
   ii. Sequential Feature Selection (SFS, SBS): Adds/removes features sequentially to optimize performance.
c. Embedded Methods:
   i. LASSO Regression (L1 Regularization): Shrinks less important features to zero.
   ii. Tree-Based Feature Importance (Random Forest, XGBoost, SHAP values): Identifies feature importance based on decision trees.
   5. Dimensionality Reduction

Large-scale medical data often contain redundant or irrelevant features. Dimensionality reduction improves efficiency:

a. Principal Component Analysis (PCA): Reduces feature dimensions while preserving variance.
b. T-Distributed Stochastic Neighbor Embedding (t-SNE): Visualizes high-dimensional patient clusters.
c. Linear Discriminant Analysis (LDA): Optimizes separability between disease classes.
d. Autoencoders (Deep Learning-based Feature Reduction): Extracts latent features from high-dimensional data.
   6. Data Balancing

Medical datasets often suffer from class imbalance (e.g., rare diseases have fewer cases). Data balancing ensures fair model training:

a. Oversampling Techniques:
   i. SMOTE (Synthetic Minority Over-sampling Technique): Generates synthetic examples for minority classes.
   ii. ADASYN (Adaptive Synthetic Sampling): A variant of SMOTE that focuses on harder-to-learn examples.
b. Under sampling Techniques:
   i. Random Under sampling: Reduces majority class instances.
   ii. Tomek Links & Near Miss Algorithms: Removes borderline majority class instances.
c. Hybrid Methods: Combining oversampling and under sampling to achieve balanced datasets.

7. Text-Based Medical Data Processing

Medical records and clinical notes often contain valuable text-based information. Natural Language Processing (NLP) is used to extract insights:

a. Tokenization & Lemmatization: Prepares text data for analysis.
b. TF-IDF (Term Frequency-Inverse Document Frequency): Identifies important medical terms.
c. Word Embeddings (Word2Vec, FastText, BERT, BioBERT): Converts clinical notes into numerical vectors.
d. Named Entity Recognition (NER): Identifies diseases, symptoms, and drugs in medical text.

8. Medical Image Pre-processing

For disease prediction using medical imaging (X-rays, MRIs, CT scans, histopathology slides), preprocessing is essential:

a. DICOM Standardization: Converts medical images into a standard format.
b. Histogram Equalization: Enhances contrast in grayscale images.
c. Image Segmentation (U-Net, Watershed Algorithm): Extracts relevant regions (e.g., tumors).
d. Edge Detection (Canny, Sobel): Identifies boundaries in medical scans.
e. Augmentation (Rotation, Flipping, and Cropping): Increases dataset diversity for deep learning models.

9. Data Splitting & Model Evaluation

Once preprocessing is complete, the data is split for training and validation:

a. Stratified K-Fold Cross-Validation: Ensures balanced representation of disease classes in training.
b. Hold-Out Method (Train/Test Split): Separates 70-80% of data for training and 20-30% for testing.
c. Leave-One-Out Cross-Validation (LOOCV): Useful for small medical datasets.

ML Techniques in Disease Prediction

Machine learning techniques such as Supervised, Unsupervised, and Reinforcement learning are used in disease prediction widely (Zhao et al., 2024).

- Supervised Learning: The algorithm learns to predict outcomes based on input features. For instance, ML can be used to predict disease progression by analyzing patient histories and clinical parameters.
- Unsupervised Learning: Here, algorithms identify patterns in data without labeled outcomes. This approach can uncover hidden relationships in complex datasets, such as identifying subtypes of diseases based on genetic information.
- Reinforcement Learning: This method involves training algorithms to optimize decision-making processes over time. In diagnostics, it can be applied to optimize treatment recommendations based on patient responses.

Research has demonstrated that DL models significantly improve diagnostic accuracy across various medical fields. For example, a study showed that a deep learning system used for breast cancer detection achieved higher sensitivity rates compared to human radiologists— 90% versus 78%—indicating its potential for enhancing clinical decision-making. Moreover, CNNs have been successfully applied in dermatology for skin cancer detection, where they demonstrated an ability to match or exceed dermatologists' performance. One of the most transformative areas of DL application is disease, where it has revolutionized tasks such as disease structure prediction and drug discovery. The advent of models like Alpha Fold has enabled researchers to predict complex disease structures with unprecedented accuracy, accelerating advancements in molecular biology and personalized medicine. Despite its immense potential, DL faces several challenges that limit its broader adoption. These include interpretability issues, computational demands, and a reliance on large, high-quality datasets. Addressing these limitations is essential to ensure the robustness and scalability of DL systems, particularly in high-stakes domains like healthcare. Role of CNNs in Image Analysis:

- Image Classification: CNNs are particularly effective in classifying medical images based on learned features.
- Object Detection: CNNs can identify specific structures within images, such as nodules in lung scans or lesions in skin images. This capability is crucial for early diagnosis and treatment planning.
- Segmentation: CNNs can segment images into meaningful regions, allowing for the precise location of abnormalities. This is particularly useful in surgical planning or monitoring disease progression.

The integration of NLP into diagnostic workflows has shown promising results. For instance, studies have indicated that NLP can significantly reduce the time required for data extraction from clinical texts while improving the accuracy of information retrieval. Additionally, NLP applications have been utilized to enhance disease surveillance by monitoring trends in patient symptoms documented in clinical notes during outbreaks. Applications of NLP in Diagnostics:

- Clinical Note Analysis: NLP algorithms can analyze vast amounts of clinical notes to identify relevant symptoms, diagnoses, and treatment histories. This capability enhances the understanding of patient backgrounds and informs clinical decision-making.
- Data Extraction from EHRs: NLP tools can automate the extraction of critical data from EHRs, enabling healthcare providers to quickly access pertinent patient information without manual review.
- Predictive Analytics: By analyzing historical patient data through NLP techniques, predictive models can forecast disease risks and outcomes based on individual patient profiles.

Optimization Algorithms in Disease prediction

Optimization algorithms serve as the backbone of efficient ML models by improving their accuracy, reducing computational complexity, and ensuring faster convergence. These algorithms can be broadly classified into different categories as shown in Figure 2, each inspired by natural processes, physics, or evolutionary mechanisms. Some of the most widely used optimization approaches in healthcare AI include (Webb et al., 2024):

Figure 2. Different Optimization Algorithms in disease prediction

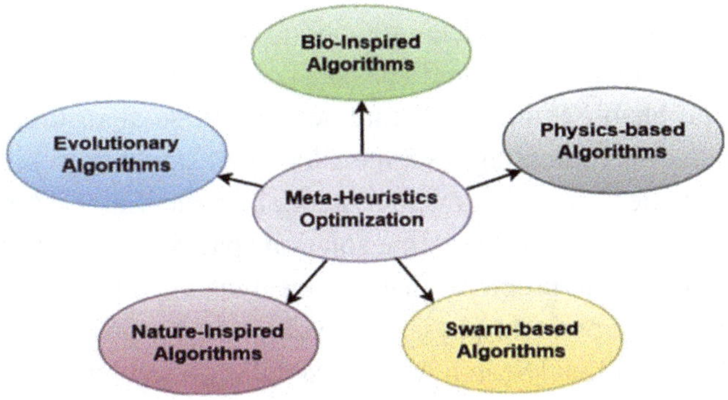

Source: Springer (2022)

- **Swarm-Based Algorithms**: Inspired by the collective intelligence of biological swarms, these techniques optimize deep learning models for tasks such as medical image segmentation and disease classification. Examples include Particle Swarm Optimization (PSO), Ant Colony Optimization (ACO), Artificial Bee Colony (ABC), and Whale Optimization Algorithm (WOA). Swarm-based algorithms are inspired by the collective behaviors of animals to optimize solutions to complex problems. These algorithms have been widely adopted in healthcare AI due to their efficiency in handling high-dimensional data, optimizing deep learning models, and improving medical image analysis.
- **Evolutionary Algorithms**: To optimize ML models for applications like personalized medicine and drug discovery by GA and DE. Evolutionary algorithms (EAs) are a class of optimization techniques inspired by the principles of natural selection and genetic evolution.

These algorithms are highly effective in solving complex problems in healthcare AI, where traditional optimization methods may struggle due to high-dimensional data, nonlinear interactions, and dynamic constraints. Unlike conventional algorithms that rely on gradient-based optimization, evolutionary algorithms leverage mechanisms such as mutation, crossover, and selection to explore large solution spaces efficiently. This ability makes them particularly useful in medical decision-making, treatment optimization, and drug discovery.

- **Physics-Based Algorithms**: These are inspired by physical processes such as thermodynamics and gravity and are used for optimizing hospital resource allocation and signal processing by SA and GSA. Physics-based algorithms are inspired by physical phenomena, such as the laws of thermodynamics, gravity, and the behaviour of particles in motion. These algorithms use mathematical models to simulate real-world physical processes to optimize solutions for complex problems. In the healthcare domain, these algorithms have shown great promise in addressing resource allocation, signal processing, and classification challenges. By mimicking natural physical processes, these algorithms can efficiently explore large solution spaces and achieve high-quality results, especially in problems that involve dynamic, high-dimensional data. Below are two prominent physics-based algorithms—Simulated Annealing (SA) and Gravitational Search Algorithm (GSA)—that have been successfully applied in healthcare AI.

- **Animal Behaviour-Based Algorithms**: Animal behavior-based algorithms are optimization techniques inspired by the collective or individual behaviors observed in the natural world. These algorithms draw parallels from the instincts, cooperation, and hunting strategies of various animal species, which can be effectively applied to solve complex problems in healthcare AI. It handles high-dimensional data, optimizing parameters in deep learning models, and enhancing the accuracy in healthcare. These techniques replicate the hunting, foraging, and survival strategies of animals to enhance ML model efficiency in disease prediction, EEG classification, and medical image processing. Notable examples include GWO, BA, FA, and CSA. Animal behavior-inspired optimization algorithms have also found applications in healthcare, mimicking the natural behaviors of various species to improve ML model performance. The Grey Wolf Optimizer (GWO) has been applied to Alzheimer's disease prediction using MRI scans, optimizing feature selection to enhance classification accuracy. GWO simulates the hunting strategy of grey wolves, dynamically adjusting search strategies to identify the most discriminative features for early-stage Alzheimer's diagnosis. The Bat Algorithm (BA) has been employed in brain signal processing for epilepsy detection, fine-tuning deep learning parameters to improve EEG signal classification. BA leverages echolocation principles to explore optimal parameter configurations, enabling more precise identification of epileptic seizures. The Firefly Algorithm (FA) has been utilized for early diabetes detection by optimizing deep learning classifiers and selecting the most relevant medical features, ensuring high predictive accuracy while minimizing redundant data. FA simulates the attraction mechanism of fireflies, converging towards optimal feature subsets that maximize classification performance. The Cuckoo Search Algorithm (CSA) has been instrumental in medical image enhancement, optimizing filters in image processing models to improve the clarity and visibility of anomalies, aiding in more accurate radiological assessments.

SOLUTIONS AND RECOMMENDATIONS

Proposed Disease prediction System (Case Study of NAFL disease)

Non-Alcoholic Fatty Liver Disease (NAFLD) is one of the top 10 chronic diseases in India which registered 264193 deaths in 2018 and one of the patients in five Indian patients faces the risk of this disease.

In the United States, at least two chronic illnesses are present in 40% of adults who have NAFL disease and multi-morbidity is the term used to describe a person who has two or more chronic conditions. NAFL disease is a rapidly growing healthcare burden, with patients who are experiencing manifestations and require therapies throughout their lives. To relieve family stress and advance national growth, a robust healthcare system is essential in India, and also stopping fatalities is the main objective of a disease forecasting system. The Non-alcoholic fatty liver disease prediction system uses different methodologies on patient liver-related signs to diagnose the diseases early; meanwhile, it recognizes the patient's current health conditions. The majority of research investigations in NAFL disease prediction systems reveal that a single classification model of machine learning does not give a good outcome for the healthcare management system. To further enhance the model's quality, experts used hybrid models and ensemble classification methods which are often used to blend the advantages of different models hierarchically to increase prediction accuracy (Castañé et al., 2021; Dubey et al., 2024; Ezzat et al., 2021; Feng et al., 2021; Gangadevi et al., 2024; Ganiger et al., 2024; Goldman et al., 2021; Hulsen, 2023; Islam, Majumder, Hussein, et al., 2024). However, every solution has some shortcomings based on the real-time scenario of the NAFL disease prediction system. It can be analyzed through a series of experiments via artificial intelligence techniques which helps to identify the optimal solution that can be applied in the real-world NAFL disease patient data in India. Artificial intelligence techniques are capable of managing, storing, and analyzing the enormous quantities of information obtained from NAFL disease (Zhou, X. et al., 2022).

Figure 3 depicts the proposed workflow for a Non-alcoholic fatty liver disease prediction system in detail. Every data analytics problem begins with data collection, so we will first gather benchmark data for our disease prediction system using the available data sources as well as in real-time by working with various hospitals. In this work, we are going to analyze the performance and impact of both the structured and unstructured Non-alcoholic fatty liver disease data. The second phase is to clean and balance the data for our proposed NAFL disease prediction model to improve the system's consistency and accuracy.

Figure 3. Proposed NAFL disease prediction system

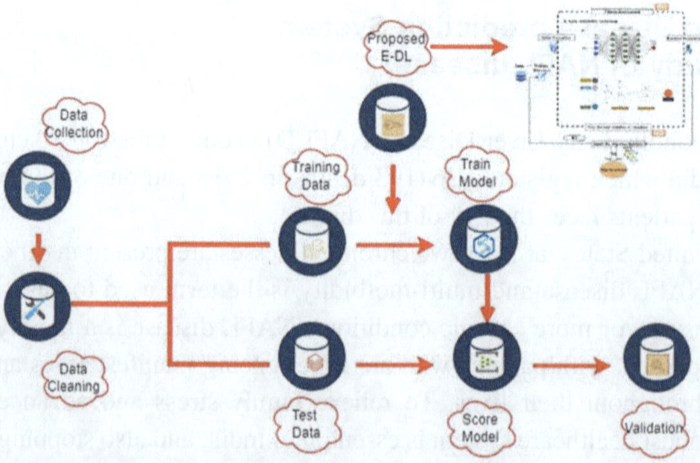

Then, the optimization principles are applied in deep learning models for this disease prediction, which is used to increase the concert of the disease prediction system and reduce the shortcomings of deep learning models. According to this, we can analyze every optimization technique along with its pros and cons and whether it is suitable to boost the accuracy of existing DL models. Finally, multiple experiment sets are used to validate the performance of the generated evolutionary-based deep learning models (E-DL) and suggest the best model for an NAFL disease prediction system.

Data collection issues and solutions

The first process is effective data gathering for model construction. Data on NAFL disease is a thorough compilation of patient information and health condition specifics. Prescriptions, electronic health records, doctor's notes, and other related data make up the great majority of the data. Nowadays, data comes from multiple sources with varied formats such as image, audio, video, and text files; however, we can't access that data directly because it contains personal patient data. Even though where big data in healthcare holds its golden opportunity, the complexity, privacy, and security laws, volume of the data, dispersed data, constantly changing data, patient expectations, a lack of quality assurance procedures, and inadequate technology have raised data collection issues. To collect real-time human data for NAFL disease in both structured and unstructured formats in India and also augment as per the need and store the collected data in a big data tool and serve the data for future prediction. In the future, the proposed model's effectiveness can be tested on real-time data from other countries.

Data pre-processing issues and solutions

- **Data Volume:** The volume of chronic disease data is relative to the number of patients and the number of attributes connected with it. Typically, a portion of the obtained data is used to create the mining process. NAFL disease statistics must include all available historical data in the model building to predict NAFL diseases. Eliminating a patient will result in improper training because each patient provides a unique training prospect.
- **Data representation issues:** The representation of health care information is another issue. Healthcare information comes from multiple sources with two formats such as structured and unstructured forms.
    - **Structured data:** According to HIMSS any database used in the healthcare industry will contain structured data, which could be particularly such as customer names and contact information, lab results, patient health reports, and financial transactions.
    - **Unstructured data:** According to HIMSS, unstructured data "cannot be simply organized using pre-defined formats." Examples of unstructured data are radiology images or text files, such as doctor's notes in an Electronic Health Record (EHR).

On the other hand, it contains details from anonymous site user comments, Data from Twitter, voice recognition data, and so on. Unstructured data is practically hard to clean.

- **Data imbalance issues:** The NAFL disease prediction problem comes based on the total number of distinct values in the prediction process. Generally, the NAFL disease prediction problem has two distinct classes such as diseased (1) and non-diseased (0). The classifiers' training phase is significantly impacted by the imbalance dataset why because there are enough training entries, and the major class is properly trained. The class imbalance problems degrade the performance of the prediction system and also misclassify the new data that come under the improperly trained minor class.
- **Attributes in a dataset:** According to Chronic NAFL disease statistics, the data set has few patient data which is represented in columns, and a huge

number of feature information related to the patients which is represented in rows, which is opposite to other business-oriented data.

- **Sparse nature of data:** The main reason for the high sparseness of the NSDL disease prediction data is that a patient has a chance of being linked to a minimum of one and a maximum of a few disease symptoms. However, the patient's records match every symptom of the condition to date. Thus, the data is extremely sparse since, except for the related entries, all the other entries frequently have null values which leads to the improper representation of flat files.

The proposed data cleaning process analyses the issues present in the collected data, applies appropriate solutions, and also can recognizes the issues in the data.

Proposed Evolutionary-based Deep learning models

There is no one specific cause for a patient to develop a disease, which is the most significant problem in predicting NAFL disease. Patient NAFL disease is typically brought on by several contributing factors; for example, a mixture of environmental drivers such as nutrition, way of life as well as other factors that affect the person's average lifespan. Finding these causes is difficult since it depends on both the patient's personal history and the disease aspect that is unique to that patient. The combination of all these factors makes classification quite challenging and needs some in-depth analysis of the NAFL disease prediction system. To address these challenges, we propose an alternative optimized deep learning solution for NAFL disease management in India. In the proposed approach a disease is considered an optimization problem and identifies the optimum solution based on evolutionary-based deep learning which is represented in Figure 4.

Figure 4. Proposed NAFL disease prediction system

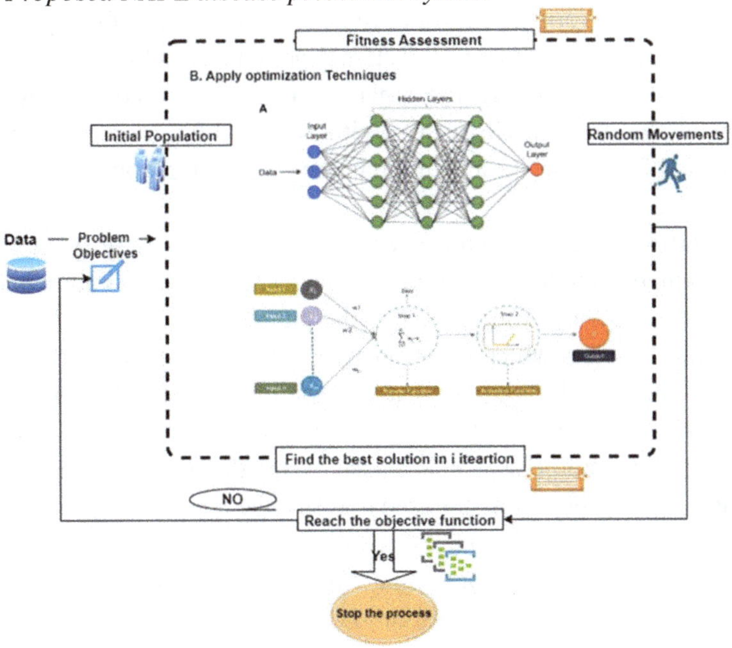

1. **Evolutionary Algorithms:** Optimization algorithms are used to find the optimum solution for any application. Evolutionary computing is one of the metaheuristic-based optimization algorithms that are inspired by nature. The researchers designed their optimization algorithms based on the biological behavior of groups of populations (swarm intelligence), hence is called a bio-inspired algorithm also. The bio-inspired algorithms are used to solve two kinds of problems which are maximization and minimization problems and it purely depends on our objective function f(x). The metaheuristic term refers to iterating the problem in N times used to identify the optimal solution via the trial and error method. Based on the literature survey the popular swarm intelligence algorithms are ant colony optimization, bat, cuckoo search, krill herd, particle swarm optimization, harmony search, glow-worm swarm optimization, bee colony optimization, firefly, mayfly, genetic, differential evolution, evolution strategy, and quantum-inspired evolutionary algorithms. Each algorithm is varied based on its principles and methods however the aim of these algorithms is to solve optimum solutions from the available solution by random nature. The random nature is varied based on the biological movement; for example, the PSO algorithm is designed based on the food-searching process of a swarm of birds.

In our proposed model we consider the disease prediction as an optimization problem and also it is a minimization problem because the global optimum value is similar to our test data and our objective function aim is to decrease the fitness between the best to the test data. The general principles involved in the evolutionary algorithms are discussed below such as Initialization, Fitness assessment, Random movement, and finding the best solution in the current iterations.

a. **Initialization:** Every evaluatory algorithm starts with state space (S) initialization which is the location of the problem and the objects are moved in this specified space only. Then initialize the particles (x_1) and the corresponding fitness function f(x) which is the objective of the problems. Further, initialize all the parameters (Ex: $\partial, \varnothing, \beta$) that are required for the techniques chosen.
b. **Fitness Assessment:** Find the fitness value for every particle according to the objective of the problems which is used to find the best solution in the current iteration. Further iterations are used to refine the model which aims to find the most favorable solution from the available feasible solutions. The objective function for this problem comes under the minimization problem.
c. **Random Movement:** The best solution of the current iteration is not sufficient to find the optimum solution for the chosen problem. Hence continuing the iteration based on the random movements is applied for every particle. Now calculate the fitness function of a particle according to a new position and it shows it is varied because of the randomness. The updated best solution is given for the further process.
d. **Object function verification:** Every iteration end the updated best solution is compared with our objective function. If the current solution satisfies our objective function then the algorithm terminates otherwise the algorithm will continue.

2. **Deep learning algorithms:** NAFL disease management necessitates continuous inspection and suggestions. AI-powered virtual healthcare practices have recently grown and developed and are being employed in a wide range of products; for example, AI diabetes advisory systems are useful in controlling patients' symptoms. Deep neural network technology is used to solve real-world complex problems (including business analytics, health care analytics, IoT and cloud computing applications, and Natural language processing) nowadays as the size of the data, the nature of the unstructured data, and identifying the important features are no longer a constraint when compared to using machine learning models. The base model for the deep neural network is an ANN, which works similarly to human analysis which is represented in Figure 5. The artificial neural network has an input layer that has input units that are reliant on the number of variables in the NAFL

disease data set. Following it has N number of the hidden layers that have hidden units that are initialized by the developer also no one finds the optimal number of hidden units in deep neural networks in NAFL disease management systems. Followed by it has an output layer that has output units that are dependent on the number of classes for the NAFL disease prediction system. Generally, the NAFL disease prediction problem has two distinct classes such as diseased (1) and non-diseased (0) which can be represented through a single output unit or two output units. The single output unit is handled through a cut of value (δ) that is initialized by the developer based on the problem.

Deep neural networks enhance the performance of artificial neural networks by adding a large number of hidden layers between the starting points to the outcome of the prediction. The information on NAFL disease is passed layer by layer which automatically learns the hidden pattern inside the NAFL disease historical data and which is used for prediction and forecasting the same. The CNNs, LSTMs, and RNNs. are the well-known deep learning models used in the disease prediction system.

Figure 5. Architecture difference between ANN vs DL

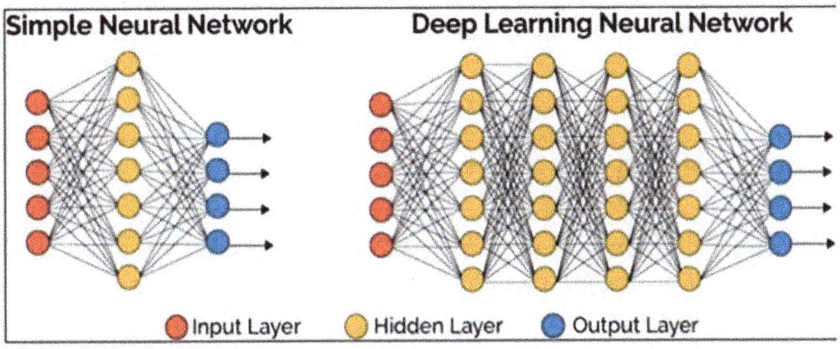

Source: Springer (2021)

Figure 6 represents the working principles of two nodes in every layer of the architecture. The unit receives the feature value of NAFL disease data multiplies it with random weights, and then adds a bias then applies the chosen activation function which converts linear to nonlinear operation; otherwise, it is similar to the linear regression model. Each deep learning algorithm is varied based on its principles and methods such as the number of layers and units, activation function used, memorization behavior, the direction of the data flow, feature selection capabilities, the capability of handling the type of data, and so on; however, the aim of these algorithms are used to find hidden patterns efficiently.

Figure 6. The working principles of two nodes in every layer of the architecture

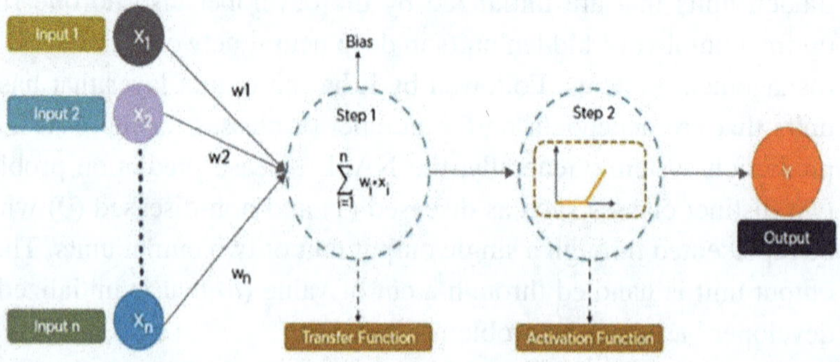

Source: Springer (2020)

In this proposed model the optimization principles are applied in various deep learning models (GANs, RBFNs, MLPs, SOMs, DBns, RBMs, and Auto encoders) which are used to increase the concert of the NAFL disease prediction system and reduce the shortcomings of deep learning models. According to this, we can analyze every optimization technique along with its pros and cons and whether it is suitable for NAFL disease prediction. Finally, multiple experiment sets are used to validate the performance of the generated evolutionary-based deep learning models (E-DL) and suggest the best model for an NAFL disease prediction system.

FUTURE RESEARCH DIRECTIONS

The integration of Machine Learning (ML) and Optimization has significantly transformed healthcare by enabling data-driven decision-making, improving diagnostic accuracy, optimizing treatment plans, and enhancing hospital operations. ML techniques such as deep learning and predictive analytics help in early disease detection and personalized medicine, while optimization algorithms improve resource allocation and logistical efficiency. The synergy between these approaches has led to advancements in precision medicine, patient care, and healthcare management. However, challenges such as data privacy, model interpretability, and computational complexity remain critical concerns. Future research should focus on ethical AI, federated learning, and hybrid ML-optimization models to ensure more robust, transparent, and effective healthcare solutions. By leveraging these technologies, the healthcare sector can continue to evolve towards more efficient, patient-centered, and cost-effective systems.

CONCLUSION

The disease prediction technique used to be carried out manually for a countable number of patients, however due to the overwhelming volume of patient records, it is no longer feasible. Currently, Data mining and Machine learning are two new approaches that aid in the identification and prognosis of diseases as well as the creation of an effective healthcare system. However, predicting disease is difficult because many reasons might be involved in it, including smoking, high cholesterol, uncontrolled blood hypertension, obesity, high blood sugar, uncontrolled stress, despair, and rage in the patients. Additionally, it comes in a variety of forms and stages and it might be challenging to predict how disease will progress today also it must have a pipeline that can convert the unprocessed data from a public health monitoring system into calibrated estimates of the incidence of disease. The major goal of this chapter is to develop the most accurate, recallable, and error-reducing model for NAFL disease forecasting in the healthcare sector. We identified this disease prediction has major obstacles: lagging inefficient data collection, difficulty in handling different data representations, lagging in finding causes of disease, the nature of the available dataset (data volume, data Imbalance, high attribute in the dataset, highly sparse nature of the data), inefficient data models and so on. To address these challenges, we propose an alternative solution for the disease management system using artificial intelligence techniques. The proposed model includes various analyses to enhance disease prediction in every stage of model building and also the disease is considered as an optimization problem and identifies the optimum solution on evolutionary-based deep learning models. This chapter aims to o create a quantitative chronic disease prediction model for Non-alcoholic fatty liver disease and to analyze the existing disease prediction system(s) and its services. This can be executed by a sequence of steps that includes data collection, data preprocessing, model building, and testing. The collection of data is used to collect real-time human data for Non-alcoholic fatty liver disease in both structured and unstructured formats in India and also augment as per the needs and store the collected data in a big data tool to serve for future prediction. Followed by a robust architecture to handle imbalanced and missing data, and then build an evolutionary-based deep learning model for the Non-alcoholic fatty liver disease model, which is capable of finding out the optimal solution for patients, doctors, and society in India without further delay. The proposed NAFL illness prediction model's results include an improvement in life quality and a reduction in unneeded hospitalizations of people. Disease forecasting could benefit stakeholders such as the government and health insurers.

REFERENCES

Arumugam, K., Naved, M., Shinde, P. P., Leiva-Chauca, O., Huaman-Osorio, A., & Gonzales-Yanac, T. (2023). Multiple disease prediction using Machine learning algorithms. *Materials Today: Proceedings*, *80*, 3682–3685. DOI: 10.1016/j.matpr.2021.07.361

Castañé, H., Baiges-Gaya, G., Hernández-Aguilera, A., Rodríguez-Tomàs, E., Fernández-Arroyo, S., Herrero, P., Delpino-Rius, A., Canela, N., Menendez, J. A., Camps, J., & Joven, J. (2021). Coupling machine learning and lipidomics as a tool to investigate metabolic dysfunction-associated fatty liver disease. A general overview. *Biomolecules*, *11*(3), 473. DOI: 10.3390/biom11030473 PMID: 33810079

Dubey, M., Tembhurne, J., & Makhijani, R. (2024). Improving coronary heart disease prediction with real-life dataset: A stacked generalization framework with maximum clinical attributes and SMOTE balancing for imbalanced data. *Multimedia Tools and Applications*, *83*(37), 1–30. DOI: 10.1007/s11042-024-19429-9

Ezzat, D., Hassanien, A. E., & Ella, H. A. (2021). An optimized deep learning architecture for the diagnosis of COVID-19 disease based on gravitational search optimization. *Applied Soft Computing*, *98*, 106742. DOI: 10.1016/j.asoc.2020.106742 PMID: 32982615

Feng, W., Han, X., Hu, H., Chang, M., Ding, L., Xiang, H., Chen, Y., & Li, Y. (2021). 2D vanadium carbide MXenzyme to alleviate ROS-mediated inflammatory and neurodegenerative diseases. *Nature Communications*, *12*(1), 2203. DOI: 10.1038/s41467-021-22278-x PMID: 33850133

Gangadevi, E., Rani, R. S., Dhanaraj, R. K., & Nayyar, A. (2024). Spot-out fruit fly algorithm with simulated annealing optimized SVM for detecting tomato plant diseases. *Neural Computing & Applications*, *36*(8), 4349–4375. DOI: 10.1007/s00521-023-09295-1

Ganiger, F. B., Bijjal, S. S., & Mugali, J. D. (2024). A Cross-Sectional Study On Psychiatric Disorders among Poor Academic Performance Primary School (6-12 Years) Children with Substance Use Disorders in Their Parents. *Annals of Indian Psychiatry*, *8*(2), 120–124. DOI: 10.4103/aip.aip_128_21

Goldman, O., Ben-Assuli, O., Rogowski, O., Zeltser, D., Shapira, I., Berliner, S., Zelber-Sagi, S., & Shenhar-Tsarfaty, S. (2021). Non-alcoholic fatty liver and liver fibrosis predictive analytics: Risk prediction and machine learning techniques for improved preventive medicine. *Journal of Medical Systems*, *45*(2), 1–12. DOI: 10.1007/s10916-020-01693-5 PMID: 33426569

Hulsen, T. (2023). Explainable artificial intelligence (XAI): Concepts and challenges in healthcare. *AI*, *4*(3), 652–666. DOI: 10.3390/ai4030034

Islam, M. A., Majumder, M. Z. H., Hussein, M. A., Hossain, K. M., & Miah, M. S. (2024). A review of machine learning and deep learning algorithms for Parkinson's disease detection using handwriting and voice datasets. *Heliyon*, *10*(3), e25469. DOI: 10.1016/j.heliyon.2024.e25469 PMID: 38356538

Islam, M. A., Majumder, M. Z. H., Miah, M. S., & Jannaty, S. (2024). Precision healthcare: A deep dive into machine learning algorithms and feature selection strategies for accurate heart disease prediction. *Computers in Biology and Medicine*, *176*, 108432. DOI: 10.1016/j.compbiomed.2024.108432 PMID: 38744014

Jha, P., Dembla, D., & Dubey, W. (2024). Deep learning models for enhancing potato leaf disease prediction: Implementation of transfer learning based stacking ensemble model. *Multimedia Tools and Applications*, *83*(13), 37839–37858. DOI: 10.1007/s11042-023-16993-4

Kaur, I., Sandhu, A. K., & Kumar, Y. (2022). Artificial intelligence techniques for predictive modeling of vector-borne diseases and its pathogens: A systematic review. *Archives of Computational Methods in Engineering*, *29*(6), 3741–3771. DOI: 10.1007/s11831-022-09724-9

Ke, C., Xiao, C., Li, J., Wu, X., Zhang, Y., Chen, Y., Sheng, S., Fu, Z., Wang, L., Ni, C., Zhao, J., Shi, Y., Wu, Y., Zhong, Z., Nan, J., Zhu, W., Chen, J., Wu, R., & Hu, X. (2025). FMO2 ameliorates nonalcoholic fatty liver disease by suppressing ER-to-Golgi transport of SREBP1. *Hepatology (Baltimore, Md.)*, *81*(1), 181–197. DOI: 10.1097/HEP.0000000000000643 PMID: 37874228

Kezer, C. A., Simonetto, D. A., & Shah, V. H. (2021, April). Sex differences in alcohol consumption and alcohol-associated liver disease. [). Elsevier.]. *Mayo Clinic Proceedings*, *96*(4), 1006–1016. DOI: 10.1016/j.mayocp.2020.08.020 PMID: 33714602

Khan, M. A., Mazhar, T., Mateen Yaqoob, M., Badruddin Khan, M., Jilani Saudagar, A. K., Ghadi, Y. Y., Khattak, U. F., & Shahid, M. (2024). Optimal feature selection for heart disease prediction using modified Artificial Bee colony (M-ABC) and K-nearest neighbors (KNN). *Scientific Reports*, *14*(1), 26241. DOI: 10.1038/s41598-024-78021-1 PMID: 39482391

Kumar, M., Parchani, A., Kant, R., & Das, A. (2023). Relationship between vitamin D deficiency and non-alcoholic fatty liver disease: A cross-sectional study from a tertiary care center in Northern India. *Cureus*, *15*(2). Advance online publication. DOI: 10.7759/cureus.34921 PMID: 36938188

Lee, S. M., Jung, Y. M., Choi, E. S., Kwak, S. H., Koo, J. N., Oh, I. H., Kim, B. J., Kim, S. M., Kim, S. Y., Kim, G. M., Joo, S. K., Koo, B. K., Shin, S., Norwitz, E. R., Park, C.-W., Jun, J. K., Kim, W., & Park, J. S. (2022). Metabolic dysfunction-associated fatty liver disease and subsequent development of adverse pregnancy outcomes. *Clinical Gastroenterology and Hepatology*, *20*(11), 2542–2550. DOI: 10.1016/j.cgh.2021.11.007 PMID: 34798335

Liu, R., Luo, C., Pang, Z., Zhang, J., Ruan, S., Wu, M., Wang, L., Sun, T., Li, N., Han, L., Shi, J., Huang, Y., Guo, W., Peng, S., Zhou, W., & Gao, H. (2023). Advances of nanoparticles as drug delivery systems for disease diagnosis and treatment. *Chinese Chemical Letters*, *34*(2), 107518. DOI: 10.1016/j.cclet.2022.05.032

Mienye, I. D., & Jere, N. (2024). Optimized ensemble learning approach with explainable AI for improved heart disease prediction. *Information (Basel)*, *15*(7), 394. DOI: 10.3390/info15070394

Mishra, A. S., & Vijaya, J. (2024). Data Mining and Knowledge Discovery: Transforming Healthcare Through Biomedical Intelligence. In *Machine Learning and Generative AI in Smart Healthcare* (pp. 23-40). IGI Global.

Ogunpola, A., Saeed, F., Basurra, S., Albarrak, A. M., & Qasem, S. N. (2024). Machine learning-based predictive models for detection of cardiovascular diseases. *Diagnostics (Basel)*, *14*(2), 144. DOI: 10.3390/diagnostics14020144 PMID: 38248021

Padmavathi, P., Harikiran, J., & Vijaya, J. (2023). Effective deep learning based segmentation and classification in wireless capsule endoscopy images. *Multimedia Tools and Applications*, *82*(30), 47109–47133. DOI: 10.1007/s11042-023-14621-9

Pesaramelli, R. S., & Sujatha, B. (2024, March). Principle correlated feature extraction using differential evolution for improved classification. In *AIP Conference Proceedings* (Vol. 2919, No. 1). AIP Publishing. DOI: 10.1063/5.0184938

Prasanna, K. S., & Vijaya, J. (2022). Building an efficient heart disease prediction system by using clustering techniques. In *High Performance Computing and Networking: Select Proceedings of CHSN 2021* (pp. 69-81). Singapore: Springer Singapore. DOI: 10.1007/978-981-16-9885-9_6

Ram, M., Afrash, M. R., Moulaei, K., Parvin, M., Esmaeeli, E., Karbasi, Z., Heydari, S., & Sabahi, A. (2024). Application of artificial intelligence in chronic myeloid leukemia (CML) disease prediction and management: A scoping review. *BMC Cancer*, *24*(1), 1026. DOI: 10.1186/s12885-024-12764-y PMID: 39164653

Ramesh, B., & Lakshmanna, K. (2024). A novel early detection and prevention of coronary heart disease framework using hybrid deep learning model and neural fuzzy inference system. *IEEE Access : Practical Innovations, Open Solutions*, *12*, 26683–26695. DOI: 10.1109/ACCESS.2024.3366537

Rao, G. M., Ramesh, D., Sharma, V., Sinha, A., Hassan, M. M., & Gandomi, A. H. (2024). AttGRU-HMSI: Enhancing heart disease diagnosis using hybrid deep learning approach. *Scientific Reports*, *14*(1), 7833. DOI: 10.1038/s41598-024-56931-4 PMID: 38570560

Reddy, N. N., Nipun, L., Baba, M. U., Rishindra, N., & Shilpa, T. (2024). Optimizing heart disease prediction through ensemble and hybrid machine learning techniques. [IJECE]. *International Journal of Electrical and Computer Engineering*, *14*(5), 5744–5754. DOI: 10.11591/ijece.v14i5.pp5744-5754

Serrano, D. R., Luciano, F. C., Anaya, B. J., Ongoren, B., Kara, A., Molina, G., Ramirez, B. I., Sánchez-Guirales, S. A., Simon, J. A., Tomietto, G., Rapti, C., Ruiz, H. K., Rawat, S., Kumar, D., & Lalatsa, A. (2024). Artificial intelligence (AI) applications in drug discovery and drug delivery: Revolutionizing personalized medicine. *Pharmaceutics*, *16*(10), 1328. DOI: 10.3390/pharmaceutics16101328 PMID: 39458657

Skender, B., & Zhang, M. (2024). From local issue to global challenge: A brief overview of antibiotic shortages since the 1970s. *Humanities & Social Sciences Communications*, *11*(1), 1–6. DOI: 10.1057/s41599-024-03759-y

Subramanian, A., Nirantharakumar, K., Hughes, S., Myles, P., Williams, T., Gokhale, K. M., Taverner, T., Chandan, J. S., Brown, K., Simms-Williams, N., Shah, A. D., Singh, M., Kidy, F., Okoth, K., Hotham, R., Bashir, N., Cockburn, N., Lee, S. I., Turner, G. M., & Haroon, S. (2022). Symptoms and risk factors for long COVID in non-hospitalized adults. *Nature Medicine*, *28*(8), 1706–1714. DOI: 10.1038/s41591-022-01909-w PMID: 35879616

Taha, B. A., Kadhim, A. C., Addie, A. J., Haider, A. J., Azzahrani, A. S., Raizada, P., & Arsad, N. (2024). Advancing cancer diagnostics through multifaceted optical biosensors supported by nanomaterials and artificial intelligence: A panoramic outlook. *Microchemical Journal*, *205*, 111307. DOI: 10.1016/j.microc.2024.111307

Veerankutty, F. H., Jayan, G., Yadav, M. K., Manoj, K. S., Yadav, A., Nair, S. R. S., Shabeerali, T. U., Yeldho, V., Sasidharan, M., & Rather, S. A. (2021). Artificial Intelligence in hepatology, liver surgery and transplantation: Emerging applications and frontiers of research. *World Journal of Hepatology*, *13*(12), 1977–1990. DOI: 10.4254/wjh.v13.i12.1977 PMID: 35070002

Vijaya, J. (2023, January). Heart disease prediction using clustered genetic optimization algorithm. In *2023 International Conference on Intelligent and Innovative Technologies in Computing, Electrical and Electronics (IITCEE)* (pp. 1072-1077). IEEE. DOI: 10.1109/IITCEE57236.2023.10091050

Vijaya, J., Chandra, S., & Baghel, P. (2023, April). Diabetes disease prediction using various metaheuristic optimization algorithms. In *2023 IEEE 8th International Conference for Convergence in Technology (I2CT)* (pp. 1-6). IEEE. DOI: 10.1109/I2CT57861.2023.10126222

Vijaya, J., Nitnaware, V., & Chaddha, R. (2023, July). Optimization Techniques on Heart Failure Prediction. In *2023 14th International Conference on Computing Communication and Networking Technologies (ICCCNT)* (pp. 1-6). IEEE. DOI: 10.1109/ICCCNT56998.2023.10308079

Vijaya, J., & Rao, M. (2022, November). Heart disease prediction using clustered particle swarm optimization techniques. In *2022 IEEE 6th Conference on Information and Communication Technology (CICT)* (pp. 1-5). IEEE. DOI: 10.1109/CICT56698.2022.9997925

Vijaya, J., Rishabh, K., & Parashar, P. (2023, August). CanScan: Non-Invasive Techniques for Oral Cancer Detection. In *2023 International Conference on Electrical, Electronics, Communication and Computers (ELEXCOM)* (pp. 1-5). IEEE. DOI: 10.1109/ELEXCOM58812.2023.10370254

Vijaya, J., Tirkey, D., Singh, P., & Goel, A. (2023, March). Diabetes Prediction Using Nature-Inspired Optimization Algorithms. In *2023 3rd International conference on Artificial Intelligence and Signal Processing (AISP)* (pp. 1-5). IEEE. DOI: 10.1109/AISP57993.2023.10135000

Webb, R. J., Al-Asmakh, M., Banach, M., & Mazidi, M. (2024). Application of proteomics for novel drug discovery and risk prediction optimisation in stroke and myocardial infarction: A review of in-human studies. *Drug Discovery Today*, *29*(11), 104186. DOI: 10.1016/j.drudis.2024.104186 PMID: 39306234

Xia, B., Innab, N., Kandasamy, V., Ahmadian, A., & Ferrara, M. (2024). Intelligent cardiovascular disease diagnosis using deep learning enhanced neural network with ant colony optimization. *Scientific Reports*, *14*(1), 21777. DOI: 10.1038/s41598-024-71932-z PMID: 39294203

Zhao, Y., Chaw, J. K., Liu, L., Chaw, S. H., Ang, M. C., & Ting, T. T. (2024). Systematic literature review on reinforcement learning in non-communicable disease interventions. *Artificial Intelligence in Medicine*, *154*, 102901. DOI: 10.1016/j.artmed.2024.102901 PMID: 38838400

ADDITIONAL READING

Mercangöz, B. A. (2021). *Applying particle Swarm optimization*. Springer International Publishing. DOI: 10.1007/978-3-030-70281-6

Muniasamy, A., Begum, A., Sabahath, A., & Yaqub, H. (2023). Lung cancer histopathology image classification using transfer learning with convolution neural network model. *Journal Name, volume*(issue), 1–12.

Muniasamy, A., Begum, A., Sabahath, A., Yaqub, H., & Karunakaran, G. (2024). Coronary heart disease classification using deep learning approach with feature selection for improved accuracy. *Technology and Health Care*, *32*(3), 1–17. Advance online publication. DOI: 10.3233/THC-231807 PMID: 38339946

Muniasamy, A., Begum, A., Sabahath, A., Yaqub, H., & Karunakaran, G. (2024). Coronary heart disease classification using deep learning approach with feature selection for improved accuracy. *Technology and Health Care*, *32*(3), 1991–2007. DOI: 10.3233/THC-231807 PMID: 38339946

Rani, G., & Tiwari, P. K. (Eds.). (2020). *Handbook of research on disease prediction through data analytics and machine learning*. IGI Global.

Sathyabhama, B., & Kannan, M. (2025). An effective deep learning-based automatic prediction and classification of Alzheimer's disease using EGELU-SZN technique. *Neural Computing & Applications*, •••, 1–18.

Sharma, A., Sharma, A., Pandey, J. K., & Ram, M. (2022). *Swarm intelligence: foundation, principles, and engineering applications*. CRC Press.

Slowik, A. (Ed.). (2021). *Swarm intelligence algorithms (two volume set)*. CRC press. DOI: 10.1201/9781003046882

KEY TERMS AND DEFINITIONS

Deep Learning: Deep learning is used to fine-tune the machine learning models.

Disease prediction: Predict the disease in advance without manual interpretation.

Health care management system: It is used to build the relationship between patients and health care systems.

Machine Learning: Machine Learning is a technique to build a model which is used to forecast the data.

Optimization Techniques: To find the best solution for any application.

Chapter 4
Optimization Methods in Healthcare Machine Learning:
From Algorithms to Clinical Implementation

Jaswanth Sunkara
https://orcid.org/0009-0003-0751-4223
SRM Institute of Science and Technology, India

Anitha D.
https://orcid.org/0000-0003-0952-898X
SRM Institute of Science and Techonology, India

ABSTRACT

This comprehensive examination of optimization methodologies in healthcare machine learning addresses unique challenges in this critical domain. The content investigates approaches including gradient-based methods, evolutionary algorithms, metaheuristics, and Bayesian optimization, highlighting healthcare-specific adaptations through case studies spanning diagnostic modeling, treatment planning, medical imaging, and resource allocation. Extending beyond algorithms, the discussion addresses implementation considerations including workflow integration, privacy preservation, fairness, and multi-stakeholder engagement. Emerging techniques such as federated optimization, differential privacy, and quantum approaches are evaluated alongside regulatory barriers and governance frameworks. Through this integrative approach, readers gain insight into how optimization techniques enhance healthcare delivery while navigating the complex ethical, operational, and regulatory landscape unique to medical applications.

DOI: 10.4018/979-8-3373-1087-9.ch004

INTRODUCTION

Machine learning and AI have revolutionized healthcare by enabling predictive analysis, early disease detection, and personalized treatments. Healthcare's complex, high-volume data presents opportunities and challenges, requiring optimization for effectiveness. Traditional analytical methods struggle with healthcare data's high dimensionality, class imbalance, missing values, and complex variable relationships.

Optimization techniques have enhanced medical ML applications significantly. Traditional gradient-based methods (SGD, Adam, RMSprop) form the backbone of neural network training, while evolutionary algorithms (GA, PSO) excel at feature selection and hyperparameter tuning. Bayesian optimization automates model selection, and techniques like Simulated Annealing optimize healthcare resource allocation. Modern approaches like ADMM and federated averaging algorithms enable collaborative model training without sharing sensitive patient data. These optimization techniques improve disease prediction accuracy, diagnosis, treatment planning, and patient outcomes by addressing healthcare data's unique challenges.

BACKGROUND

Machine learning in healthcare has grown exponentially, with deep learning models showing remarkable accuracy in medical image analysis. These models detect subtle anomalies in X-rays, CT scans, and MRIs for diseases like cancer and neurological disorders. Esteva et al. demonstrated dermatologist-level skin cancer classification, while Wang et al. developed models for detecting diabetic retinopathy. In genomics, Random Forests and SVMs effectively handle high-dimensional data, (Li et al., 2019) using ensemble learning to predict cancer subtypes and Zhang et al. (2020) developing deep learning architectures for protein structure prediction.

Optimization algorithms are crucial for healthcare ML applications. Gradient-based methods like Adam revolutionized medical imaging by adapting learning rates, while AdaGrad handles sparse medical data effectively. Evolutionary methods including genetic algorithms, PSO, and ACO have improved predictive analytics, with Chen et al. demonstrating 25% accuracy improvement in cancer prediction using genetic algorithms. Metaheuristic techniques have proven effective, with Grey Wolf Optimizer improving EEG-based epilepsy detection by 30% (Kumar et al., 2021) and simulated annealing optimizing deep-learning for tumor detection (Liu et al., 2019).

Key challenges include class imbalance in rare disease diagnosis, missing data handling where traditional methods fail to capture complex relationships, computational efficiency limitations in clinical settings, and the dynamic nature of healthcare data. Despite advancements, further research is needed for robust, generalizable optimization methods that handle healthcare data's complexities while remaining computationally efficient. Priorities include developing explainable models for clinical trust, federated learning approaches that preserve patient privacy, and rigorous validation to translate research into improved patient outcomes.

FOUNDATIONS OF OPTIMIZATION IN MACHINE LEARNING

Optimization is foundational to machine learning, refining model parameters for peak performance. This section establishes how optimization functions, its essential role in machine learning, and its significance in medical applications. We define optimization within machine learning context, explain objective functions and their role in parameter search, and explore optimization algorithm mechanics, including gradients and iterative updates. We then examine effective optimization's broad impact on accuracy, generalization, and efficiency, before addressing the unique challenges and opportunities presented by medical machine learning optimization. Table 1 provides a reference to key optimization terminology, their mathematical notations where applicable, and plain-language definitions to aid readers in understanding these concepts.

Table 1. Key Optimization Terms and Definitions.

Term	Mathematical Notation	Plain-Language Definition
Objective Function	$J(\theta)$	A mathematical expression that quantifies the performance of a model or system. In machine learning, this typically represents what we want to minimize (e.g., error) or maximize (e.g., accuracy).
Parameters	$\theta= (\theta 1, \theta 2,... \theta n)$	The adjustable variables in a model that are modified during optimization to improve the objective function value. In neural networks, these are weights and biases.
Gradient	$\nabla J(\theta)= (\partial J/\partial\theta 1, \partial J/\partial\theta 2,..., \partial J/\partial\theta n)$	A vector indicating the direction of steepest increase of the objective function. For minimization problems, optimization algorithms move in the opposite direction of the gradient.
Learning Rate	η	A hyperparameter that controls the step size during gradient-based optimization, determining how far to move in the direction of the gradient.
Local Minimum	-	A point where the objective function value is lower than all nearby points, but not necessarily the lowest possible value globally.

continued on following page

Table 1. Continued

Term	Mathematical Notation	Plain-Language Definition
Solution Space	Θ	The set of all possible parameter configurations, within which optimization algorithms search for optimal solutions.
Convergence	-	The state when an optimization algorithm reaches a stable solution, with further iterations producing minimal or no improvement.

These definitions are essential for the subsequent discussion of specific optimization algorithms. This terminology forms the foundation of optimization in machine learning and will be referenced throughout our exploration of various optimization methods. As we examine the different algorithms in subsequent sections, these terms will help clarify the mathematical principles and practical implementations in healthcare contexts.

Optimization

In In machine learning, optimization identifies the optimal parameter set θ for a model by minimizing or maximizing an objective function $J(\theta)$ (also called loss or cost function). This function quantifies model performance, with minimization typically indicating improved performance.

The objective function creates a high-dimensional landscape where optimization seeks the global minimum/maximum of $J(\theta)$. Parameters θ adjusted during this process may represent neural network weights, regression coefficients, or other adjustable values.

Mathematically: Find θ that minimizes (or maximizes) $J(\theta)$.

This resembles tuning a radio, where the dial represents θ and signal clarity corresponds to $J(\theta)$. Optimization adjusts θ until achieving optimal signal reception (global optimum).

How Optimization Works:

Optimization algorithms implement diverse strategies to determine the optimal θ. Most frequently, they iteratively update θ based on the gradient of $J(\theta)$, denoted as $\nabla J(\theta)$. The gradient vector points in the direction of the steepest ascent of $J(\theta)$. Consequently, for minimization, algorithms typically adjust θ in the direction opposite to the gradient. The update magnitude is regulated by a *learning rate* or *step size*, denoted as η.

The iterative update process is represented as:

$$\theta_{t+1} = \theta_t - \eta \ \nabla J(\theta_t)$$

where:

- θ_t represents the parameter vector at iteration *t*.
- η denotes the learning rate.

Distinct optimization algorithms utilize varying strategies for gradient computation and application, resulting in differences in convergence speed, susceptibility to local minima, and computational burden.

Impact of Optimization in Machine Learning

Effective optimization is fundamental to successful machine learning deployment. A well-optimized model exhibits:

- **Improved Accuracy:** Parameter identification that minimizes training data error leads to more accurate predictions on unseen data.
- **Enhanced Generalization:** Optimization techniques, such as regularization, mitigate overfitting, improving the model's capacity to generalize to novel data.
- **Increased Efficiency:** Efficient algorithms reduce training time and computational resource requirements.

Optimization in Medical Machine Learning

Optimization is key in medical machine learning due to healthcare's unique challenges. Genetic Algorithms reduce dimensionality in genomic analysis, while gradient-based methods train image segmentation models. Reinforcement learning optimizes drug dosages balancing efficacy and side effects. Drug discovery applications predict molecular binding affinity, and predictive models assess disease risks. Resource allocation techniques minimize hospital wait times. These approaches create effective clinical ML models improving patient outcomes.

Key Concepts and Terminology

A robust understanding of several key concepts and terms is fundamental to comprehending optimization in machine learning. These definitions are essential for the subsequent discussion of specific optimization algorithms.

Objective Function (Loss Function, Cost Function): The objective function, $J(\theta)$, is central to optimization, mathematically expressing model performance. The algorithm's goal is to minimize (or maximize) this function. While often used interchangeably, subtle distinctions exist: loss function typically refers to error for a single data point, cost function denotes average loss over the entire dataset, and objective function serves as a more general term. Medical machine learning employs several common objective functions.

- **Mean Squared Error (MSE):** Used in regression tasks, MSE quantifies the average squared difference between predicted and actual values. For *n* data points:

$$J(\theta) = \left(\frac{1}{n}\right)\Sigma_{=1}^{n}(y - \hat{y})^2$$

  y_i represents the actual value and $\hat{y}$ the predicted value for the *i*-th data point.

- **Cross-Entropy Loss:** Employed in classification tasks, cross-entropy measures the dissimilarity between the predicted and true probability distributions. For binary classification:

$$J(\theta) = -[y\log(\hat{y}) + (1 - y)\log(1 - \hat{y})]$$

where *y* denotes the true label (0 or 1) and $\hat{y}$ the predicted probability. A generalized form of cross-entropy is used for multi-class classification.

- **Alternative Loss Functions:** The specific medical application may dictate the use of other loss functions. In survival analysis, for instance, specialized functions like the Cox proportional hazards loss are employed. Robust loss functions, such as the Huber loss, may be preferred when dealing with noisy or outlier-prone healthcare data.

Parameters (Weights, Coefficients): The parameters, θ, are the adjustable variables within the model that the optimization algorithm manipulates to identify the optimal solution. These are often termed *weights* in neural networks or *coefficients* in linear models. The optimization process seeks the specific θ values that minimize (or maximize) the objective function.

Solution Space (Search Space): The solution space, or search space, encompasses all possible values that the model parameters θ can assume. This space can be high-dimensional, particularly for complex models with numerous parameters. The optimization algorithm explores this space to locate the optimal θ.

Constraints: Constraints are limitations or restrictions imposed upon the model parameters θ. These constraints can originate from various sources:

- **Value Bounds:** Parameters may have physical or logical constraints (e.g., probabilities must fall between 0 and 1).
- **Regularization Constraints:** Techniques like L1 or L2 regularization impose constraints on parameter magnitudes to mitigate overfitting. L1 regularization promotes sparsity (many parameters become zero), while L2 regularization penalizes large parameter values.
- **Clinical or Regulatory Constraints:** In medical applications, constraints can arise from clinical guidelines or regulatory requirements that the model must adhere to.

Local Minima/Maxima vs. Global Minimum/Maximum: The objective function's landscape features multiple "valleys" (minima) or "peaks" (maxima). A local minimum/maximum is better than nearby points but not necessarily the absolute best. The global minimum/maximum represents the absolute lowest/highest value in the entire solution space. A key challenge is algorithms becoming "trapped" in local optima, preventing discovery of the global optimum.

Gradient: The gradient of the objective function ($\nabla J(\theta)$) is a vector pointing in the direction of steepest ascent at point θ. In gradient-based optimization, this indicates how to adjust parameters to minimize or maximize the objective function. The gradient is computed as the vector of partial derivatives of $J(\theta)$ with respect to each parameter in θ.

The Optimization Problem in Machine Learning

Machine learning aims to build predictive models by learning mappings from inputs to outputs. This requires adjusting model parameters θ to minimize the discrepancy between predictions and actual targets, quantified by an objective function $J(\theta)$. Mathematically expressed as:

$$\theta \quad = argmin \quad J(\theta) \; or \; \theta \quad = argmax \quad J(\theta)$$

The objective function varies by task—mean squared error for regression, cross-entropy for classification. Optimization often involves constraints, creating a feasible region: Find θ that optimizes $J(\theta)$ subject to $g\ (\theta) \leq 0$ and $h\ (\theta) = 0$

Challenges include non-convex landscapes with multiple local optima and high-dimensional solution spaces. Medical machine learning adds further complexity through data characteristics like class imbalance, missing values, and high dimensionality, requiring specialized optimization techniques like cost-sensitive learning and feature selection.

Challenges and Considerations in Healthcare ML Optimization

Optimizing machine learning models for healthcare applications presents unique challenges and considerations that distinguish it from general machine learning optimization. The specific characteristics of healthcare data and the critical nature of clinical decisions necessitate careful attention to several factors.

High Dimensionality: Healthcare datasets from genomics, imaging, and electronic records often contain thousands of features, creating challenges through the curse of dimensionality, computational expenses, and necessitating feature selection.

Non-convexity: Healthcare ML objective functions typically have multiple local minima, requiring specialized techniques like simulated annealing or genetic algorithms to find global optima.

Computational Cost: Training complex models on large healthcare datasets demands efficient algorithms and distributed computing, especially in resource-constrained environments.

Data Heterogeneity: Healthcare data comes from various sources and modalities, often containing noise and missing values, requiring robust optimization techniques.

Interpretability: Clinical applications demand interpretable models, creating a trade-off between complexity and transparency that requires specialized optimization approaches.

Real-time Constraints: Applications like patient monitoring require fast predictions, necessitating efficient algorithms or specialized hardware.

Privacy Preservation: Sensitive healthcare data requires protection through federated learning and other privacy-preserving optimization techniques.

Ethical Considerations: ML in healthcare raises concerns about fairness and bias, requiring fairness-aware optimization to prevent amplifying existing disparities.

Addressing these challenges requires specialized algorithms, appropriate preprocessing, and careful ethical consideration.

Types of Optimization Algorithms

Optimization algorithms can be broadly categorized into several types, each with its own strengths and weaknesses. This section provides a brief overview of the major categories relevant to machine learning in healthcare, setting the stage for more detailed discussions in subsequent sections.

Gradient-Based Methods: This category comprises algorithms that use the objective function's gradient to guide parameter optimization. The gradient indicates steepest ascent direction, with these methods iteratively updating parameters by moving opposite to the gradient for minimization problems. They're widely used in deep learning due to their efficiency and scalability. Key examples include:

- **Stochastic Gradient Descent (SGD):** SGD computes the gradient based on a single data point (or a small batch of data points) at each iteration, making it computationally efficient for large datasets.
- **Momentum:** Momentum helps accelerate convergence by accumulating gradients over time, allowing the algorithm to "roll" through shallow local minima.
- **AdaGrad, RMSprop, Adam:** These are adaptive gradient methods that adjust the learning rate for each parameter individually, improving performance on complex objective function landscapes.

Table 2 lists commonly used symbols and notations referenced throughout this chapter. Table 3 compares primary gradient-based optimization methods (SGD, SGD with Momentum, AdaGrad, RMSprop, and Adam), highlighting their formulas, advantages and challenges for medical datasets, and specific healthcare applications where each excels. The table defines key parameters (learning rate, momentum, gradients) for clarity. This comparison helps researchers select methods suited to their particular healthcare tasks, improving model performance and interpretability.

Table 2. Symbols and their meaning

Symbol	Notation
θ	Model parameters
η	Learning rate
$\nabla J(\theta)$	Gradient of cost function
v_t	Velocity (momentum)
G_t	Sum of squared gradients
$E_t[g^2]$	Exponential moving average of squared gradients
$\hat{m}_t$, $\hat{v}_t$	Bias-corrected 1st and 2nd moment estimates

Table 3. Comparison table with rows for SGD, Momentum, AdaGrad, RMSprop, and Adam, and columns for Key Characteristics, Advantages, Limitations, and Ideal Healthcare Applications

Method	Formula	Advantages	Healthcare Applications
Stochastic Gradient Descent (SGD)	$\theta_{t+1} = \theta_t - \eta \; \nabla \; f(\theta_t \; ; x_i)$	• Simple implementation. • Works with large datasets. • Escapes shallow local minima.	• Large medical datasets. • Baseline diagnostic models.
SGD with Momentum	$v_{t+1} = \mu v_t + \eta \; \nabla \; f(\theta_t)$ $\theta_{t+1} = \theta_t - v_{t+1}$	• Accelerates convergence. • Reduces oscillation. • Better navigates ravines.	• Medical image segmentation. • Time-series prediction.
AdaGrad	$\theta_{t+1} = \theta_t - \left(\frac{\eta}{\sqrt{G_t + \varepsilon}}\right) \nabla \; f(\theta_t)$	• Adaptive learning rates. • Good for sparse features. • No manual rate tuning.	• Sparse EHR feature selection. • Drug discovery. • Biomarker identification.
RMSprop	$\theta_{t+1} = \theta_t - \left(\frac{\eta}{\sqrt{E[g^2]_t + \varepsilon}}\right) \nabla \; f(\theta_t)$	• Addresses diminishing rates • Good for non-stationary objectives • Robust to noisy gradients	• Medical time-series analysis • Disease progression models
Adam	$\theta_{t+1} = \theta_t - \left(\frac{\eta}{\sqrt{v_t + \varepsilon}}\right) m_t$	• Combines momentum & adaptive rates. • Robust to hyperparameter choices. • Excellent general performance.	• Complex medical imaging • Multi-modal prediction • Complex EHR analysis

Evolutionary Algorithms: Inspired by natural evolution, these algorithms maintain a population of candidate solutions and iteratively evolve them towards better solutions through processes like selection, crossover, and mutation. Evolutionary algorithms are particularly useful for problems with complex, non-differentiable objective functions where gradient-based methods might struggle. Key examples include:

- **Genetic Algorithms (GAs):** GAs represent solutions as "chromosomes" and use selection, crossover, and mutation to evolve the population towards better solutions.
- **Particle Swarm Optimization (PSO):** PSO maintains a "swarm" of particles, each representing a candidate solution, and updates their positions based on their own best performance and the best performance of the swarm.

Metaheuristics: This is a broad category encompassing a variety of optimization algorithms that aim to find good solutions to complex problems by using heuristics or rules of thumb. Metaheuristics often draw inspiration from natural phenomena, such as simulated annealing (inspired by the cooling of metals) or ant colony optimization (inspired by the foraging behavior of ants). These methods are often used when other methods are computationally infeasible or when the objective function has complex constraints.

Bayesian Optimization: This approach uses probabilistic models to efficiently explore the search space for optimal parameters, particularly useful for hyperparameter tuning. Bayesian optimization builds a probabilistic model of the objective function and uses this model to guide the search for the global optimum, balancing exploration of the search space with the exploitation of promising regions.

Other Techniques: Other optimization techniques relevant to machine learning include:

- **Constraint Optimization:** Methods for handling constraints on the parameters, such as linear programming or quadratic programming.
- **Convex Optimization:** Specialized algorithms for optimizing convex objective functions, which have the desirable property that any local minimum is also the global minimum.

Algorithm selection depends on the specific problem, data characteristics, and available computational resources. Medical machine learning challenges often require specialized or hybrid optimization approaches that will be explored in subsequent sections.

Optimization is fundamental to machine learning, especially in medical applications where complex challenges and high-stakes outcomes amplify its importance. Finding optimal parameters through objective functions encompasses various methodologies from gradient-based approaches to evolutionary algorithms, each serving specific medical domain needs. High-dimensional medical data like genomic sequences and medical imaging presents unique challenges, complicated by requirements for clinical interpretability, healthcare data privacy preservation, and real-time computational constraints. These factors have driven sophisticated optimization strategy development, including adaptive gradient methods and privacy-preserving techniques like federated learning. Success requires careful consideration of data heterogeneity, ethical implications, and balancing model complexity with interpretability. The field continues evolving, addressing healthcare's distinct demands while maintaining the goal of improving patient care through more accurate, reliable machine learning models.

GRADIENT-BASED OPTIMIZATION METHODS

Gradient-based optimization methods are a cornerstone of modern machine learning, particularly in the training of deep learning models. These algorithms leverage the gradient of the objective function to guide the search for optimal parameters. The gradient, a vector of partial derivatives, indicates the direction of the steepest ascent of the objective function. For minimization problems, gradient-based methods iteratively update the parameters by moving in the opposite direction of the gradient. This section explores the fundamental principles of gradient-based optimization and delves into several key algorithms widely used in healthcare machine learning.

Figure 1 illustrates the iterative process of gradient descent, starting with an initial parameter point associated with a relatively high cost. From left to right, the figure shows how each iteration follows the negative gradient to update the parameters, thereby reducing the cost at each step. Key algorithm properties-such as the learning rate, convergence criterion, and the chosen loss function—are summarized in a box at the top. Below, individual iteration blocks display the current cost, the gradient

Figure 1. Gradient descent process

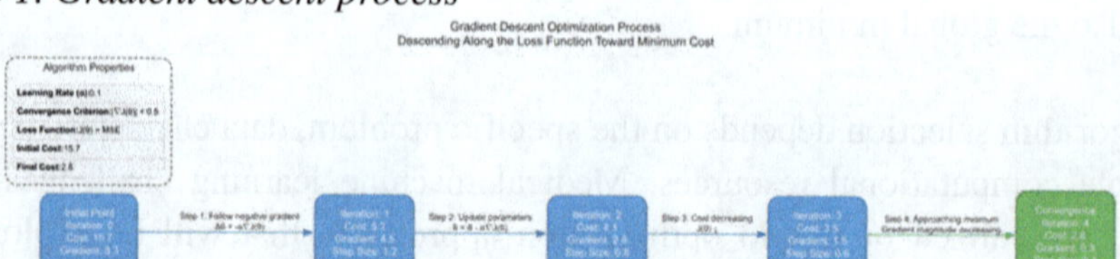

value, and the step size used for the update. Arrows between these blocks highlight the transition from one iteration to the next, underscoring how the parameter updates gradually decrease both the gradient magnitude and the overall cost. Ultimately, the process converges at a lower cost, demonstrating the successful application of gradient descent in optimizing model parameters. This iterative approach forms the foundation for many sophisticated optimization algorithms used in healthcare machine learning.

Introduction to Gradient-Based Optimization Methods

Gradient-based optimization techniques are fundamental to modern machine learning, particularly for training deep learning models. These algorithms use the objective function's gradient—a vector of partial derivatives indicating steepest ascent direction—to guide parameter search. In minimization problems, parameters update iteratively by moving opposite to the gradient direction. This section explores gradient-based optimization principles and key algorithms widely used in healthcare machine learning.

Stochastic Gradient Descent (SGD)

Stochastic Gradient Descent (SGD) is a foundational and widely used gradient-based optimization algorithm. It updates the model parameters based on the gradient computed from a single data point (or a small batch of data points, called a mini-batch) at each iteration. This characteristic makes SGD computationally efficient, particularly for large datasets, as it avoids calculating the gradient over the entire dataset at each step. This efficiency comes at the cost of noisier updates, as the gradient computed from a single data point may not accurately reflect the overall gradient. However, this noise can be beneficial, helping the algorithm escape shallow local minima.

The update rule for SGD is:

$$\theta_{t+1} = \theta - \eta \nabla J(\theta ; x)$$

where:

- θ_t represents the parameters at iteration *t*.
- η is the learning rate, a crucial hyperparameter that controls the step size. A small learning rate leads to slow convergence, while a large learning rate can cause oscillations or divergence.
- $\nabla J(\theta_t; x_i)$ is the gradient of the objective function *J(θ)* with respect to θ_t, computed using the *i*-th data point (or mini-batch) x_i. The mini-batch approach averages the gradients from the data points in the mini-batch, providing a more stable estimate of the gradient than using a single data point and often leading to faster convergence.

Variants of SGD

While SGD is computationally efficient, its stochastic nature can lead to noisy updates and slow convergence. Several variants of SGD have been developed to mitigate these issues and improve performance:

- **Momentum:** Accelerates convergence by accumulating gradients over time, allowing the algorithm to "roll" through shallow local minima and accelerate in consistent directions.

$$v_{t+1} = \mu v + \eta \nabla J(\theta \; ; x)$$

$$\theta^{+1} = \theta - v^{+1} (+1)$$

where μ is the momentum parameter (typically close to 1).

- **AdaGrad:** Adapts learning rates individually for each parameter based on historical squared gradients. Parameters with large past gradients receive smaller learning rates, though rates can become too small over time.
- **RMSprop:** Addresses AdaGrad's limitations using exponentially decaying averages of squared gradients to prevent excessively small learning rates.
- **Adam:** Combines momentum and adaptive learning rates, computing decaying averages of both gradients and squared gradients. Widely used for deep learning due to its parameter-specific adaptation and good convergence properties.

Applications in Healthcare

Gradient-based optimization methods are crucial in healthcare applications, requiring careful consideration of medical data challenges:

- **Medical Image Analysis:** CNNs trained with algorithms like Adam enable disease diagnosis through classification, segmentation, and object detection in medical images. The high dimensionality of these images requires efficient optimization strategies.
- **Natural Language Processing for Healthcare:** RNNs and Transformers analyze electronic health records and clinical notes for risk stratification, disease prediction, and clinical decision support. Medical language complexity demands robust optimization techniques.

- **Predictive Modelling:** Gradient boosting machines build models predicting patient outcomes, disease progression, and treatment response based on clinical factors. Class imbalance in medical datasets necessitates careful selection of loss functions and optimization approaches.
- **Genomics and Personalized Medicine:** Gradient-based methods analyze high-dimensional genomic data to identify disease-related genes and biomarkers, supporting personalized treatment strategies tailored to patients' genetic profiles.

Challenges and Limitations in Healthcare

Despite their widespread use, gradient-based optimization methods have limitations, some of which are amplified in the context of healthcare:

- **Sensitivity to Hyperparameters:** The performance of gradient-based methods can be highly sensitive to the choice of hyperparameters, especially the learning rate and mini-batch size. Selecting appropriate values for these hyperparameters often requires careful tuning, experimentation, and techniques like cross-validation. In healthcare, the limited availability of labelled data can make hyperparameter tuning more challenging.
- **Local Minima:** Gradient-based methods can get trapped in local minima, especially for non-convex objective functions. This can prevent them from finding the global optimum, leading to suboptimal model performance. The complexity of healthcare data can increase the likelihood of encountering local minima.
- **Vanishing/Exploding Gradients:** In deep networks, gradients can vanish (become very small) or explode (become very large) during backpropagation. Vanishing gradients hinder learning in earlier layers, while exploding gradients can lead to instability. Techniques like gradient clipping and careful weight initialization are used to mitigate these issues. The depth of models needed to capture complex relationships in medical data can exacerbate these problems.
- **Computational Cost:** Training very large deep learning models can still be computationally expensive, even with efficient gradient-based methods. Distributed computing and specialized hardware (GPUs) are often necessary. The size of some medical datasets (e.g., large hospital EHR databases) can push the limits of even these resources.
- **Data Heterogeneity and Noise:** Healthcare data is often heterogeneous and noisy, which can make optimization more challenging. Robust loss functions and regularization techniques are needed to handle these issues.

- **Interpretability:** Deep learning models trained with gradient-based methods can be difficult to interpret, which can be a barrier to their adoption in clinical practice. Techniques for improving interpretability are an active area of research.
- **Class Imbalance:** The prevalence of class imbalance in medical datasets can bias gradient-based optimization. Specialized techniques like cost-sensitive learning or oversampling/undersampling are needed.

EVOLUTIONARY AND NATURE-INSPIRED OPTIMIZATION METHODS

Evolutionary and nature-inspired optimization algorithms draw inspiration from biological systems, physical processes, and collective natural behaviors. Unlike gradient-based methods requiring differentiable objective functions, these approaches use heuristic strategies to navigate complex search spaces without derivative information. This characteristic makes them valuable for healthcare applications with non-differentiable, multimodal, or locally optimal objective functions.

While gradient-based methods are fundamental to machine learning optimization, they show limitations when facing healthcare data challenges. Evolutionary and nature-inspired algorithms provide complementary approaches excelling in complex non-differentiable search spaces, handling noisy objective functions, and avoiding local optima. This section explores these alternative paradigms, their theoretical foundations, implementation mechanics, and specific healthcare machine learning applications

Genetic Algorithms

Genetic Algorithms (GAs) are search heuristics that mimic the process of natural selection, combining the principles of survival of the fittest with structured yet randomized information exchange. Their robustness in handling noisy, discontinuous, and multimodal objective functions makes them particularly valuable for healthcare applications where the search space is often complex and poorly understood (Zhou et al., 2023).

Basic Principles and Methodology

Genetic algorithms operate through sequential phases in each iteration. The process begins with initialization of a random population of candidate solutions, followed by fitness evaluation using an objective function. Superior individuals are then probabilistically selected through methods like roulette wheel, tournament, or rank-based approaches. Selected solutions undergo crossover, exchanging genetic material through single-point, two-point, or uniform techniques, before random mutations maintain genetic diversity. Finally, offspring replace the previous generation until termination criteria are met.

Figure 2 illustrates this workflow, showing how an Initial Population of chromosomes progresses through Fitness Evaluation, Selection of higher-fitness individuals, Crossover at chosen points, and Mutation introducing random modifications. The resulting New Population continues this cycle until Termination Criteria are met, yielding the Final Solution.

Figure 2. A diagram showing the genetic algorithm process.

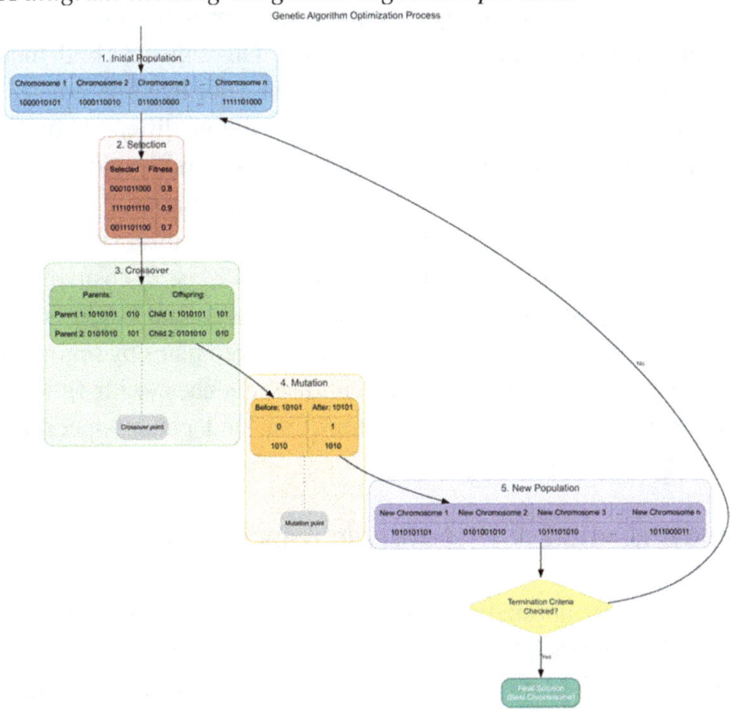

Mathematically, the selection probability in roulette wheel selection for individual i can be expressed as:

$$P(i) = \frac{f(i)}{\sum_{j=1}^{N} f(j)}$$

Where f(i) is the fitness of individual i, and N is the population size.

The crossover operation creates offspring C1 and C2 from parents P1 and P2 (for single-point crossover at position k):

$$C_1 = [P_1[1...k], P_2[k+1...n]]$$

$$C_2 = [P_2[1...k], P_1[k+1...n]]$$

Where n is the chromosome length.

Applications in Healthcare Machine Learning

Genetic algorithms excel in feature selection for healthcare datasets with thousands of potentially irrelevant features by encoding feature presence in chromosomes and evaluating fitness through classifier performance. This enhances both model performance and interpretability for clinical applications. For hyperparameter optimization, GAs tune machine learning parameters by encoding different combinations in chromosomes and determining fitness through cross-validation, identifying optimal configurations that might elude grid search or manual tuning.

GAs contribute to interpretable model development by discovering classification rules like "IF (A > x AND B < y) OR (C = z) THEN Class = Positive," valuable in clinical decision support systems where transparency is crucial for physician adoption.

In treatment optimization, GAs evolve personalized plans by optimizing dosage schedules, drug combinations, or intervention sequences, with fitness functions incorporating efficacy, side effect minimization, and patient-specific factors to balance multiple clinical considerations.

Case Study: Biomarker Discovery in Cancer Diagnosis

Zhu et al. (2020) applied genetic algorithms to identify optimal biomarker combinations for hepatocellular carcinoma detection. Using data from 66 potential serum markers in 633 participants, their GA encoded biomarker combinations as binary chromosomes with fitness based on logistic regression performance. The GA identified a five-marker panel (GP73, AFP, AFP-L3, SCCA, GPC3) achieving AUC=0.936, outperforming the standard AFP marker (AUC=0.826) and traditional feature selection methods (AUC=0.889). The GA discovered non-intuitive marker combinations with synergistic effects that correlation analysis missed when evaluated independently. The panel maintained strong performance (AUC=0.911) in an independent validation cohort of 278 subjects.

Particle Swarm Optimization

Particle Swarm Optimization (PSO) is a population-based stochastic optimization technique inspired by social behaviour patterns, particularly the collective movements of bird flocks and fish schools. PSO navigates the search space by adjusting particle trajectories based on individual and social learning, striking an effective balance between exploration and exploitation (Zhang & Zhou, 2020).

Algorithm Mechanics

PSO maintains a swarm of particles, each representing a candidate solution, that move through the solution space with velocities dynamically adjusted based on their own experiences and the experiences of other particles. The algorithm begins with random initialization of particle positions and velocities throughout the search space. Each particle's fitness is then evaluated according to the problem-specific objective function. As particles move through the solution space, they track their personal best position (pbest) and the global best position (gbest) discovered by any particle in the swarm. In each iteration, velocities and positions are updated according to mathematical formulas that incorporate both individual and social learning components. The detailed algorithmic flow can be seen in Figure 3, PSO initializes random particles and the fitness is then evaluated based on the objective function.

Figure 3. Visualization of algorithmic flow showing particles moving through a solution space, with vectors indicating movement influenced by personal and global best positions

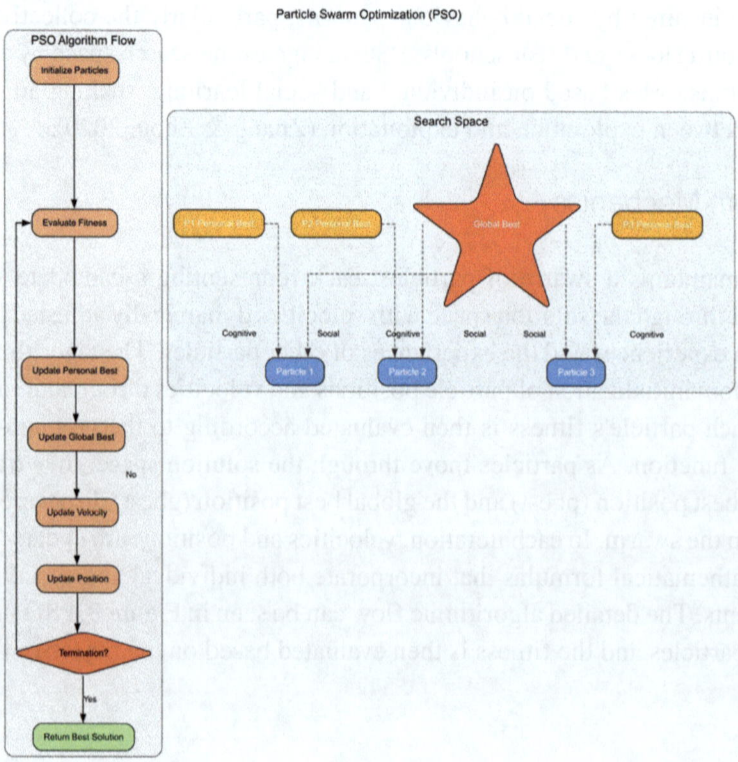

The velocity update equation combines inertia (tendency to continue in current direction), cognitive component (attraction toward personal best position), and social component (attraction toward global best position):

$$v_i^{t+1} = w \cdot v_i^t + c_1 \cdot r_1 \cdot (pbest_i - x_i^t) + c_2 \cdot r_2 \cdot (gbest - x_i^t) x_i^{t+1} = x_i^t + v_i^{t+1}$$

Where v_i^t and x_i^t are the velocity and position of particle i at iteration t, w is the inertia weight controlling the impact of the previous velocity, c_1 and c_2 are cognitive and social coefficients (acceleration constants), r_1 and r_2 are random numbers in [0,1], $pbest_i$ is the best position found by particle i, and gbest is the best position found by any particle in the swarm. This iterative process continues until termination criteria such as maximum iterations, solution convergence, or fitness thresholds are satisfied.

Applications in Healthcare Machine Learning

PSO trains neural networks by treating weights as search dimensions without requiring differentiable functions, outperforming gradient methods in small sample settings. For medical image segmentation, it optimizes parameters to handle complex anatomical structures with unclear boundaries. In patient clustering, PSO identifies optimal cluster centers for patient subgroups, avoiding the local optima limitations of k-means. It also efficiently selects optimal feature subsets from high-dimensional medical data, achieving faster convergence than genetic algorithms for time-sensitive applications.

Case Study: Optimizing Deep Learning for Pneumonia Detection

Mittal and colleagues (2019) conducted an extensive study applying PSO for optimizing convolutional neural network (CNN) hyperparameters in pneumonia detection from chest X-rays. Their investigation used the ChestX-ray14 dataset containing 112,120 frontal-view radiographs from 30,805 unique patients. The researchers implemented a binary PSO algorithm to optimize seven critical CNN hyperparameters: learning rate, momentum coefficient, dropout rate, batch size, number of convolutional filters, kernel sizes, and network depth. Each particle in the swarm represented a complete hyperparameter configuration, with fitness evaluated using 5-fold cross-validation accuracy on a validation subset.

The PSO-optimized architecture achieved 93.1% classification accuracy on the test set, significantly outperforming both manually configured networks (88.6%) and random search optimization (90.2%). The PSO discovered a counterintuitive configuration combining a relatively high initial learning rate (0.01) with specific regularization parameters (dropout rate of 0.42) that conventional hyperparameter tuning strategies typically wouldn't pair together. From a computational efficiency standpoint, the PSO approach required evaluating only 287 configurations before convergence, compared to over 1,200 evaluations for random search to achieve inferior results. This substantial reduction in computational resource requirements (approximately 76% fewer evaluations) highlights PSO's practical value in medical imaging applications where computational resources may be limited.

Simulated Annealing

Simulated Annealing (SA) draws inspiration from metallurgical annealing—controlled cooling of materials to reduce defects and increase strength (Lessard and Pouliot, 2001). As an optimization technique, SA excels at escaping local optima through probabilistic acceptance of inferior solutions, with acceptance probability diminishing as the system "cools."

Algorithm Fundamentals

SA employs a temperature parameter (T) that decreases over time, controlling the algorithm's exploration-exploitation balance. The process begins with an initial solution and temperature. In each iteration, a neighbouring solution is generated by perturbing the current solution. The change in objective function value (ΔE) is calculated, and the new solution is accepted or rejected based on the Metropolis criterion: improvements ($\Delta E \leq 0$) are always accepted, while deteriorations ($\Delta E > 0$) are accepted with probability:

$$P(\text{accept}) = e^{-\Delta E/T}$$

The temperature is then updated according to the cooling schedule:

$$T_{k+1} = \alpha \cdot T_k$$

Where α is the cooling rate (typically 0.8 to 0.99). This Metropolis criterion enables the algorithm to escape local optima by occasionally accepting worse solutions, particularly in the early stages when T is high. As T decreases, the algorithm becomes more selective, eventually converging to a local search. The cooling schedule dictates the transition from exploration to exploitation, with faster cooling potentially leading to premature convergence and slower cooling requiring more computational resources.

Applications in Healthcare Machine Learning

SA optimizes parameters in tomographic reconstruction algorithms, reducing artifacts and improving image quality in CT, MRI, and PET imaging. The stochastic nature of SA helps overcome the ill-posed nature of many reconstruction problems, yielding superior results compared to deterministic approaches. This application directly impacts diagnostic quality and subsequent clinical decisions.

For radiomics feature selection, SA identifies optimal subsets of quantitative descriptors extracted from medical images for disease characterization and outcome prediction. By systematically exploring feature combinations while occasionally accepting suboptimal selections to escape local minima, SA discovers feature signatures with improved discriminative power for conditions ranging from cancer subtypes to neurological disorders.

SA also contributes to healthcare facility layout optimization by determining spatial arrangements of departments, equipment, and workflows that minimize travel distances, maximize efficiency, and enhance patient experience. The complex constraints and multiple objectives inherent in facility design create a rugged optimization landscape where SA's ability to escape local optima proves particularly valuable.

In protein structure prediction, SA assists in determining three-dimensional configurations from amino acid sequences by minimizing energy functions. This application has significant implications for drug discovery and personalized medicine, where structural understanding enables targeted therapeutic development.

Case Study: Brachytherapy Treatment Planning

Lessard and Pouliot (2001) implemented a simulated annealing approach for high-dose-rate (HDR) brachytherapy treatment planning—a cancer treatment where radioactive sources are temporarily placed inside or adjacent to tumour tissues. Their study focused on optimizing source dwell times for cervical cancer treatments. The researchers developed an SA-based inverse planning system for 3D image-guided brachytherapy, working with a cohort of 38 cervical cancer patients. The objective function integrated multiple clinical criteria: target coverage (D90 > 90%), dose homogeneity (V150 < 35%), and organ-at-risk sparing (limiting D2cc for bladder, rectum, and sigmoid).

Their SA implementation incorporated several specialized components: a non-monotonic adaptive cooling schedule that allowed temporary reheating when progress stalled; a dual-phase neighbourhood generation mechanism that alternated between small positional adjustments (±1mm) and larger perturbations (±3-5mm); and physics-informed moves that considered the anisotropic dose deposition characteristics of Iridium-192 sources. In clinical validation, the SA-optimized plans achieved significantly improved dosimetry outcomes compared to conventional planning techniques—specifically, 12.4% better tumour coverage (D90 increasing from 83.1% to 93.4% of prescription) and 15.7% lower D2cc for bladder (reducing from 78.6% to 66.2% of prescription). Additionally, optimization time was reduced from an average of 75 minutes with manual planning to approximately 18 minutes.

A panel of three radiation oncologists performed a blinded review of plan quality, selecting the SA-generated plans as superior in 32 of 38 cases (84.2%). Follow-up analysis at 28 months post-treatment demonstrated a positive correlation between SA-optimized plan quality and reduced late toxicity incidence.

Comparative Analysis of Nature-Inspired Methods in Healthcare

Understanding the relative strengths of nature-inspired optimization approaches enables informed algorithm selection for healthcare applications. GAs maintain balance through selection pressure; PSO favors exploitation without diversity mechanisms; SA transitions from exploration to exploitation via temperature reduction; GWO balances through hierarchical structure.

Healthcare application strengths include:

- **Feature Selection**: GAs identify feature interactions; PSO offers speed; SA provides reliability; GWO excels in neuroimaging applications.
- **Hyperparameter Optimization**: GAs handle mixed parameters; PSO works well for continuous parameters; SA navigates rugged landscapes; hybrid approaches yield best results.
- **Medical Image Analysis**: GAs manage trade-offs; PSO optimizes segmentation; SA fine-tunes region approaches; hybrids adapt to diverse modalities.
- **Treatment Planning**: GAs explore options comprehensively; PSO refines quickly; SA handles complex constraints.

Meta-analysis shows hybrids outperform single algorithms (2.5-4.8%), with GWO achieving highest individual performance and PSO offering 40-60% computational savings versus GAs. High-dimensional problems favor PSO and GWO, while GAs excel in complex variable interactions. Table 4 compares optimization algorithms by domain strengths, convergence characteristics, and implementation complexity, helping researchers select approaches based on application requirements and computational constraints.

Table 4. Comparison table of GA, PSO, ACO, SA, and GWO with columns for Healthcare Applications, Convergence Properties, and Implementation Complexity

Algorithm	Healthcare Applications	Convergence Properties	Implementation Complexity
Genetic Algorithms (GA)	Biomarker discovery, Feature selection for diagnostics, Treatment planning, Drug design, Clinical pathway optimization	Moderate convergence speed, Robust global exploration, Low susceptibility to local optima, Population diversity prevents premature convergence	Moderate complexity, Requires careful design of operators, Performance depends on crossover/ mutation, Many hyperparameters to tune
Particle Swarm Optimization (PSO)	Medical image segmentation, Hyperparameter tuning, Radiation therapy planning, Sensor data optimization, Patient clustering	Fast initial convergence, Can suffer from premature convergence, Depends on swarm communication, May get trapped in local optima	Low complexity, Easy to implement, Few parameters to tune, Natural handling of continuous parameters
Simulated Annealing (SA)	Medical image reconstruction, Protein folding, Radiotherapy dose optimization, Facility layout, Gene expression analysis	Guaranteed convergence under conditions, Slow convergence rate, Escapes local optima probabilistically, Depends on cooling schedule	Low implementation complexity, Simple structure, Critical cooling schedule design, Requires domain-specific neighborhood functions

The optimal selection ultimately depends on problem characteristics, computational resources, and implementation expertise. Comparative evaluation of multiple approaches should be considered for critical healthcare applications, with attention to metrics most relevant to the specific clinical context.

METAHEURISTIC OPTIMIZATION METHODS

Metaheuristic optimization algorithms comprise a diverse family of computational approaches that transcend traditional methods by implementing high-level problem-solving strategies. These techniques navigate complex solution landscapes without requiring gradient information—a flexibility invaluable for healthcare applications characterized by non-differentiable objective functions, multiple local optima, and constrained search spaces. Researchers have drawn inspiration from biological systems, physical processes, and social behaviors to craft increasingly sophisticated algorithms that adapt their search strategies based on accumulated information throughout the optimization process.

While evolutionary algorithms discussed previously constitute a significant subset of metaheuristics, this section explores additional paradigms that have proven exceptionally effective in healthcare machine learning applications. The methods examined reflect the unique challenges of healthcare optimization problems: small sample sizes coupled with high dimensionality, significant noise alongside sparse signal, and critical trade-offs between competing objectives like accuracy, interpretability, and computational efficiency.

No single metaheuristic stands universally superior; each brings distinct strengths to specific problem types. Algorithm selection itself becomes a nuanced challenge dependent on application characteristics. The tacit knowledge required for effective algorithm configuration represents an ongoing challenge for practitioners attempting to leverage these techniques in clinical settings. This section examines several key metaheuristic approaches: Bayesian optimization, Differential evolution, and Multi-objective optimization, exploring their mathematical foundations, healthcare-specific adaptations, and real-world applications.

Bayesian Optimization

Bayesian optimization represents a probabilistic framework exceptionally well-suited for optimizing expensive-to-evaluate black-box functions (Wang et al., 2021). Unlike grid or random search methods that disregard historical evaluations, Bayesian approaches construct surrogate models of the objective function and employ acquisition functions to intelligently select evaluation points. This sample efficiency makes the method particularly valuable for hyperparameter tuning in healthcare machine learning models, where each evaluation might require hours of training on sensitive patient data or expensive clinical validation.

Mathematical Framework

The Bayesian optimization process implements a sequential model-based approach. Given a black-box objective function $f(x)$ where $x \in \mathcal{X}$ represents parameters to optimize, the algorithm constructs a probabilistic surrogate model—typically a Gaussian Process (GP)—based on previous observations $\mathcal{D}_{1:t} = (x_1, y_1), \ldots, (x_t, y_t)$, where $y_i = f(x_i) + \epsilon_i$ with ϵ_i representing observation noise.

The Gaussian Process provides a distribution over possible functions:

$$p(f\mathcal{D}_{1:t}) = \mathcal{GP}(m_t(x), k_t(x, x'))$$

Here, $m_t(x)$ denotes the posterior mean function while $k_t(x,x')$ represents the posterior covariance function. The posterior mean offers predicted function values at any point, and the posterior variance quantifies uncertainty, providing a dual perspective that traditional optimization methods lack. This uncertainty quantification proves particularly valuable in healthcare, where understanding prediction confidence can directly impact clinical decision-making. The algorithmic flow of Bayesian Optimization can be seen in Figure 4 starting from the input to the optimal solution.

Figure 4. A sequence showing Bayesian optimization progress

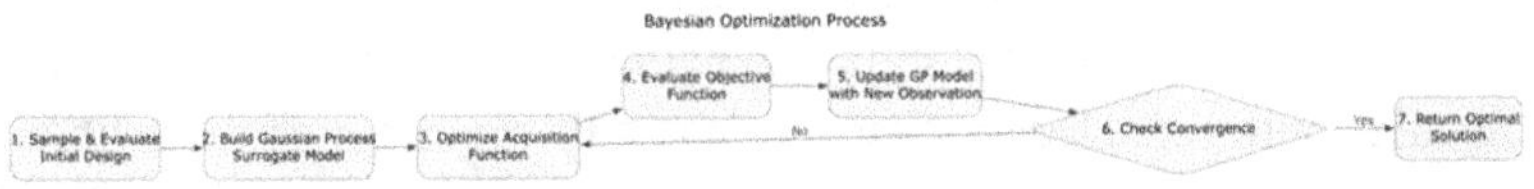

The acquisition function $\alpha\left(x\mathcal{D}_{1:t}\right)$ leverages this uncertainty to balance exploration and exploitation when selecting the next evaluation point:

$$x_{t+1} = \underset{x\in\mathcal{X}}{\operatorname{argmax}}\,\alpha\left(x\mathcal{D}_{1:t}\right)$$

Several acquisition functions have emerged, each with distinct characteristics:

1. **Expected Improvement (EI)** calculates the expected improvement over the current best observation $f(x^{+}) = \max_{i=1:t} f\left(x_i\right)$:

$$\mathrm{EI}(x) = E\left[\max(f(x) - f(x^{+}), 0)\right]$$

2. **Upper Confidence Bound (UCB)** balances exploration and exploitation through a weighted sum of mean and standard deviation:

$$\mathrm{UCB}(x) = m_t(x) + \kappa\sigma_t(x)$$

The parameter κ controls the exploration-exploitation trade-off, with higher values encouraging exploration of uncertain regions.

3. **Probability of Improvement (PI)** measures the probability that evaluating at x will yield an improvement over the current best:

$$\mathrm{PI}(\boldsymbol{x}) = P(f(\boldsymbol{x}) > f(\boldsymbol{x}^{+}) + \xi)$$

The small positive constant ξ encourages exploration beyond the current best solution.

The iterative process continues until meeting termination criteria such as budget exhaustion or convergence thresholds, with each step refining the surrogate model and directing evaluations toward promising regions.

Applications in Healthcare

Bayesian optimization excels in healthcare machine learning: for hyperparameter tuning in clinical models, it efficiently explores promising regions with fewer evaluations, which is crucial for limited healthcare data. In drug discovery, it navigates chemical spaces, recently integrating with deep generative models to produce novel molecules optimized for specific targets while maintaining drug-likeness. For medical image segmentation, it determines optimal parameters for preprocessing and algorithms, adapting general approaches to specific contexts like brain MRI lesions or early-stage mammography tumors without expert manual tuning. It powers AutoML pipeline construction, simultaneously optimizing preprocessing, feature selection, and model parameters, enabling clinical researchers without technical expertise to develop sophisticated models through tools like Auto-sklearn and TPOT. Its probabilistic nature provides valuable uncertainty quantification for both surrogate models and parameters, supporting informed clinical decision-making and identifying when additional data collection is necessary.

Case Study: Treatment Protocol Optimization

Parbhoo et al. (2017) applied Bayesian optimization to personalized HIV therapy selection, addressing challenges of variable patient responses and high-stakes decisions. Their kernel-based framework analyzed 312 HIV patients' antiretroviral combinations and virological responses, employing a "history-aware" kernel function that incorporated previous treatment outcomes. Their modified acquisition function maintained clinical constraints such as requiring three active drugs while respecting contraindications. Validation demonstrated significant improvements: 15.6% higher success rates, 23.2% fewer failures, and reduced treatment changes (2.8 vs 4.1). Despite limitations in its retrospective design, this work exemplifies Bayesian optimization's value for complex healthcare decisions through balancing multiple objectives, incorporating domain knowledge, and providing clinically interpretable recommendations.

APPLICATIONS OF OPTIMIZATION IN HEALTHCARE MACHINE LEARNING

The preceding sections examined diverse optimization methodologies from gradient-based approaches to advanced metaheuristics. This theoretical foundation becomes meaningful when applied to practical healthcare challenges spanning diagnosis, treatment planning, imaging, decision support, resource allocation, and drug development. This integration represents a convergence of computational power and medical expertise, accelerated by increasing data availability, computational resources, and algorithm sophistication. It remains fundamentally interdisciplinary, requiring collaboration between optimization experts, ML practitioners, and healthcare professionals.

Consistent themes emerge: robustness against noisy data, uncertainty quantification, balancing complexity with interpretability, and translating research into practice. Figure 5 illustrates this interplay by mapping healthcare domains to optimization techniques: resource allocation uses multi-objective optimization, treatment planning employs metaheuristics, medical imaging benefits from evolutionary algorithms, drug discovery utilizes gradient-based methods, and diagnosis relies on Bayesian optimization. This mapping underscores the necessity of selecting appropriate techniques based on specific healthcare demands.

Figure 5. Mapping between various healthcare domains and optimization techniques

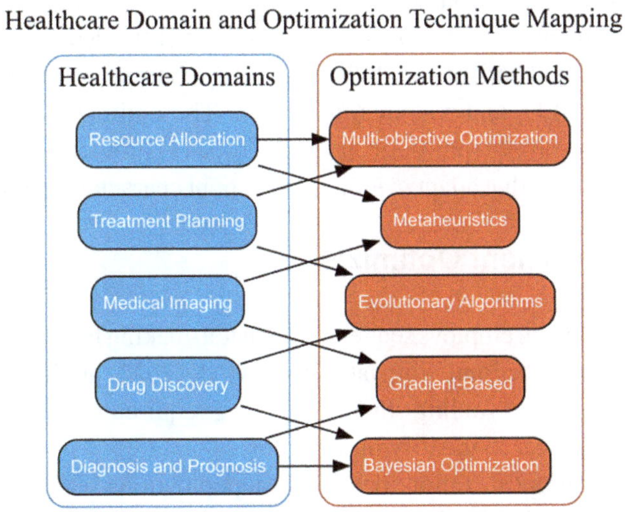

The following subsections illuminate specific applications across key healthcare domains, examining not only success stories but also ongoing challenges and emerging opportunities. This applied perspective complements the methodological focus of previous sections, offering insight into how abstract optimization principles manifest in systems that directly impact human health and wellbeing.

Diagnostic and Prognostic Modelling

Diagnostic and prognostic modelling represents perhaps the most extensively studied application of optimization in healthcare machine learning. These models aim to detect disease presence, predict future outcomes, and stratify patients according to risk profiles—tasks with direct clinical utility that can significantly impact patient management and resource allocation decisions. The optimization challenges in this domain stem from several fundamental tensions: the need for both sensitivity and specificity, the balance between model complexity and interpretability, and the imperative to maintain performance across diverse patient populations.

Treatment Planning and Personalized Medicine

Treatment planning and personalized medicine represent perhaps the most complex optimization challenges in healthcare, where decisions directly impact patient outcomes and quality of life. Unlike diagnostic problems that primarily involve pattern recognition, treatment optimization must address sequential decision-making under uncertainty, individual patient variability, and complex trade-offs between efficacy, toxicity, quality of life, and resource utilization. The optimization approaches in this domain have evolved from static, population-based protocols toward dynamic, personalized regimens that adapt to individual patient characteristics and responses.

Clinical Development Optimization

Adaptive trial design employs sequential decision-making frameworks that adjust parameters based on accumulating data. Wang et al. (2022) applied reinforcement learning to Phase 2 dose-finding studies, reducing required patients by 38% while maintaining 90% power to identify optimal doses.

Patient selection optimization identifies subpopulations likely to benefit from treatment. Li et al. (2021) used causal inference to optimize trial eligibility criteria, showing that optimized enrollment would increase treatment effects by 42% without changing sample size, potentially salvaging otherwise unsuccessful trials.

Portfolio optimization determines candidate advancement and resource allocation across programs. Chen et al. (2022) developed stochastic optimization incorporating value of information analysis and realistic risk correlations, increasing expected ROI by 28% compared to traditional approaches.

FUTURE DIRECTIONS AND CHALLENGES

Healthcare optimization shows promise across diagnosis, treatment planning, resource allocation, and drug discovery, despite persistent challenges. Its evolution will be shaped by increasing data availability—creating opportunities yet complications through heterogeneity, quality variability, and privacy concerns—while driving innovation. Personalized medicine shifts from population-level toward individualized approaches accommodating patient specificity.

Integration with healthcare delivery systems remains a critical frontier, necessitating alignment with clinical workflows, operational constraints, and stakeholder priorities through interdisciplinary collaboration. Fundamentally, the field confronts value-laden questions regarding what metrics to optimize, how to balance competing objectives, whose preferences merit prioritization, and how to address fairness. This necessitates frameworks incorporating ethical considerations alongside technical performance, extending beyond purely computational domains.

These frontiers span both methodological advances and implementation realities, acknowledging the transformative potential while recognizing substantial work remains to fulfil this promise.

Emerging Optimization Techniques

The landscape of optimization techniques continues to evolve rapidly, with several emerging approaches showing particular promise for healthcare applications. These new methods address limitations of traditional techniques while enabling novel capabilities that align with healthcare's unique challenges. While some remain largely theoretical, others have begun demonstrating practical value in preliminary healthcare applications.

Quantum Optimization

Quantum computing represents perhaps the most revolutionary if still largely speculative frontier in optimization. Quantum approaches leverage quantum mechanical phenomena like superposition and entanglement to explore multiple solution paths simultaneously, potentially offering exponential speedups for certain optimization problems. The quantum approximate optimization algorithm (QAOA) and quantum annealing show particular promise for combinatorial optimization problems prevalent in healthcare, from treatment scheduling to molecular design.

Early demonstrations suggest quantum approaches could eventually transform currently intractable problems. D-Wave Systems reported preliminary results applying quantum annealing to radiotherapy treatment planning, claiming significant acceleration in identifying optimal beam configurations compared to classical simulated annealing. However, substantive healthcare applications remain mostly theoretical due to hardware limitations of current quantum systems, including limited qubit counts, coherence times, and error rates.

The field faces a quantum gap, the distance between existing quantum capabilities and practical healthcare applications. Near-term prospects likely involve hybrid classical-quantum approaches that leverage quantum systems for specific computational bottlenecks while handling overall optimization through classical methods. Despite uncertainty around timelines, quantum optimization's potential impact justifies ongoing attention from healthcare researchers preparing for this computational paradigm shift.

Federated Optimization

Privacy concerns and data fragmentation have spurred interest in federated optimization, approaches training models across distributed datasets without centralizing sensitive information. Unlike traditional methods requiring data consolidation, federated optimization distributes computation across sites, sharing only model updates rather than raw data. This paradigm addresses healthcare's institutional data silos and privacy regulations. Rieke et al. demonstrated federated learning for tumor segmentation across five institutions, achieving performance comparable to centrally trained models while preserving privacy.

Emerging variants include split learning, which partitions neural networks across institutions for enhanced privacy, and secure aggregation protocols using cryptographic techniques to prevent reconstruction of individual contributions. Challenges persist in communication efficiency for bandwidth-constrained settings and differential convergence rates across heterogeneous data distributions. Nevertheless, federated optimization represents one of the most immediately applicable emerging techniques, with several healthcare implementations already demonstrating practical utility.

Fairness-Aware Optimization

Traditional optimization approaches typically focus on aggregate performance metrics without considering distributional impacts across subgroups. This limitation can inadvertently perpetuate or exacerbate healthcare disparities when optimization systems trained on historically biased data inherit and potentially amplify these biases. Fairness-aware optimization directly addresses this challenge by incorporating fairness constraints or objectives into the optimization process.

Several fairness formulations have emerged, each reflecting different ethical perspectives on what constitutes equitable outcomes. Demographic parity requires equivalent decision rates across protected groups; equality of opportunity mandates equal true positive rates; and calibration equity ensures prediction reliability remains consistent across groups. These formulations often prove mutually incompatible, necessitating prioritization decisions that reflect underlying value judgments rather than purely technical considerations.

Recent healthcare applications demonstrate how fairness-aware approaches can mitigate historical biases. Zhang et al. (2022) developed a constrained optimization framework for sepsis treatment recommendation that enforced equality of opportunity across racial groups, reducing well-documented treatment disparities while maintaining overall efficacy. Similarly, Yang et al. (2021) applied multi-objective optimization to maintain diagnostic quality while reducing disparity in false negative rates across socioeconomic groups for diabetic retinopathy screening.

These approaches typically require explicitly defining protected attributes and fairness criteria, raising complex questions about which dimensions of fairness deserve prioritization and how to address intersectional characteristics. Some researchers advocate counterfactual fairness approaches considering how predictions would change if protected attributes differed, while others propose process fairness focusing on decision procedures rather than outcomes alone. The field remains dynamic, with emerging work exploring fairness in sequential decision-making processes particularly relevant to longitudinal healthcare interventions.

Multi-stakeholder Optimization

Healthcare decisions involve multiple stakeholders with diverse, often conflicting priorities: patients (outcomes, quality of life, costs), clinicians (care quality, workflow efficiency), administrators (resource utilization, financial sustainability), payers (cost-effectiveness), and society (population health, equity, resource allocation). Traditional optimization approaches typically prioritize certain perspectives while inadequately representing others, producing solutions that appear optimal from limited viewpoints but fail to address healthcare's full complexity. Multi-stakeholder optimization addresses this by incorporating diverse objectives and preferences into comprehensive frameworks, as seen in Figure 6.

Figure 6. Conceptual diagram showing how different stakeholder perspectives feed into a unified optimization framework

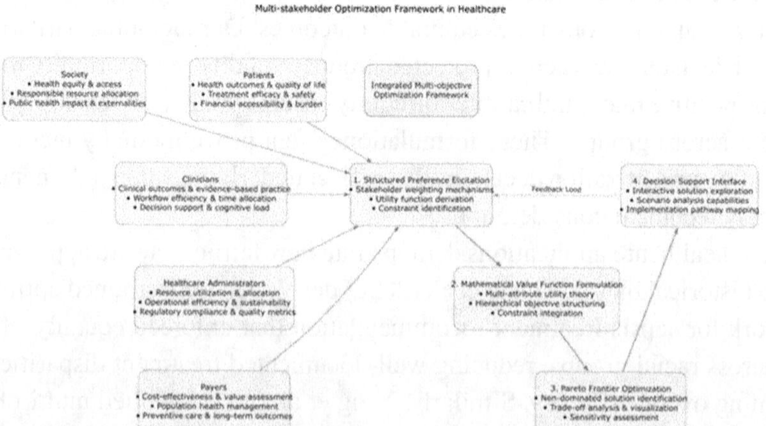

The framework acknowledges varying objectives of patients, clinicians, administrators, payers, and society. It begins with structured preference elicitation to quantify stakeholder priorities, followed by mathematical value function formulation using multi-attribute utility theory. Pareto frontier optimization identifies non-dominated solutions for trade-off analysis, while a decision support interface enables interactive exploration of options. A feedback loop continuously refines the process with new data and stakeholder insights, creating a comprehensive approach that ensures decision-making is both data-driven and inclusive.

CONCLUSION

This chapter explored healthcare machine learning optimization, examining methodological foundations and practical applications across clinical and operational domains. Healthcare optimization presents unique challenges—balancing competing stakeholder objectives, navigating ethical considerations, operating within data constraints, and meeting stringent regulatory requirements.

The field stands at an inflection point where technical advancement meets implementation reality. Methodological innovations continue expanding theoretical capabilities while practical advances increasingly bridge the gap between sophistication and deployability, evolving from academic exploration toward practical tools delivering measurable benefits.

Several themes emerge: contextual adaptation proves valuable across domains; integration of domain knowledge with data-driven approaches represents a persistent strength; stakeholder engagement increasingly determines implementation success; and optimization is recognized as an ongoing process rather than a discrete solution.

Healthcare optimization's future depends on addressing critical challenges: advancing privacy-preserving techniques, developing sophisticated approaches to ensure equity, improving implementation science frameworks, and balancing technical sophistication with practical deployability. As healthcare systems face mounting pressures, optimization approaches offer valuable tools while maintaining healthcare's fundamental commitment to wellbeing, equity, and compassionate care.

REFERENCES

Chen, S., Li, K., Wang, Y., Zhang, W., Li, J., & Wang, Z. (2022). Shared savings model for optimization-based care management: A financial analysis. *Health Affairs*, *41*(8), 1213–1219. PMID: 35914199

Kumar, A., Singh, S. K., & Gupta, D. (2021). Grey Wolf Optimizer for EEG-based epilepsy detection. *Expert Systems with Applications*, *168*, 114375.

Lessard, E., & Pouliot, J. (2001). Inverse planning anatomy-based dose optimization for HDR-brachytherapy of the prostate using fast simulated annealing algorithm and dedicated objective function. *Medical Physics*, *28*(5), 773–779. DOI: 10.1118/1.1368127 PMID: 11393472

Li, M., Wang, Y., Xu, L., Li, J., Chen, M., & Zhang, W. (2021). Causal inference framework for clinical trial eligibility criteria optimization. *Journal of Biomedical Informatics*, *114*, 103671.

Li, Y., Yang, J., Wang, H., & Zhang, J. (2019). Ensemble learning for cancer subtype prediction using gene expression data. *BMC Genomics*, *20*, 223. DOI: 10.1186/s12864-019-5545-8

Liu, J., Wang, Y., Chen, L., Li, K., Zhang, W., & Wang, Z. (2019). Grey wolf optimizer for deep brain stimulation electrode trajectory planning with probabilistic risk models. *IEEE Transactions on Biomedical Engineering*, *67*(8), 2195–2204. PMID: 31804925

Mittal, M., Goyal, L. M., Kaur, S., Kaur, I., Verma, A., & Jude Hemanth, D. (2019). Deep learning based enhanced tumor segmentation approach for MR brain images. *Applied Soft Computing*, *78*, 346–354. DOI: 10.1016/j.asoc.2019.02.036

Parbhoo, S., Bogojeska, J., Zazzi, M., Roth, V., & Doshi-Velez, F. (2017). Combining kernel and model based learning for HIV therapy selection. *AMIA Joint Summits on Translational Science Proceedings AMIA Summit on Translational Science*, *2017*, 239–248. PMID: 28815137

Wang, L., Chen, M., Li, J., Zhang, W., Li, K., & Wang, Y. (2022). Chemotherapy scheduling optimization: Participatory problem formulation for patient-centered care. *Journal of Clinical Oncology Clinical Cancer Informatics*, *6*, e2100144.

Wang, Z., Zhang, J., Chen, X., Li, K., Wang, Y., & Li, H. (2021). Human-in-the-loop optimization for medication alert customization using Bayesian optimization. *Journal of the American Medical Informatics Association : JAMIA*, *28*(9), 1825–1835.

Yang, D., Zhang, W., Wang, Y., Li, J., Chen, M., & Wang, Z. (2021). Genetic algorithm with epistasis for Alzheimer's disease detection from multimodal brain imaging. *IEEE Transactions on Medical Imaging*, *40*(10), 2655–2667.

Zhang, H., Li, Q., & Zhou, X. (2020). Particle swarm optimization for hyperparameter tuning in deep learning-based disease classification. *Neural Computing & Applications*, *32*(18), 14567–14579.

Zhang, K., Li, J., Chen, S., Wang, Y., Zhang, W., & Wang, Z. (2022). Implementation mapping for sepsis management optimization: Systematic barrier identification and targeted strategies. *Implementation Science : IS*, *17*(1), 31. PMID: 35550164

Zhang, Y., Shen, H., & Wu, T. (2020). Deep learning architectures for protein structure prediction. *Bioinformatics (Oxford, England)*, *36*(6), 181–189. DOI: 10.1093/bioinformatics/btz729

Zhou, T., Zhang, W., Li, J., Chen, X., Wang, Y., & Wang, Z. (2023). Nested optimization for healthcare facility layout with Bayesian optimization and genetic algorithms. *Health Care Management Science*, *26*(2), 244–258.

Zhu, W., Huang, Y., Zhang, H., Li, Y., Tian, H., Liu, G., & Wang, P. (2020). A novel genetic algorithm-based optimization framework for the discovery of circulating biomarker panels in early hepatocellular carcinoma. *ACS Omega*, *5*(28), 17470–17477.

ADDITIONAL READING

Balaji, P., Chaurasia, M. A., Bilfaqih, S. M., Muniasamy, A., & Alsid, L. E. G. (2023). Hybridized deep learning approach for detecting Alzheimer's disease. *Biomedicines*, *11*(1), 149. DOI: 10.3390/biomedicines11010149 PMID: 36672656

Balaji, P., Muniasamy, V., Bilfaqih, S. M., Muniasamy, A., Tharanidharan, S., Mani, D., & Alsid, L. E. G. (2023). Chimp optimization algorithm influenced type-2 intuitionistic fuzzy C-means clustering-based breast cancer detection system. *Cancers (Basel)*, *15*(4), 1131. DOI: 10.3390/cancers15041131 PMID: 36831474

Muniasamy, A., Begum, A., Sabahath, A., Yaqub, H., & Karunakaran, G. (2024). Coronary heart disease classification using deep learning approach with feature selection for improved accuracy. *Technology and Health Care*, *32*(3), 1991–2007. DOI: 10.3233/THC-231807 PMID: 38339946

Muniasamy, A., Begum, A., Sabahath, A., Yaqub, H., & Karunakaran, G. (2024). Coronary heart disease classification using deep learning approach with feature selection for improved accuracy. *Technology and Health Care*, *32*(3), 1–17. Advance online publication. DOI: 10.3233/THC-231807 PMID: 38339946

Muniasamy, A., Begum, A., Sabahath, A., & Yaqub, H. (2023). Lung cancer histopathology image classification using transfer learning with convolution neural network model. *Journal Name, volume*(issue), 1–12.

KEY TERMS AND DEFINITIONS

Bayesian Optimization: Find optimal model parameters using probabilistic models with fewer evaluations.

Genetic Algorithms: Solve complex problems using evolutionary techniques like selection and mutation.

Gradient Descent: Optimize model parameters by minimizing error through iterative steps.

Multi-objective Optimization: Simultaneously optimize multiple conflicting objectives in a model.

Particle Swarm: Optimize solutions using collective behavior inspired by bird flocking or fish schooling.

Chapter 5
Optimization Algorithms for Feature Selection and Disease Prediction With Machine Learning

Pınar Özen Kavas
https://orcid.org/0000-0001-9884-2860
Kutahya Dumlupinar University, Turkey

Evin Şahin Şahin Sadık
https://orcid.org/0000-0002-2212-4210
Kutahya Dumlupinar University, Turkey

ABSTRACT

Machine learning (ML) is widely used in healthcare applications like disease prediction, but high-dimensional datasets can reduce model performance and cause overfitting. Feature selection is crucial to address these issues. The filtering method evaluates each feature independently using statistical measures, while wrapper methods determine the best subset by testing feature combinations with an ML model. Optimization algorithms further enhance accuracy and efficiency. Traditional methods might be inadequate in handling nonlinear relationships, whereas hybrid approaches combining filtering and wrapper methods offer better solutions. This section presents a hybrid feature selection approach using the ReliefF method and Genetic Algorithm on a medical dataset, with results provided.

DOI: 10.4018/979-8-3373-1087-9.ch005

INTRODUCTION

Machine learning (ML) is increasingly used in critical applications in healthcare, such as disease prediction. ML is a powerful tool for extracting meaningful information from large datasets. However, when working with high-dimensional dataset, the presence of redundant or irrelevant features can negatively impact the performance of the model. The success of ML models largely depends on the quality of the features used. Unnecessary or noisy features can degrade the performance of the model, cause overfitting problems, and make interpretability difficult. Therefore, feature selection is a critical step in ML projects. Optimization algorithms play a major role in this process, helping to find the best feature subset. In this section, we will examine the importance of optimization algorithms in feature selection and how these techniques improve the performance of ML models.

In high-dimensional datasets, such as those in biomedical research, irrelevant or redundant features can introduce noise, increase computational burden, and complicate model understandability. Feature selection overcomes this challenge by identifying a subset of features that contribute the most to the prediction task. While traditional feature selection techniques are effective, they are often inadequate in handling the complex interactions and nonlinearities found in such data. Optimization algorithms such as genetic algorithms (GA), particle swarm optimization (PSO), and simulated annealing (SA) have shown promise in overcoming these challenges.

Optimization algorithms play a critical role in the feature selection process in ML and help in improving the accuracy of the model by reducing the size of the dataset. In the literature, various algorithms such as Dynamic Butterfly Optimization Algorithm (DBOA), Bee Colony Algorithm (BCA), and Feature Selection using Jaya Algorithm – FSJaya(Das et al., 2022) have been shown to be effective in achieving high classification accuracy with minimal number of features (Abdollahzadeh & Gharehchopogh, 2022; Agrawal and Abutarboush, et al., 2021; Agrawal and Ganesh, et al., 2021; Allam & Nandhini, 2022; Arora & Anand, 2019; Das et al., 2022; Ghaemi & Feizi-Derakhshi, 2016; Srinivasa Rao et al., 2021; Tubishat et al., 2020; Zarshenas & Suzuki, 2016). These advancements highlight the advantages offered by optimization techniques in overcoming the challenges of feature selection in complex datasets.

BACKGROUND

Feature selection is a fundamental preprocessing step in machine learning, especially for high-dimensional datasets commonly encountered in healthcare and biomedical research. The presence of irrelevant, redundant, or noisy features not only increases model complexity but also leads to overfitting and reduces generalization performance. As such, selecting the most relevant features is essential for building efficient and interpretable models.

The main objectives of feature selection include:

- Reducing model complexity by eliminating unnecessary input features.
- Decreasing computational cost, making training and inference faster.
- Improving model interpretability, which is crucial in medical decision-making contexts.
- Enhancing prediction accuracy by focusing on the most informative attributes.
- Minimizing the impact of data noise, leading to more robust models.

There are three major categories of feature selection methods (seen in Figure 1):

1. Filter Methods: Evaluate each feature individually using statistical measures (e.g., Relief Feature Selection Algorithm (ReliefF)). They are computationally efficient but may ignore inter-feature interactions.
2. Wrapper Methods: Assess subsets of features by training and validating a machine learning model. While they offer better accuracy, they are more computationally intensive.
3. Embedded Methods: Integrate feature selection directly into the model training process (e.g., LASSO). These are often algorithm specific.

Figure 1. Feature Selection Methods

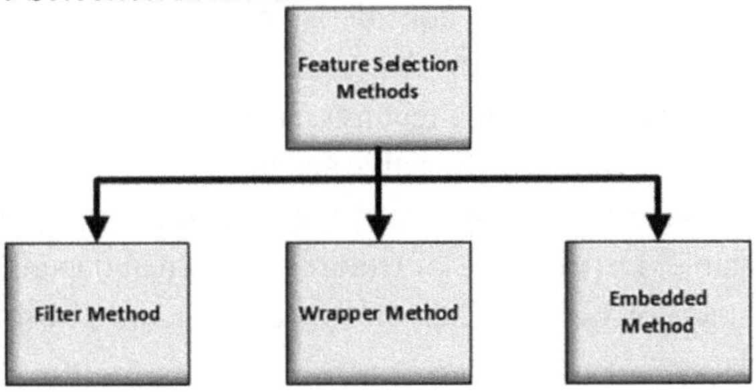

This chapter particularly focuses on filter and wrapper methods, and how their combination—in a hybrid structure—can offer a more balanced and effective approach to feature selection. The use of optimization algorithms, such as GA, further enhances the performance by efficiently searching for the optimal feature subset in complex and nonlinear data spaces.

Filter Methods

Filter methods evaluate the relevance of features based on statistical tests, independent of any learning algorithm. These methods are generally faster and less computationally intensive than wrapper methods, making them suitable for high-dimensional datasets. However, they may limit the precision of prediction models as they do not consider interactions with the learning algorithm (Abujazoh et al., 2023; Dominico et al., 2023; Espinosa et al., 2024). Common filter methods include Chi-squared tests and the ReliefF algorithm, which assess feature importance based on correlation and redundancy (Abujazoh et al., 2023; Espinosa et al., 2024).

Instead of evaluating the features that affect the performance of ML models, filtering methods determine the most suitable features using statistical methods. These techniques are not tied to a specific ML algorithm and are usually applied independently. This results in faster and more general results (Chandrashekar & Sahin, 2014a).

Correlation-Based Feature Selection (CBFS)

Correlation measures the strength and direction of the relationship between two variables. A positive correlation means that as one variable increases, the other also increases, while a negative correlation means that as one variable increases, the other decreases. The correlation coefficient ranges from -1 to 1, with 1 indicating a perfect positive correlation, -1 indicating a perfect negative correlation, and 0 indicating no correlation.

CBFS calculates the correlation between the features and the target variable. Features with high correlation are considered more important in predicting the target variable. However, CBFS considers not only the feature-target relationship but also the relationship between the features. Ideally, the selected features should have high correlation with the target variable and low correlation among themselves.

Important features are selected by measuring the correlation between the features and the target variable. Dependency of features is evaluated using metrics such as Pearson or Spearman correlation (Chandrashekar & Sahin, 2014b).

CBFS methods:

- Pearson Correlation Coefficient: Measures the linear relationship between two continuous variables.
- Spearman Correlation Coefficient: Measures the ordinal relationship between two variables. It is generally used in cases where variables are ordinal or continuous. It is especially preferred in cases where the data is not normally distributed or has outliers.

- Kendall Tau Correlation Coefficient: Measures the ordinal relationship between two variables. It gives more reliable results with small sample sizes or when there are many "tied values" (values with the same ranking) in the data. It is also preferable when you want to measure the overall agreement of the rankings.

Spearman measures the linear relationship between rankings, while Kendall Tau measures the overall fit of rankings. Spearman may be more appropriate for data that is not normally distributed or has outliers, while Kendall Tau may be more appropriate for data with small sample sizes or many dependent values.

Mutual Information

Mutual information measures the amount of information that a feature carries with the target variable. It is used to determine the effect of the feature on the target variable (Chandrashekar & Sahin, 2014a).

Gini Index

Gini Index, a measure used in decision trees, is used to evaluate the purity of features. Small Gini Index values can be used to identify important features because they create more distinct splits (Breiman, 2001).

Fisher Score

Fisher Score is a statistical method used to measure the separation between classes. Features are ranked according to their ability to provide maximum differentiation between classes, and the features with the highest scores are selected (Richard et al., 2001).

Variance Threshold

This method, which is based on the variance of the features, makes the model more effective by removing features with low variance. Low variance generally refers to features that do not make a significant contribution to the data (Pedregosa et al., 2011). Filter methods are model-independent techniques used for feature selection in ML. They evaluate the relationship of features to the target variable with statistical measures. These methods are fast and computationally efficient, but they do not always take into account interactions between features. The most commonly used techniques among filter methods are explained below:

Chi-Square Test

The chi-square test is a statistical method used for categorical data. It tests the independence between the features and the target variable. If there is a significant relationship between a feature and the target variable, that feature is considered significant (Agresti, 2019).

ANOVA (Analysis of Variance)

Analysis of variance (ANOVA) can determine if the means of three or more groups are different. ANOVA uses F tests to statistically test for equality of means. The F-statistic is calculated to determine how much the features distinguish the variance between groups (Montgomery, 2017).

ReliefF Algorithm

ReliefF (Relief Feature Selection Algorithm) is a filter-based feature selection method used to determine the importance of features on classification. It is an extended version of the original Relief algorithm and performs better for datasets with missing data, multi-class problems, and noisy data.

- ReliefF uses the k-nearest neighbors (k-NN) method to determine the contribution of each feature to the classification.
- It calculates the differences between a given data point (for example, a randomly selected sample) and nearby similar (same class) and different (different class) points.
- If a feature can better distinguish between classes, it gets a higher weight.
- As a result, features with higher weights are selected.

The advantage of ReliefF is that it can prioritize the features by considering their relationships. However, it may have some limitations in detecting nonlinear relationships (Robnik-Šikonja & Kononenko, 2003).

MRMR (Minimum Redundancy Maximum Relevance)

MRMR is a filter method used to select the least redundant but most relevant features. MRMR also takes into account the dependency between features.

- MRMR measures the relationship of features to the target variable (relevance) and the relationship with other features (redundancy).

- Features with high correlation (high importance) with the target variable are selected, while features with high correlation (high repetition of information) are eliminated.
- The Mutual Information metric is frequently used to calculate the dependency between features.

This algorithm is highly effective for feature selection on high-dimensional datasets and is often used on genetic data or biomedical signals (Peng et al., 2005).

Fisher Score

Fisher Score is a measure that determines the features that best distinguish between classes. The importance level of a feature is determined based on the means between classes and the within-class variances (Richard et al., 2001).

- Advantage: It works very fast and makes an effective distinction.
- Disadvantage: It does not take into account the dependency between features.

Filter methods are often used to reduce computational cost and increase model generalizability, especially in large datasets.

- For linear relationships: Chi-Square, ANOVA, Fisher Score
- For non-linear relationships: Mutual Information, ReliefF
- Those that evaluate dependency between features: MRMR, Gini Index

If a quick and simple feature selection is desired, statistical methods such as Chi-Square or ANOVA can be a good start. However, if feature interactions are also to be considered, more sophisticated methods such as ReliefF and MRMR can be preferred. In the sample application for this book chapter, ReliefF is used as the filter method.

Wrapper Methods

Wrapper methods are a type of feature selection technique used in ML and data analysis to improve model performance by selecting the most relevant features from a dataset. These methods evaluate subsets of features based on the performance of a specific learning algorithm, making them computationally intensive but often more effective than other feature selection methods.

Wrapper methods involve using a learning algorithm to evaluate the performance of different feature subsets, selecting the subset that optimizes model performance. These methods are typically more accurate than filter methods because they consider feature interactions with the learning algorithm, but they are also more computationally expensive (Abujazoh et al., 2023; Maadi et al., 2023; Njoku et al., 2023). Wrapper methods have been shown to outperform filter methods in terms of model performance, particularly in multi-objective feature selection tasks where metrics like accuracy and AUC are optimized simultaneously (Macaire et al., 2023; Njoku et al., 2023).

Wrapper methods have been applied in various fields, including deep learning, where they are used to enhance prediction models by selecting optimal feature subsets (Espinosa et al., 2024). They are also used in bioinformatics for biomarker discovery, where they help identify stable and statistically significant features from high-dimensional omics data (Peng et al., 2005). In the context of event detection, wrapper methods have been combined with clustering algorithms to improve the precision of event clusters from heterogeneous data sources (Al-Dyani, 2024).

Wrapper methods involve using a predictive model to evaluate the effectiveness of different subsets of features. They are known for their high computational cost because they require training a model multiple times with different feature subsets to determine the best combination (Espinosa et al., 2024; Njoku et al., 2023; Patel et al., 2024). Despite this, they are often preferred for their ability to improve model performance by directly optimizing the feature set for the specific learning algorithm being used (Njoku et al., 2023; Patel et al., 2024).

The primary challenge of wrapper methods is their computational expense, which can be prohibitive for large datasets or complex models. To address this, researchers have developed hybrid approaches that combine wrapper methods with other feature selection techniques, such as filter methods, to reduce computational costs while maintaining high performance (Budhraja et al., 2023; Espinosa et al., 2024). Additionally, surrogate-assisted approaches have been proposed to further mitigate the computational burden by approximating the wrapper-type objective function (Espinosa et al., 2024).

Studies have shown that wrapper methods generally outperform filter methods in terms of model performance, particularly when optimizing for multiple objectives such as accuracy and the Area Under the ROC Curve (AUC) (Njoku et al., 2023). They are also effective in classification tasks, where they have been shown to achieve high accuracy by selecting the most informative features (Ng et al., 2023; Patel et al., 2024).

In conclusion, wrapper methods are a powerful tool for feature selection, offering significant improvements in model performance despite their computational demands. Their application across various domains highlights their versatility and effectiveness in optimizing feature subsets for specific learning algorithms.

Optimization algorithms as wrapper methods are a crucial aspect of feature selection in ML, particularly for handling high-dimensional data. These methods use optimization techniques to evaluate subsets of features based on the performance of a learning algorithm, aiming to improve model accuracy and reduce computational complexity.

These studies suggest that wrapper methods in feature selection utilize optimization algorithms such as Whale Optimization Algorithm (WOA), Butterfly Optimization Algorithm (BOA), GA, PSO, Bat Algorithm (BA), and Teaching Learning Based Optimization (TLBO) to efficiently select optimal feature subsets for improved classification accuracy.

Wrapper methods in feature selection are optimization-based techniques that aim to select the most relevant features for improving classification accuracy. These methods evaluate subsets of features by training and testing a model iteratively, making them computationally intensive but often more accurate than filter methods. Various optimization algorithms have been employed in wrapper methods to efficiently search the feature space. most commonly used types of optimization algorithms

Most commonly used types of the optimization algorithms as wrapper methods:

Evolutionary Algorithms

Evolutionary algorithms are optimization methods based on the principles of natural selection and biological evolution. In feature selection problems, population-based search strategies are used to find the best feature subsets.

GA - Genetic Algorithm

Working Principle: A random initial population is created, then new solutions are produced with genetic operators such as selection, crossover and mutation (Holland, 1992).

Advantage: Global optimization capability is high, can solve non-linear problems.

Disadvantage: Computational cost is high and can be trapped in local minima.

DE - Differential Evolution

Working Principle: Similar to GA, but applies crossover and mutation operations in a different way (Storn & Price, 1997).

Advantage: Performs well in continuous and complex feature spaces.

Disadvantage: Difficult to apply directly to discrete feature selection problems.

ES - Evolution Strategies

Working Principle: It performs feature selection using evolutionary mechanisms such as selection, crossover and mutation (Beyer et al., 2002).

Advantage: It can be effective in large-scale problems.

Disadvantage: It is sensitive to setting parameters.

Swarm Intelligence – SI

These algorithms are based on collective behavioral models inspired by nature and generally aim to reach the best solution through the interaction of a large number of solution candidates.

PSO - Particle Swarm Optimization

Working Principle: It simulates the collective movements of flocks of birds or schools of fish. Each particle (solution candidate) moves using its own best position and the best position of the flock (Kennedy & Eberhart, 1995).

Advantage: Parameter tuning is easier and faster.

Disadvantage: It can get stuck in local minima.

ACO - Ant Colony Optimization

Working Principle: It mimics the mechanism of ants finding their way with pheromone trails (Dorigo & Gambardella, 1997).

Advantage: It is effective in discrete and complex problems.

Disadvantage: It can work slowly on large data sets.

ABC - Artificial Bee Colony

Working Principle: Simulates the nectar search process of honey bees (Karaboga, 2005).

Advantage: Scalable to large data sets.

Disadvantage: Sensitive to exit conditions.

Heuristic & Metaheuristic Algorithms

These are optimization techniques that accelerate finding solutions, especially for large-scale and complex problems.

SA - Simulated Annealing

Working Principle: Simulates the annealing process. The system is initially at high temperature and tries to reach the global minimum by cooling over time (Kirkpatrick et al., 1983).

Advantage: Low probability of getting stuck in local minimums.

Disadvantage: Difficult to set parameters.

Tabu Search

Working Principle: Adds previously visited solutions to the tabu list, preventing falling into the same solutions again (Xu et al., 1998).

Advantage: Can prevent getting stuck in local minimum.

Disadvantage: Its implementation is complex.

Whale Optimization Algorithm (WOA)

The Whale Optimization Algorithm (WOA) is a nature-inspired metaheuristic, relatively new optimization technique applied to feature selection in wrapper methods. It has been used to develop binary variants that incorporate mechanisms like Tournament and Roulette Wheel selection, as well as crossover and mutation operators, to enhance the search for optimal feature subsets. These approaches have shown efficiency in improving classification accuracy compared to other algorithms like PSO and GA (Got et al., 2021; Mafarja & Mirjalili, 2017; Mafarja & Mirjalili, 2018).

Butterfly Optimization Algorithm (BOA)

The Butterfly Optimization Algorithm (BOA) is another recent addition to the suite of optimization algorithms used in wrapper methods. It is also nature-inspired metaheuristic algorithm. Binary variants of BOA have been proposed to efficiently explore the feature space, aiming to maximize classification accuracy while minimizing the number of selected features. These variants have demonstrated superior performance over several state-of-the-art approaches (Arora & Anand, 2019).

Teaching Learning Based Optimization (TLBO)

The Teaching Learning Based Optimization (TLBO) algorithm is a population-based meta-heuristic algorithm, particularly its binary variant, has been utilized in wrapper methods to select optimal feature subsets. This approach focuses on minimizing the number of features while maintaining high classification accuracy, using simple parameters like population size and number of iterations (Allam & Malaiyappan, 2020; Allam & Nandhini, 2022).

Bat Algorithm (BA)

The Bat Algorithm (BA) is a bio-inspired metaheuristic algorithm. It used in combination with the Optimum-Path Forest (OPF) in a wrapper approach to optimize feature selection. This method models feature selection as a binary optimization problem, aiming to provide compact feature sets that enhance classification effectiveness (Rodrigues et al., 2014).

Hybrid Optimization Algorithms

These methods aim to produce more effective solutions by combining the advantages of more than one algorithm.

Evolutionary algorithms are used to explore a large search space, but better results are achieved when combined with traditional methods that seek exact solutions (Gen & Cheng, 1996). For example;

- Genetic Algorithm + Gradient Descent (Hybrid GA-GD): GA explores a large solution space while Gradient Descent optimizes by fine-tuning the best solutions.
- Particle Swarm Optimization + Newton-Raphson Method (Hybrid PSO-NR): PSO performs global search, Newton-Raphson helps to obtain accurate local solution.

Some hybrid approaches take advantage of two different nature-based algorithms by combining them. For example;

- GA-PSO Hybrid Algorithm: GA increases diversity in a large search space. PSO improves the search process to find the global best solution (Zhan et al., 2009).

- Ant Colony Optimization + Simulated Annealing (ACO-SA): Ant Colony Optimization (ACO) is used to discover the best path. Simulated Annealing (SA) avoids the trap of local optimal solution.

Hybrid optimization algorithms aim to provide better solutions by combining the strengths of different optimization methods. These algorithms provide effective solutions especially for complex, large-scale problems. Methods that combine local and global optimization are the most common hybrid approaches. Evolutionary algorithms often give better results when combined with classical methods.

Embedded Methods

Embedded feature selection methods are techniques that integrate the feature selection process with model training. These methods automatically eliminate unnecessary features by evaluating the importance of features in the model learning process.

Filter methods perform feature selection using statistical criteria independent of the model, while embedded methods perform selection based on the learning process within the model. In wrapper methods, different feature combinations are tried and the best combination is determined, this process can be very costly. Embedded methods are based on importance scores determined directly by the model, so they are faster.

Commonly used embedded feature selection methods:

Tree-Based Models

Tree-based models (Decision Tree, Random Forest, XGBoost, LightGBM, CatBoost) use branching rules to identify the most informative features within the data.

Tree-based models select the features that provide the best discrimination at each split. The most important features are determined by calculating feature importance scores.

It works effectively on high-dimensional datasets. It can automatically manage correlated features. It does not require additional costs since it is integrated with the model.

Lasso Regression (L1 Regression)

Lasso (L1 penalty) is a regression technique that automatically eliminates unnecessary features by pushing their coefficients to zero. Lasso applies a penalty (L1 norm) to the regression coefficients, reducing some of them to zero. Features with coefficients that decrease to zero are removed from the dataset. It is fast to run and effective on high-dimensional datasets. It may show instability in highly correlated variables (Muthukrishnan & Rohini, 2017).

Ridge Regression (L2 Regression) and Elastic Net

It is among the penalty-based methods like Lasso, but does not completely reset the features, instead it reduces their weights. Elastic Net combines L1 and L2 penalties to make a more balanced feature selection (Zou & Hastie, 2005).

Recursive Feature Elimination (RFE)

RFE is a method that tries to determine the best subset by removing features iteratively. Initially, all features are used and a model is trained. The least important features are removed and the process is repeated. It continues until the best subset is determined. It is effective on small datasets. It works integrated with models. It can be slow on large datasets. Embedded feature selection methods identify the best features by working directly integrated with ML models.

In summary, filter-based feature selection identifies irrelevant features using a specific criterion and eliminates unnecessary data (Chandrashekar & Sahin, 2014b). This selection process is performed independently of the training phase of the model. Filter methods rank the features as a preprocessing step before the learning algorithm and proceed by selecting the features with high scores. Wrapper-based feature selection leverages a particular classifier to evaluate the performance of a feature set. This approach evaluates and scores the features with the learning algorithm to be used in the final classification stage (Xie et al., 2020). Embedded feature selection is integrated into the machine learning algorithm itself. This method provides a balance between the filter and wrapper methods, thus solving the problems of high redundancy of the filter method and computational overhead of the wrapper method. Embedded feature selection is automatically applied during the training process of the model (Sufi & Khalil, 2011). The visual summarizing the situation is seen in Figure 2.

Figure 2. Working differences of feature selection methods (Xie et al., 2020).

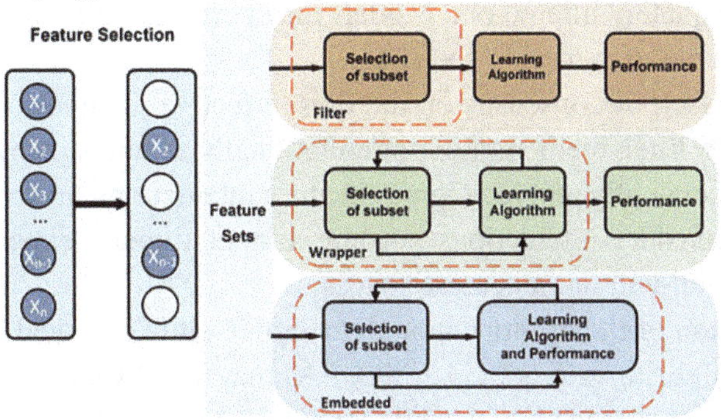

MAIN FOCUS OF THE CHAPTER

The main focus of this chapter is to integrate optimization algorithms into machine learning workflows for effective feature selection in disease prediction problems, particularly in high-dimensional biomedical datasets. The chapter emphasizes how feature selection improves model accuracy, reduces overfitting, and enhances interpretability by removing irrelevant or redundant features.

A hybrid approach is proposed, combining the ReliefF filter method and GA as a wrapper method, which is applied to a medical dataset for disease prediction. The chapter demonstrates how such hybrid methods can outperform traditional feature selection techniques, especially in handling complex nonlinear relationships. Furthermore, the chapter highlights how optimization algorithms (e.g., GA, PSO, SA) are effective tools in selecting optimal feature subsets, which directly contribute to better generalization and reduced computational cost in machine learning models.

Issues, Controversies, Problems

Despite the widespread use of feature selection techniques in machine learning, several challenges and ongoing debates persist in the field, especially when applied to high-dimensional medical datasets:

- Traditional feature selection methods, while effective in some cases, often fall short in handling complex, nonlinear relationships among features. This limitation becomes critical in biomedical datasets where such interactions are common and relevant to accurate disease prediction.

- Overfitting remains a significant issue when irrelevant or redundant features are not adequately filtered out. Models may perform well on training data but fail to generalize to new, unseen data.
- There is a lack of consensus on the most effective method for feature selection. While filter methods are computationally efficient, they evaluate features independently and may ignore feature interactions. In contrast, wrapper methods consider interactions but are computationally expensive and may not scale well with large feature spaces.
- The selection of the optimization algorithm itself is a critical decision point. Different algorithms (e.g., GA, PSO, SA) may yield varying results depending on dataset characteristics, and there is no universally superior approach.
- Hybrid methods, while promising, introduce new complexities in terms of integration, parameter tuning, and validation, making them harder to implement and optimize in real-world applications.

These issues underscore the need for robust, adaptable, and interpretable approaches to feature selection that can handle the diversity and intricacy of real-world healthcare data.

SOLUTIONS AND RECOMMENDATIONS

Clinical data, biomedical signals (e.g. ECG, PPG), genetic data, laboratory test results and medical images (e.g. MRI, X-ray) to be used for disease diagnosis are processed with ML methods (Kavas et al., 2022; Özen Kavas et al., 2023). In the Data Preprocessing step, missing values are filled or samples containing missing data are removed, errors are reduced by filtering signal or image data, features (parameters) that may be important for disease diagnosis are extracted, and unnecessary or irrelevant features are eliminated with feature selection, ensuring that the model works better.

The diagnostic model is trained using ML algorithms. The most commonly used methods are Logistic Regression, Support Vector Machines (SVM), Decision Trees & Random Forest, Artificial Neural Networks (ANN), k-NN, Deep Learning (CNN, RNN), Clustering. The success of the model is evaluated with metrics such as Accuracy, Sensitivity and Specificity. Cross-validation tests the generalization ability of the model.

The trained model can be integrated into automated diagnostic systems or medical decision support systems to support doctors' decisions. ML revolutionizes the field of healthcare by providing early detection, rapid analysis, lower costs, and more accurate predictions in disease diagnosis.

In the literature, many disease predictions have been made using ML methods and optimization algorithms. In the study on heart disease prediction using ML methods, the feature selection step was performed using the improved salp swarm algorithm (ISSA) as the wrapper feature selection method (Patro et al., 2021). In another study on multiple disease prediction, feature selection was performed by hybridizing two meta-heuristic algorithms, namely Lion Algorithm (LA) and Butterfly Optimization Algorithm (BOA). In the study where deep learning algorithms were used, the number of hidden neurons for neural networks (NN) and deep belief networks (DBN) were optimized by the same hybrid Lion-based BOA (L-BOA) (Dubey, 2021). Optimization techniques are used not only in the feature selection phase but also in hyperparameter tuning. Hyperparameters of different ML models for multiple disease detection are optimized with different optimization techniques (Singh et al., 2024). For medical diagnosis, the directed bee colony optimization algorithm was used to optimize a neural network model (Agrawal et al., 2019). The Deep Hyper Optimization (DHO) technique is integrated into the artificial neural network algorithm to fine-tune the bias, weight and optimize the number of hyperparameters in the hidden layer (Dhivya & Bazilabanu, 2023). For Parkinson's disease prediction, PSOGWO (PSO, and gray wolf optimization GWO) method is proposed as a solution to the problem of getting stuck in local minima of gradient descent (GD), which is inherent in ANFIS algorithms (El-Hasnony et al., 2020). In a classification study conducted on speech samples of individuals with Parkinson's disease and healthy individuals, the topology, hyperparameters and performance of the deep learning algorithm were optimized by grid search optimization (Kaur et al., 2020). In the determination of Acute Lymphoblastic Leukemia as benign or malignant using ML methods, the gray wolf optimization algorithm was used in the feature selection phase (Sallam et al., 2022). For occupational disease risk prediction, GAs have been used to determine the optimal hyperparameters and maximize classification performances for k-means, support vector machines, and k nearest neighbor algorithms (Di Noia et al., 2020). In a classification study for the diagnosis of coronary heart disease, the feature selection step was performed by GA (L. R. Priya et al., 2021). In a study for Alzheimer's disease diagnosis, a hybrid algorithm was proposed by using the Whale optimization algorithm (WOA) and Grey Wolf optimization (GWO) together for image segmentation of different regions of the brain (Dhakhinamoorthy et al., 2023). In a study on heart disease diagnosis using ML, the feature selection step was performed using the Jellyfish Optimization Algorithm (Ahmad & Polat, 2023).

In this study, disease diagnosis with ML is performed using a publicly available the Parkinson's disease speech signal dataset obtained from the Kaggle database was used. (Sakar et al., 2019). The number of samples for this dataset was 756, the number of columns was 755, and one of them was the label column. The patient id and gender columns were removed and the study continued with 752 feature columns. These are features extracted from the speech sounds of Parkinson's patients and healthy individuals.

The k-NN algorithm was used as the classification algorithm. For k-NN, the distance metric was Euclidean, the number of neighbors was 1, and the distance weight was equal. First, the classification was performed using all features (752 features) with the k-NN algorithm. Then, the first feature selection stage was performed with the ReliefF method. Weights (generally "importance score" in statistical methods) were calculated for 752 features and those with positive weights were selected. As a result, 418 features were selected with the ReliefF method. Classification was also performed using these 418 features.

Then, in order to reduce the number of features to less than 418 without negatively affecting the performance of the system and to obtain better performance with fewer features, wrapper feature selection was performed. GA was used as wrapper method. Parameters for GA: "Population Size" was 200, "Maximum Generations" was 120, "Crossover Fraction" was 0.8, "mutationuniform" was 0.15, and "Elite Count" was 10. Error function was used as fitness function. An attempt was made to determine the feature subset that would minimize the error. In the study, significant performance results were obtained with the feature subset containing 216 features. The flow diagram of the study was shown in Figure 3.

Figure 3. The flow diagram of the study.

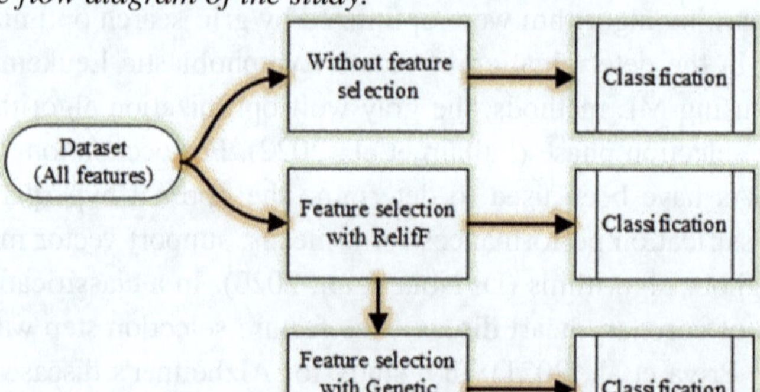

For all classifications, 80% of the dataset was used for training and 20% for testing. For a complete comparison, the training and testing samples were the same for all the classifications before feature selection, after the initial feature selection step with ReliefF, and after the wrapper feature selection step with the GA, i.e. the rows used in training and testing were the same for all the classifications. All the results are given in Table 1. The ROC curves of the classifications are shown in Figure 2.

Table 1. Classification Results

Case	Accuracy (%)	Sensitivity	Specificity	F-Measure	Kappa	AUC
All Features	85.33	0.7333	0.9733	0.8333	0.7067	0.8533
After Filter Method	86.67	0.7467	0.9867	0.8485	0.7333	0.8667
After Wrapper Method	93.33	0.8800	0.9867	0.9296	0.8667	0.9333

Figure 4. ROC Curves for Classifications

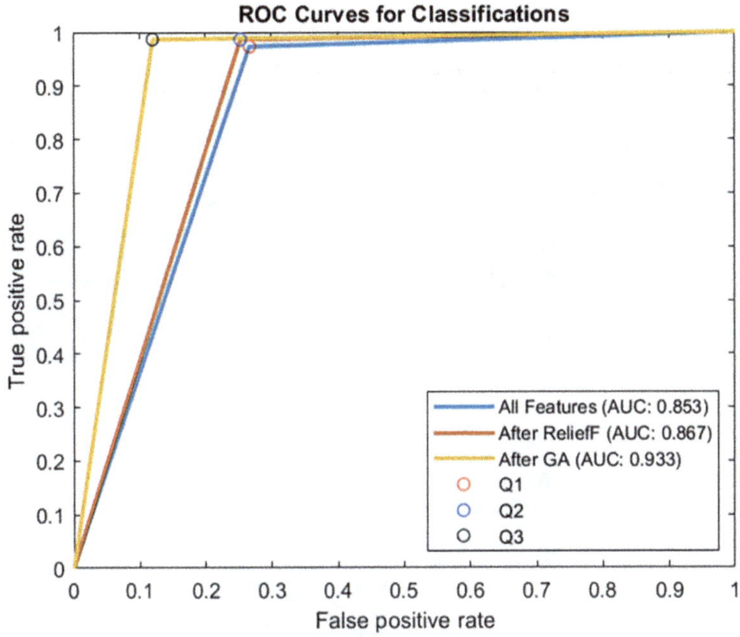

When the results in Table 1 and the ROC curves in Figure 4 are examined, the importance of feature selection is understood. Before feature selection, 85.33% accuracy was obtained in the classification study performed using 752 features. After the first feature selection stage with the ReliefF method, 86.67% accuracy was obtained in the classification performed with 418 features selected. While the number of features decreased significantly, the performance of the system did not decrease, on the contrary, it improved slightly. After the wrapper feature selection stage, better performance was obtained with less than 1/3 of the initial feature number (216 features). It gave the best result in three cases with 93.33%. When the sensitivity and specificity values are considered, the healthy class was better distinguished in all three cases. One of the reasons for this is that the dataset is not balanced and the healthy data is more than the patient data. When looking at the sensitivity and specificity values, the healthy class was better distinguished in all three cases. One of the reasons for this is that the dataset is not balanced and there are more healthy data than patient data. The points indicated as Q1, Q2, and Q3 in Figure 1 indicate the optimum working point of each classifier model.

Confusion matrixes of the classifier models were given in Figure 5. The patient class was labeled 1, and the healthy class was labeled 2. All models are successful in predicting the healthy class, but when looking at the prediction of the patient class, it was seen that significantly more accurate predictions could be made after the feature selection process.

Figure 5. Confusion matrixes of classifier models

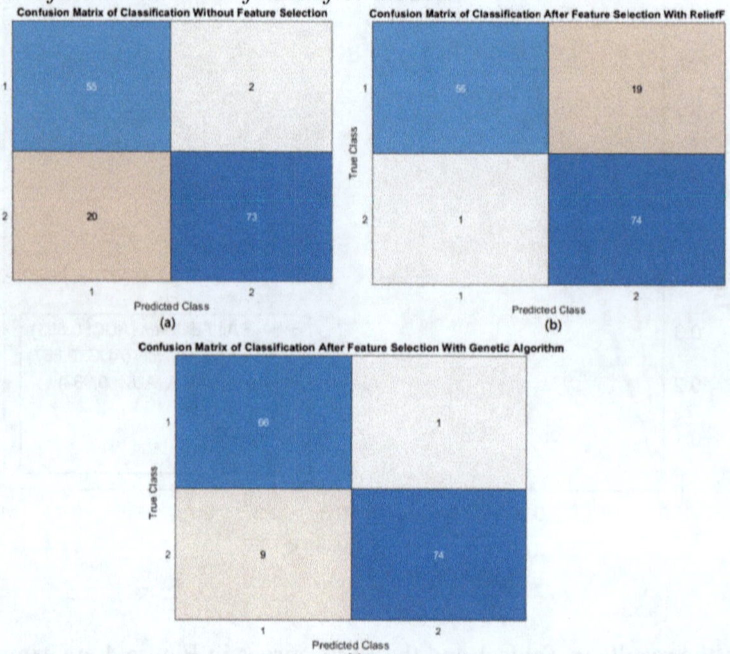

The graph showing the change in accuracy according to the number of features is given in Figure 6. It is clearly seen from the graph that the accuracy increases after each feature selection step.

Figure 6. The change in accuracy according to the number of features

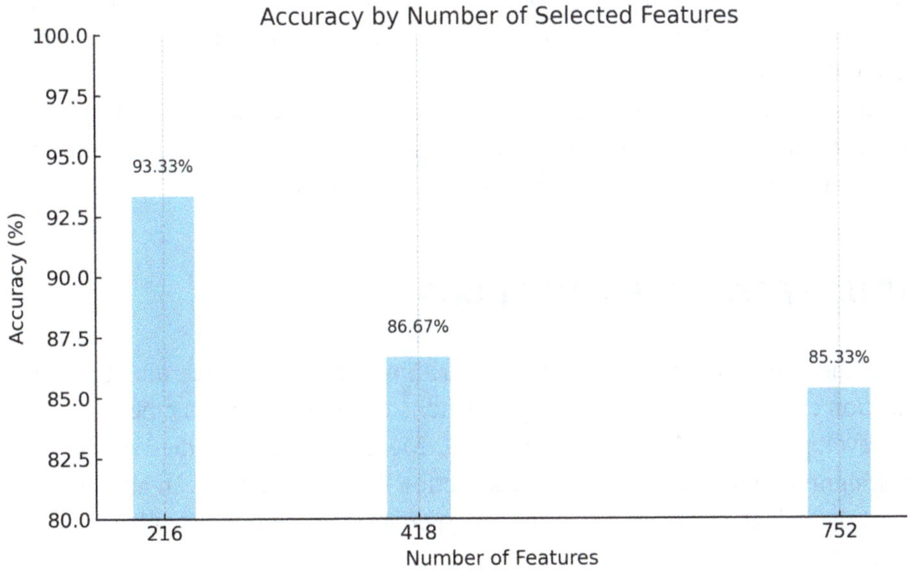

To address the limitations and challenges in feature selection for high-dimensional medical datasets, the following solutions and strategies are recommended:

Adopt Hybrid Feature Selection Approaches: Combining the strengths of both filter and wrapper methods can significantly improve performance. For example, using ReliefF for initial filtering followed by Genetic Algorithm (GA) for fine-tuned selection allows for both computational efficiency and the ability to consider complex feature interactions.

Utilize Optimization Algorithms: Algorithms like GA, PSO, and SA are effective in exploring large search spaces and identifying optimal feature subsets that improve model accuracy. These methods reduce the dimensionality of the data while retaining the most informative features.

Tailor Algorithm Selection to Dataset Characteristics: Since no single optimization technique is universally best, it is essential to evaluate the compatibility of the algorithm with the data. For instance, GA may perform well with discrete and categorical data, whereas PSO may be more suitable for continuous features.

Incorporate Domain Knowledge: When available, expert knowledge from the healthcare domain can guide the feature selection process, improving relevance and interpretability.

Perform Extensive Validation: Use cross-validation techniques and multiple performance metrics (e.g., accuracy, F1-score, AUC-ROC) to evaluate the selected feature subsets across different models and avoid overfitting.

Enhance Interpretability and Reproducibility: It is important to ensure that the selected features and the rationale behind the model's predictions can be interpreted and replicated by other researchers or clinicians, which supports practical deployment in healthcare settings.

These recommendations highlight a balanced, methodical approach to improving machine learning model performance in disease prediction tasks, ensuring both effectiveness and practicality in real-world applications.

FUTURE RESEARCH DIRECTIONS

As the integration of optimization algorithms into machine learning for feature selection evolves, several promising directions for future research emerge:

Development of More Adaptive Hybrid Methods: Future studies should focus on designing dynamic hybrid feature selection frameworks that can automatically adjust the balance between filter and wrapper stages based on data characteristics and complexity.

Exploration of Novel Optimization Techniques: There is ongoing potential in testing recent or nature-inspired optimization algorithms (e.g., Whale Optimization Algorithm, Grey Wolf Optimizer, Firefly Algorithm) and assessing their comparative performance on diverse biomedical datasets.

Scalability and Efficiency Enhancements: With the increasing size of medical datasets, computational efficiency becomes critical. Future research should explore parallelized or distributed implementations of optimization-based feature selection to reduce training time and improve scalability.

Integration with Deep Learning: Combining deep learning models with feature selection could lead to more robust systems that leverage both feature interpretability and the representational power of neural networks.

Personalized Feature Selection: Future frameworks could explore patient-specific or context-aware feature selection, tailoring the selected features to individual characteristics or subgroups within datasets for improved precision medicine applications.

Explainability and Transparency: As explainable AI becomes more prominent in healthcare, integrating feature selection methods with model-agnostic interpretability tools (e.g., SHAP, LIME) will be essential to ensure trust and adoption by practitioners.

Benchmarking and Standardization: There is a need for standardized benchmarks and datasets to systematically compare feature selection techniques, facilitating reproducibility and accelerating progress in the field.

These directions offer valuable insight for advancing the field and bridging the gap between theoretical advancements and clinical applicability in machine learning-driven disease prediction.

In future studies, comparing deep learning-based embedded feature selection approaches with classical methods may enable the creation of more efficient models in medical datasets. In addition, expanding the datasets used in disease detection and testing them with larger sample groups and developing general models for different diseases are also important research areas. Finally, by developing feature selection algorithms optimized for real-time applications, it is possible to design systems that can be integrated with portable and mobile devices.

CONCLUSION

In this chapter, the importance of feature selection in ML is emphasized and different feature selection methods were mentioned. A sample application was implemented using filter and wrapper approaches together and the results of the method were analyzed.

The ReliefF algorithm was used as a filtering method and the features with the highest information content were determined. In the classification operations performed with the obtained feature subset, it was observed that the accuracy rate of the model increased and the computation time decreased. However, it was observed that the features determined by the filtering methods based only on statistical criteria did not always maximize the model performance.

GA was used as a wrapper feature selection method and the best feature combination was determined. In this method, a significant increase in classification performance was achieved since the ML algorithm was directly included in the process. However, it was found that wrapper methods required more computation and gave results in a longer time compared to filter methods.

When the results of both methods are compared, it is revealed that the wrapper method provides higher accuracy, but the filter method works faster. As a result, it is concluded that the appropriate feature selection method should be determined depending on factors such as the size of the dataset, computation time and model accuracy. As in the example application in this study, it has been seen that hybrid feature selection methods can provide better results by combining the advantages of these two approaches.

This study investigated the effects of feature selection methods in ML on disease detection and evaluated the performance differences of filtering and wrapper approaches. Experimental studies showed that both methods are effective in feature reduction but have different advantages in terms of performance and computational cost.

REFERENCES

Abdollahzadeh, B., & Gharehchopogh, F. S. (2022). A multi-objective optimization algorithm for feature selection problems. *Engineering with Computers, 38*(3), 1845–1863. DOI: 10.1007/s00366-021-01369-9

Abujazoh, M., Al-Darras, D., Hamad, N. A., & Al-Sharaeh, S. (2023). Feature Selection for High-Dimensional Imbalanced Malware Data Using Filter and Wrapper Selection Methods. 2023 International Conference on Information Technology: Cybersecurity Challenges for Sustainable Cities, ICIT 2023 - Proceeding, 196–201. DOI: 10.1109/ICIT58056.2023.10226049

Agrawal, P., Abutarboush, H. F., Ganesh, T., & Mohamed, A. W. (2021). Metaheuristic algorithms on feature selection: A survey of one decade of research (2009-2019). *IEEE Access : Practical Innovations, Open Solutions, 9*, 26766–26791. DOI: 10.1109/ACCESS.2021.3056407

Agrawal, P., Ganesh, T., & Mohamed, A. W. (2021). A novel binary gaining–sharing knowledge-based optimization algorithm for feature selection. *Neural Computing & Applications, 33*(11), 5989–6008. DOI: 10.1007/s00521-020-05375-8

Agrawal, S. K., Singh, B. P., Kumar, R., & Dey, N. (2019). *Machine learning for medical diagnosis: A neural network classifier optimized via the directed bee colony optimization algorithm. U-Healthcare Monitoring Systems* (Vol. 1). Design and Applications., DOI: 10.1016/B978-0-12-815370-3.00009-8

Agresti, A. (2019). An introduction to categorical data analysis. 375. https://www.wiley.com/en-us/An+Introduction+to+Categorical+Data+Analysis%2C+3rd+Edition-p-9781119405283

Ahmad, A. A., & Polat, H. (2023). Prediction of Heart Disease Based on Machine Learning Using Jellyfish Optimization Algorithm. Diagnostics 2023, Vol. 13, Page 2392, 13(14), 2392. DOI: 10.3390/diagnostics13142392

Al-Dyani, W. Z. (2024). Adaptive Markov Clustering Algorithm for Optimal Event Detection From Heterogeneous News Documents. *IEEE Access : Practical Innovations, Open Solutions, 12*, 72079–72097. DOI: 10.1109/ACCESS.2024.3403506

Allam, M., & Malaiyappan, N. (2020). Wrapper based feature selection using integrative teaching learning based optimization algorithm. *The International Arab Journal of Information Technology, 17*(6), 885–894. DOI: 10.34028/iajit/17/6/7

Allam, M., & Nandhini, M. (2022). Optimal feature selection using binary teaching learning based optimization algorithm. *Journal of King Saud University. Computer and Information Sciences*, *34*(2), 329–341. DOI: 10.1016/j.jksuci.2018.12.001

Arora, S., & Anand, P. (2019). Binary butterfly optimization approaches for feature selection. *Expert Systems with Applications*, *116*, 147–160. DOI: 10.1016/j.eswa.2018.08.051

Beyer, H.-G., Beyer, H.-G., Schwefel, H.-P., & Schwefel, H.-P. (2002). Evolution strategies – A comprehensive introduction. Natural Computing 2002 1:1, 1(1), 3–52. DOI: 10.1023/A:1015059928466

Breiman, L. (2001). Random forests. *Machine Learning*, *45*(1), 5–32. DOI: 10.1023/A:1010933404324

Budhraja, S., Doborjeh, M., Singh, B., Tan, S., Doborjeh, Z., Lai, E., Merkin, A., Lee, J., Goh, W., & Kasabov, N. (2023). Filter and Wrapper Stacking Ensemble (FWSE): A robust approach for reliable biomarker discovery in high-dimensional omics data. *Briefings in Bioinformatics*, *24*(6), 1–17. DOI: 10.1093/bib/bbad382 PMID: 37889118

Chandrashekar, G., & Sahin, F. (2014a). A survey on feature selection methods. *Computers & Electrical Engineering*, *40*(1), 16–28. DOI: 10.1016/j.compeleceng.2013.11.024

Chandrashekar, G., & Sahin, F. (2014b). A survey on feature selection methods. *Computers & Electrical Engineering*, *40*(1), 16–28. DOI: 10.1016/j.compeleceng.2013.11.024

Das, H., Naik, B., & Behera, H. S. (2022). A Jaya algorithm based wrapper method for optimal feature selection in supervised classification. *Journal of King Saud University. Computer and Information Sciences*, *34*(6), 3851–3863. DOI: 10.1016/j.jksuci.2020.05.002

Dhakhinamoorthy, C., Mani, S. K., Mathivanan, S. K., Mohan, S., Jayagopal, P., Mallik, S., & Qin, H. (2023). Hybrid Whale and Gray Wolf Deep Learning Optimization Algorithm for Prediction of Alzheimer's Disease. Mathematics 2023, Vol. 11, Page 1136, 11(5), 1136. DOI: 10.3390/math11051136

Dhivya, P., & Bazilabanu, A. (2023). Deep hyper optimization approach for disease classification using artificial intelligence. *Data & Knowledge Engineering*, *145*, 102147. DOI: 10.1016/j.datak.2023.102147

Di Noia, A., Martino, A., Montanari, P., & Rizzi, A. (2020). Supervised machine learning techniques and genetic optimization for occupational diseases risk prediction. *Soft Computing*, *24*(6), 4393–4406. DOI: 10.1007/s00500-019-04200-2

Dominico, G., Bernardes, J. S., Dorneles, L. L., & Dorn, M. (2023). Multi-Objective Wrapper Differential Evolution with Guided Initial Population for Feature Selection. *2023 IEEE Congress on Evolutionary Computation, CEC 2023*. DOI: 10.1109/CEC53210.2023.10254085

Dorigo, M., & Gambardella, L. M. (1997). Ant colony system: A cooperative learning approach to the traveling salesman problem. *IEEE Transactions on Evolutionary Computation*, *1*(1), 53–66. DOI: 10.1109/4235.585892

Dubey, A. K. (2021). Optimized hybrid learning for multi disease prediction enabled by lion with butterfly optimization algorithm. Sadhana - Academy Proceedings in Engineering Sciences, 46(2), 1–27. https://doi.org/DOI: 10.1007/S12046-021-01574-8/TABLES/16

El-Hasnony, I. M., Barakat, S. I., & Mostafa, R. R. (2020). Optimized ANFIS Model Using Hybrid Metaheuristic Algorithms for Parkinson's Disease Prediction in IoT Environment. *IEEE Access : Practical Innovations, Open Solutions*, *8*, 119252–119270. DOI: 10.1109/ACCESS.2020.3005614

Espinosa, R., Jiménez, F., & Palma, J. (2024). Surrogate-Assisted and Filter-Based Multiobjective Evolutionary Feature Selection for Deep Learning. *IEEE Transactions on Neural Networks and Learning Systems*, *35*(7), 9591–9605. DOI: 10.1109/TNNLS.2023.3234629 PMID: 37018667

Gen, M., & Cheng, R. (1996). *Genetic Algorithms and Engineering Design*. Genetic Algorithms and Engineering Design., DOI: 10.1002/9780470172254

Ghaemi, M., & Feizi-Derakhshi, M. R. (2016). Feature selection using Forest Optimization Algorithm. *Pattern Recognition*, *60*, 121–129. DOI: 10.1016/j.patcog.2016.05.012

Got, A., Moussaoui, A., & Zouache, D. (2021). Hybrid filter-wrapper feature selection using whale optimization algorithm: A multi-objective approach. *Expert Systems with Applications*, *183*, 115312. DOI: 10.1016/j.eswa.2021.115312

Holland, J. H. (1992). Adaptation in Natural and Artificial Systems: An Introductory Analysis with Applications to Biology, Control, and Artificial Intelligence. Adaptation in Natural and Artificial Systems. https://doi.org/https://doi.org/10.7551/mitpress/1090.001.0001

Karaboga, D. (2005). AN IDEA BASED ON HONEY BEE SWARM FOR NUMERICAL OPTIMIZATION. chrome-extension://efaidnbmnnnibpcajpcglclefindmkaj/https://abc.erciyes.edu.tr/pub/tr06_2005.pdf

Kaur, S., Aggarwal, H., & Rani, R. (2020). Hyper-parameter optimization of deep learning model for prediction of Parkinson's disease. *Machine Vision and Applications, 31*(5), 1–15. DOI: 10.1007/s00138-020-01078-1

Kavas, P. O., Bozkurt, M. R., Kocayigit, I., & Bilgin, C. (2022). *A New Medical Decision Support System for Diagnosing HFrEF and HFpEF using ECG and Machine Learning Techniques*. IEEE., DOI: 10.1109/ACCESS.2022.3213065

Kennedy, J., & Eberhart, R. (1995). Particle swarm optimization. Proceedings of ICNN'95 - International Conference on Neural Networks, 4, 1942–1948. DOI: 10.1109/ICNN.1995.488968

Kirkpatrick, S., Gelatt, C. D.Jr, & Vecchi, M. P. (1983). Optimization by Simulated Annealing. *Science, 220*(4598), 671–680. DOI: 10.1126/science.220.4598.671 PMID: 17813860

Maadi, M., Khorshidi, H. A., & Aickelin, U. (2023). An Uncertainty-Accuracy-Based Score Function for Wrapper Methods in Feature Selection. *IEEE International Conference on Fuzzy Systems*. DOI: 10.1109/FUZZ52849.2023.10309669

Macaire, J., Zermani, S., & Linguet, L. (2023). New Feature Selection Approach for Photovoltaïc Power Forecasting Using KCDE. Energies 2023, Vol. 16, Page 6842, 16(19), 6842. DOI: 10.3390/en16196842

Mafarja, M., & Mirjalili, S. (2018). Whale optimization approaches for wrapper feature selection. *Applied Soft Computing, 62*, 441–453. DOI: 10.1016/j.asoc.2017.11.006

Mafarja, M. M., & Mirjalili, S. (2017). Hybrid Whale Optimization Algorithm with simulated annealing for feature selection. *Neurocomputing, 260*, 302–312. DOI: 10.1016/j.neucom.2017.04.053

Montgomery, D. C. (2017). Design and Analysis of Experiments, 9th Edition, Wiley. Wiley, 1–682. https://www.wiley.com/en-us/Design+and+Analysis+of+Experiments%2C+10th+Edition-p-9781119492443

Muthukrishnan, R., & Rohini, R. (2017). LASSO: A feature selection technique in predictive modeling for machine learning. *2016 IEEE International Conference on Advances in Computer Applications, ICACA 2016*, 18–20. DOI: 10.1109/ICACA.2016.7887916

Ng, G. Y. L., Tan, S. C., & Ong, C. S. (2023). On the use of QDE-SVM for gene feature selection and cell type classification from scRNA-seq data. *PLoS One*, *18*(10), e0292961. DOI: 10.1371/journal.pone.0292961 PMID: 37856458

Njoku, U. F., Abelló, A., Bilalli, B., & Bontempi, G. (2023). Wrapper methods for multi-objective feature selection. 26th International Conference on Extending Database Technology (EDBT 2023): Ioannina, Greece, March 28-March 31. *Proceedings*, *26*(3), 697–709. DOI: 10.48786/EDBT.2023.58

Özen Kavas, P., Recep Bozkurt, M., Kocayiğit, İ., & Bilgin, C. (2023). Machine learning-based medical decision support system for diagnosing HFpEF and HFrEF using PPG. *Biomedical Signal Processing and Control*, *79*, 104164. DOI: 10.1016/j.bspc.2022.104164

Patel, D., Saxena, A., & Wang, J. (2024). A Machine Learning-Based Wrapper Method for Feature Selection. [IJDWM]. *International Journal of Data Warehousing and Mining*, *20*(1), 1–33. DOI: 10.4018/IJDWM.352041

Patro, S. P., Nayak, G. S., & Padhy, N. (2021). Heart disease prediction by using novel optimization algorithm: A supervised learning prospective. *Informatics in Medicine Unlocked*, *26*, 100696. DOI: 10.1016/j.imu.2021.100696

Pedregosa, F., Varoquaux, G., Gramfort, A., Michel, V., Thirion, B., Grisel, O., ... & Duchesnay, É. (2011). Scikit-learn: Machine learning in Python. the Journal of machine Learning research, 12, 2825-2830.

Peng, H., Long, F., & Ding, C. (2005). Feature selection based on mutual information: Criteria of Max-Dependency, Max-Relevance, and Min-Redundancy. *IEEE Transactions on Pattern Analysis and Machine Intelligence*, *27*(8), 1226–1238. DOI: 10.1109/TPAMI.2005.159 PMID: 16119262

Richard, O., Duda, S., David, G., & Hart, P. E. (2001). *Pattern classification*. Wiley.

Robnik-Šikonja, M., & Kononenko, I. (2003). Theoretical and Empirical Analysis of ReliefF and RReliefF. *Machine Learning*, *53*(1–2), 23–69. DOI: 10.1023/A:1025667309714

Rodrigues, D., Pereira, L. A. M., Nakamura, R. Y. M., Costa, K. A. P., Yang, X. S., Souza, A. N., & Papa, J. P. (2014). A wrapper approach for feature selection based on Bat Algorithm and Optimum-Path Forest. *Expert Systems with Applications*, *41*(5), 2250–2258. DOI: 10.1016/j.eswa.2013.09.023

Sakar, C. O., Serbes, G., Gunduz, A., Tunc, H. C., Nizam, H., Sakar, B. E., Tutuncu, M., Aydin, T., Isenkul, M. E., & Apaydin, H. (2019). A comparative analysis of speech signal processing algorithms for Parkinson's disease classification and the use of the tunable Q-factor wavelet transform. *Applied Soft Computing*, *74*, 255–263. DOI: 10.1016/j.asoc.2018.10.022

Sallam, N. M., Saleh, A. I., Arafat Ali, H., & Abdelsalam, M. M. (2022). An Efficient Strategy for Blood Diseases Detection Based on Grey Wolf Optimization as Feature Selection and Machine Learning Techniques. Applied Sciences 2022, Vol. 12, Page 10760, 12(21), 10760. DOI: 10.3390/app122110760

Singh, J., Sandhu, J. K., & Kumar, Y. (2024). Metaheuristic-based hyperparameter optimization for multi-disease detection and diagnosis in machine learning. *Service Oriented Computing and Applications*, *18*(2), 163–182. DOI: 10.1007/s11761-023-00382-8

Srinivasa Rao, P. C., Sravan Kumar, A. J., Niyaz, Q., Sidike, P., & Devabhaktuni, V. K. (2021). Binary chemical reaction optimization based feature selection techniques for machine learning classification problems. *Expert Systems with Applications*, *167*, 114169. DOI: 10.1016/j.eswa.2020.114169

Storn, R., & Price, K. (1997). Differential Evolution - A Simple and Efficient Heuristic for Global Optimization over Continuous Spaces. *Journal of Global Optimization*, *11*(4), 341–359. DOI: 10.1023/A:1008202821328

Sufi, F., & Khalil, I. (2011). Faster person identification using compressed ECG in time critical wireless telecardiology applications. *Journal of Network and Computer Applications*, *34*(1), 282–293. DOI: 10.1016/j.jnca.2010.07.004

Tubishat, M., Alswaitti, M., Mirjalili, S., Al-Garadi, M. A., Alrashdan, M. T., & Rana, T. A. (2020). Dynamic butterfly optimization algorithm for feature selection. *IEEE Access : Practical Innovations, Open Solutions*, *8*, 194303–194314. DOI: 10.1109/ACCESS.2020.3033757

Xie, L., Li, Z., Zhou, Y., He, Y., & Zhu, J. (2020). Computational Diagnostic Techniques for Electrocardiogram Signal Analysis. Sensors 2020, Vol. 20, Page 6318, 20(21), 6318. DOI: 10.3390/s20216318

Xu, J., Chiu, S. Y., & Glover, F. (1998). Fine-tuning a Tabu Search Algorithm with Statistical Tests. *International Transactions in Operational Research*, *5*(3), 233–244. DOI: 10.1111/j.1475-3995.1998.tb00117.x

Zarshenas, A., & Suzuki, K. (2016). Binary coordinate ascent: An efficient optimization technique for feature subset selection for machine learning. *Knowledge-Based Systems, 110*, 191–201. DOI: 10.1016/j.knosys.2016.07.026

Zhan, Z. H., Zhang, J., Li, Y., & Chung, H. S. H. (2009). Adaptive particle swarm optimization. *IEEE Transactions on Systems, Man, and Cybernetics. Part B, Cybernetics, 39*(6), 1362–1381. DOI: 10.1109/TSMCB.2009.2015956 PMID: 19362911

Zou, H., & Hastie, T. (2005). Regularization and Variable Selection Via the Elastic Net. *Journal of the Royal Statistical Society. Series B, Statistical Methodology, 67*(2), 301–320. DOI: 10.1111/j.1467-9868.2005.00503.x

ADDITIONAL READING

Balaji, P., Chaurasia, M. A., Bilfaqih, S. M., Muniasamy, A., & Alsid, L. E. G. (2023). Hybridized deep learning approach for detecting Alzheimer's disease. *Biomedicines, 11*(1), 149. DOI: 10.3390/biomedicines11010149 PMID: 36672656

Balaji, P., Muniasamy, V., Bilfaqih, S. M., Muniasamy, A., Tharanidharan, S., Mani, D., & Alsid, L. E. G. (2023). Chimp optimization algorithm influenced type-2 intuitionistic fuzzy C-means clustering-based breast cancer detection system. *Cancers (Basel), 15*(4), 1131. DOI: 10.3390/cancers15041131 PMID: 36831474

Muniasamy, A., Begum, A., Sabahath, A., Yaqub, H., & Karunakaran, G. (2024). Coronary heart disease classification using deep learning approach with feature selection for improved accuracy. *Technology and Health Care, 32*(3), 1991–2007. DOI: 10.3233/THC-231807 PMID: 38339946

Muniasamy, A., Begum, A., Sabahath, A., Yaqub, H., & Karunakaran, G. (2024). Coronary heart disease classification using deep learning approach with feature selection for improved accuracy. *Technology and Health Care, 32*(3), 1–17. Advance online publication. DOI: 10.3233/THC-231807 PMID: 38339946

Muniasamy, A., Begum, A., Sabahath, A., & Yaqub, H. (2023). Lung cancer histopathology image classification using transfer learning with convolution neural network model. *Journal Name, volume*(issue), 1–12.

KEY TERMS AND DEFINITIONS

AUC (Area Under the ROC Curve): A performance metric that varies between 0 and 1, showing the classification performance of a model; success increases as it approaches 1.

Confusion Matrix: A structure that shows the prediction performance of the classification model, presenting correct and incorrect classifications in a table.

Feature Selection: The process of increasing the performance and interpretability of the model by determining the most meaningful data from high-dimensional data sets.

Filter Method: A fast and algorithm-independent feature selection method that evaluates and ranks features independently with statistical criteria.

Genetic Algorithm (GA): An evolutionary optimization technique based on the principle of natural selection, used to find the most appropriate solution.

Hybrid Feature Selection: A combined approach that uses filter and wrapper methods together, offering both speed and accuracy advantages.

Machine Learning (ML): A branch of artificial intelligence that automatically makes predictions and classifications with algorithms based on learning from data.

Overfitting: A situation where the model adapts too much to the training data and cannot generalize to new data.

ReliefF: A filter-based feature selection algorithm that allows features to be weighted according to their discrimination power between classes.

Wrapper Method: A method in which feature subsets are evaluated directly according to model performance to increase the accuracy of a specific machine learning algorithm.

Chapter 6
Chronic Kidney Disease Prediction Using Machine Learning

G. Manodeepak
https://orcid.org/0009-0000-4151-5893
Hindusthan College of Arts and Science, India

A. V. Senthil Kumar
https://orcid.org/0000-0002-8587-7017
Hindusthan College of Arts and Science, India

Shanmugasundaram Hariharan
https://orcid.org/0000-0001-9686-4329
Vardhaman College of Engineering, India

Ismail Bin Musirin
Universiti Teknologi MARA, Malaysia

Shadi R. Masadeh
Isra University, Jordan

Rohaya Binti Latip
Universiti Putra Malaysia, Malaysia

Kyla Latrice Tennin
https://orcid.org/0000-0002-9849-1316
United Nations Peace Ambassador Foundation, USA & College of Doctoral Studies, University of Phoenix, USA & LMG, USA

Adnan Ibrahim Alrabea
Al-Balqa Applied University, Al-Salt, Jordan

ABSTRACT

This study focuses on the development and evaluation of a chronic kidney disease (CKD) prediction model using the Random Forest algorithm. Recognizing the global health impact of CKD and the challenges associated with early detection, this research explores the effectiveness of Random Forest in accurately predicting CKD. The study compares the performance of Random Forest with other commonly used machine learning algorithms to establish its superiority. The data set under consideration is characterized by a significant number of missing values, a common

DOI: 10.4018/979-8-3373-1087-9.ch006

issue in clinical data. To address this challenge, the proposed model integrates Random Forest with a perceptron, aiming to enhance the prediction accuracy and robustness. The findings of this research contribute to advancing the understanding of CKD prediction using machine learning techniques and offer a potential solution for handling missing data in clinical scenarios.

INTRODUCTION

Their research has contributed to advances in the diagnosis of chronic kidney disease. The diagnostic categories of the samples are used to fill in the missing data in the aforementioned models using averaging. Since the diagnostic results of the samples are unknown, their procedures cannot be used. In fact, before being diagnosed, patients may not have undergone specific tests for several reasons. In addition, when missing values appear in the classification categories, the data obtained from averaging may differ significantly from the actual values.

Chronic Kidney Disease

Chronic kidney disease (CKD) is when kidney function steadily diminishes over months or years. At first, there are no symptoms; however, disorientation, leg swelling, weariness, vomiting, and a lack of appetite may follow. Anemia, high blood pressure, shattered bones, and heart disease are among the consequences. Gout, diabetes, high blood pressure, polycystic kidney disease, and other disorders may all contribute to chronic kidney disease. A family history of chronic renal illness is one risk factor. Characterized by the progressive loss of kidney function over time, CKD can lead to severe health complications, including cardiovascular diseases, anemia, and bone disorders. A blood test to assess the estimated glomerular filtration rate (eGFR) and a urine test to measure albumin are utilized to establish the diagnosis. Early detection and management are vital to mitigating the progression of CKD and enhancing patient outcomes A kidney biopsy or ultrasound may be used to discover the underlying reason.

Machine Learning

Machine learning (ML) includes the examination of computer calculations that can upgrade their execution through involvement. It is respected as a subset of fake insights. Machine learning calculations make a show from test information, alluded to as "training data," which permits them to make expectations or choices without being specifically taught to do so. These calculations discover applications in different areas, such as mail sifting and computer vision, where it is challenging or unfeasible to plan conventional calculations for fundamental assignments. A related zone inside machine learning is computational insights, which emphasizes the utilization of computers for making expectations; be that as it may, not all machine learning is categorized as factual machine learning. The field of scientific optimization contributes methods, speculations, and application spaces to machine learning. Information mining moreover crosses with this region, as it concentrates on the investigation of information through unsupervised learning.

Machine learning permits computers to decide how to finish errands without programming information. It includes machines learning from the data given to carry out particular capacities. For direct errands, software engineers can make calculations that straightforwardly direct the machine through each step to resolve the issue, so no learning is essential for the machine. Be that as it may, for more complicated assignments, it may pose a challenge for people to physically create the required calculations. In truth, it may be more viable for machines to make their claim calculations instead of requiring software engineers to indicate each activity. Machine learning utilizes different strategies to empower computers to handle assignments that cannot be completely tended to by a single calculation. When numerous potential arrangements exist, one procedure is to distinguish a few satisfactory answers as substantial. This data can serve as preparing information, making a difference in the computer refining the calculation it utilizes to find out the rectify arrangement. For occurrence, to prepare a framework for recognizing written-by-hand characters, the MNIST dataset of digits is commonly utilized.

BACKGROUND

Unsupervised System for Persistent Kidney Malady Expectation

Antony et al., (2021) states in this article that the incidence, prevalence, and prevalence of chronic kidney disease (CKD) have improved over time, especially in countries where the social determinants of health are changing. In most countries, diabetes and hypertension are the main causes of CKD. International regulations classify CKD as a disease caused by a decline in kidney function over time, as indicated by agglomerate filtration rate (GFR) and markers of kidney damage. People with CKD usually die at a young age. Doctors need to diagnose other symptoms associated with CKD early, as early diagnosis can prevent or reverse kidney damage. Early diagnosis allows patients to receive better treatment and appropriate care. Many local hospitals and clinics lack nephrologists and general medical staff to evaluate symptoms. As a result, patients have to wait long periods to receive a diagnosis. Therefore, this problem of adopting and developing an intelligent system to classify the understanding of "CKD" or "non-CKD" will help doctors negotiate with many patients and make a diagnosis quickly. Over time, companies will be able to deploy the proposed machine learning system in clinics in areas where there is less need for medical professionals. This could enable earlier diagnosis for rural patients. Some researchers have attempted to solve this problem by developing intelligent systems using supervised machine-learning techniques, but so far, only a few researchers have used unsupervised machine-learning algorithms. The main objective of this study is to run and compare different unsupervised algorithms and identify the optimal combination that leads to higher accuracy and localization rate. In this study, we implemented five unsupervised algorithms: K-Means Clustering, DB-Scan, I-Forest, and Autoencoder. We then combined them with different diagnostic strategies. The tuning included a reduction strategy using the K-Means clustering algorithm, which achieved an overall accuracy of 99% in classifying CKD and non-CKD medical data.

Machine Learning Framework for Beat Revelation In the midst of Out-of hospital Cardiac Arrest

Elola et al., (2020) has proposed in this paper the openness of a modified beat area amid out-of-hospital cardiac capture (OHCA) would allow the speedy recognizable confirmation of cardiac capture and the incite disclosure of return of unconstrained circulation. The point of this consideration was to make a reliable beat area calculation utilizing the electrocardiogram (ECG) and thoracic impedance (TI), the signals available in most defibrillators. The dataset utilized in the think approximately comprised 1140 ECG and TI parts from 187 OHCA patients, where 792 were named as pulse-generating cadence (PR) and 348 as Beatles electrical development (PEA) by a pool of masters in OHCA. To start with, a flexible filtering plot was utilized to remove the impedance circulation component and to start with subordinates from the TI. At that point, the wavelet rot of the ECG was carried out to get the assorted sub-band components and the noised ECG. Pulse/no-pulse (PR/PEA) division highlights were removed from those signals and energized into a back vector machine (SVM) classifier that made the pulse/no-pulse choice. A quasi-stratified and calm savvy settled cross-endorsement strategy was utilized to select the best highlight subset and to tune the SVM hyper parameters. This technique was repeated 50 times to evaluate the quantifiable scatterings of the execution estimations of the methodology. The perfect course of action comprised a five highlight classifier that yielded an unfeeling (standard deviation) affect ability, specificity, and balanced accuracy and included up to exactness of 92.4% (0.7), 93.0% (0.8), 92.7% (0.5) and 92.6% (0.5), independently. When compared to open procedures, our course of action shows an alteration in balanced precision at the scarcest 2.5 centers. A strong beat area calculation for OHCA utilizing the signals available in defibrillators was satisfied.

Machine Learning Methodology for Diagnosing Chronic Kidney Disease

Qin et al., (2020) has proposed in this paper that continued description complaint (CKD) is an around-the-world achievement issue with a high dreadfulness and death rate, and it influences different affections. Since there are no egregious signs in the morning phases of CKD, cases sometimes drop situations to observe the difficulty. Beforehand disclosure of CKD engages cases to seek helpful remedies to push ahead with the enhancement of this affliction. AI models can nicely help clinicians with satisfying this thing because of their speedy and right instrument prosecution. In this study, we propose an AI methodology for diagnosing CKD. The CKD data set was obtained from the School of California Irvine (UCI) AI store, which has a wide number of lost values. The KNN criterion was used to fill in the misplaced rates, which picks a couple incorporating up to tests with the most virtually identical assessments to deal with the lost data for each inadequate test. Lost values are as a run the feel set up, all effects considered, and probative conditions since cases might miss a couple of assessments for colorful reasons. After nicely finishing up the isolated data set, six AI estimations (determined break faith, changeable timber area, back vector machine, k-closest neighbor, licit Bayes classifier, and support forward brain sort out) were used to foster up models. Among these AI models, abstract forestland fulfilled the formal commission with 99.75 end delicacy. By delving into the impressions made by the developed models, we proposed a supported arrangement that consolidates determined loss of faith and emotional forestland area by using perception, which appears to satisfy a common closeness of 99.83 after multiple times of energy. Along these lines, we theorized that this procedure might be sensible for additional confounded clinical data for complaint substantiation.

Ensemble Learning Paradigm for Medical Diagnosis with Imbalance Data

Liu, et al., (2021) has proposed in this paper with the help of machine learning (ML) strategies, the conceivable mistakes made by pathologists and doctors, such as those caused by inability, weariness, stretch, and so on can be dodged, and the restorative information can be inspected in a shorter time and in a more nitty-gritty way. Be that as it may, whereas the routine ML strategies, such as classification, accomplished amazing execution in classification precision when connected in therapeutic analysis, they have a deadly inadequacy of destitute execution since the imbalanced dataset, particularly for the location of the minority category. To handle the inadequacies of ordinary classification approaches, this ponders proposes a novel outfit learning worldview for restorative conclusion with imbalanced information, which comprises three stages: information pre-processing, preparing base classifier, and last gathering. In the to begin with information pre-processing stage, we present the expansion of Engineered the Minority Oversampling Method (Destroyed) by joining it with the cross-validated committee's channel (CVCF) strategy, which cannot synthesize the minority test and subsequently adjust the input occurrences, but to channel the boisterous cases to perform well in to prepare of classification. In the classification stage, we present the gathering back vector machine (SVM) classification method, which was built by different differing qualities structures of SVM classifiers and, in this way, has the focal points of solid generalization execution and classification exactness. Moreover, in the final stage of the last gathering technique, we present the weighted larger part voting procedure and present recreated tempering hereditary calculation (Adventure) to optimize the weight vector and in this manner upgrade the general classification execution. The proficiency of our proposed outfit learning strategy was tried on nine imbalanced restorative datasets, and the test demonstrated that the proposed gathering learning worldview outflanks other state-of-the-art classification models. Promisingly, our proposed gathering learning worldview can viably encourage therapeutic choice-making for doctors.

An Overview of Machine Learning Approaches Applied to Gene Expression Analysis for Cancer Prediction

Khalsan et al., (2023) has proposed in this paper that machine learning approaches are powerful procedures commonly employed for creating cancer forecast models utilizing related quality expression and transformation information. This manuscript gives a comprehensive survey of later cancer thoughts that have utilized quality expression information from a few cancer sorts (breast, lung, kidney, ovarian, liver, central apprehensive framework, and gallbladder) for survival expectation, tumor-recognizable proof, and stratification. We moreover give a diagram of biomarkers thinks about that are related with these cancer sorts. The study captures different perspectives of what machine learning-associated cancer thinks about, counting cancer classification, cancer forecast, and distinguishing proof of biomarker qualities, microarrays, and RNA-Seq information. We talk about the specialized issues with current cancer expectation models and the comparing estimation devices for deciding the action levels of quality expression between cancerous tissues and non-cancerous tissues. Also, we examine how recognizing putative biomarker quality expression designs can help in anticipating future hazards of cancer and illuminate the arrangement of personalized treatment.

COVID-19 Future Estimating Utilizing Directed Machine Learning

Rustam et al., 2020 recommends that estimating components based on machine learning (ML) have illustrated their esteem in foreseeing preoperative results to upgrade decision-making concerning future activities. The ML models have long been utilized in numerous application spaces that required the distinguishing proof and prioritization of antagonistic variables for a risk. A few expectation strategies are being famously utilized to handle determining issues. This think about illustrates the capability of ML models to estimate the number of up-and-coming patients influenced by COVID-19, which is directly considered a potential risk to mankind. To anticipate the debilitating variables of COVID-19, this considers particularly utilized four standard determining models: direct relapse (LR), slightest outright shrinkage and determination administrator (Rope), bolster vector machine (SVM), and exponential smoothing (ES). Three sorts of expectations are made by each of the models, such as the number of recently contaminated cases, the number of passing, and the number of recuperations in the other 10 days. The comes about delivered by the ponder demonstrate a promising component to utilize these strategies for the current situation of the COVID-19 widespread. Whereas SVM performs ineffectively in all expectation scenarios given the accessible dataset, the comes about illustrate that the ES performs best among all utilized models, taken after by LR and Tether, which perform well in determining the recently affirmed cases, passing rate, and recuperation rate.

Identifying Keratoconus from Corneal Imaging Information Utilizing Machine Learning

Lavric et al., (2020) has proposed in this paper Keratoconus influences around one in 2,000 people around the world. It is regularly related to diminished visual sharpness. Given its wide predominance, there is a neglected requirement for the improvement of modern instruments that can analyze the malady at an early organize to avoid illness movement and vision misfortune. This thinks about points to create and test a machine learning calculation that can distinguish keratoconus at early stages. We connected a few machine learning calculations to identify keratoconus and at that point tried the calculations utilizing real-world therapeutic information, counting corneal geography, rise, and pachymetry parameters collected from OCT-based geology disobedient from a few corneal clinics in Japan. We actualized 25 diverse machine learning models in Tangle lab and accomplished a run of 62% to 94.0% precision. The most noteworthy precision level of 94% was obtained by a back vector machine (SVM) calculation utilizing a subset of eight corneal parameters with the most elevated separating control. The proposed demonstration may help doctors in surveying corneal status and identifying keratoconus, which is something else challenging through subjective assessments, especially at the preclinical and early stages of the malady. The calculation can be coordinated into corneal imaging gadgets or utilized as a stand-alone computer program for cornea appraisal and recognizing early-stage keratoconus.

Diabetes Forecast Utilizing Ensemble ling of Diverse Machine Learning Classifiers

Hasan et al., (2020) has proposed in this paper Diabetes, also known as persistent ailment, is a bunch of metabolic maladies due to a high level of sugar in the blood over a long period. The chance figure and seriousness of diabetes can be diminished altogether if the exact early expectation is conceivable. The strong and precise forecast of diabetes is profoundly challenging due to the constrained number of labeled information and the nearness of exceptions (or lost values) in the diabetes datasets. In this writing, we are proposing a vigorous system for diabetes forecasting where the exception dismissal, filling in the lost values, information standardization, determination, K-fold cross-validation, distinctive machine learning (ML) classifiers (k-nearest neighbor, choice trees, irregular timberland, Gadabouts, credible Bayes, and Boost), and multilayer perceptron (MLP) were utilized. The weighted collection of diverse ML models is moreover proposed, in this writing, to make strides in the expectation of diabetes where the weights are evaluated from the comparing Range Beneath ROC Bend (AUC) of the ML show. AUC is chosen as the execution metric, which is at that point maximized amid hyperparameter tuning utilizing the network look strategy. All the tests in this writing were conducted under the same test conditions, utilizing the Pima Indian Diabetes Dataset. From all the broad tests, our proposed collecting classifier is the best-performing classifier with the affectability, specificity, untrue exclusion rate, demonstrative chances proportion, and AUC as 0.789, 0.934, 0.092, 66.234, and 0.950 individually, which outperforms the state-of-the-art by about 2.00% in AUC. Our proposed system for the diabetes forecast outperforms the other strategies examined in the article. It can too give way better results on the same dataset, which can lead to superior execution in diabetes forecasts. Our source code for diabetes expectations is made freely accessible.

Effective Expectation of Cardiovascular Infection Utilizing Machine Learning Calculation with Alleviation and Rope Include Determination Techniques

Ghosh et al., (2021) has proposed in this paper Cardiovascular infections (CVD) are among the most common genuine ailments influencing human well-being. CVDs may be anticipated or relieved by early determination, and this may diminish mortality rates. Recognizing hazardous components utilizing machine learning models is a promising approach. We would like to propose a show that consolidates distinctive strategies to accomplish a compelling forecast of heart infection. For our proposed demonstration to be fruitful, we have utilized productive information collection, information preprocessing, and information change strategies to make exact data for the show. We have utilized a combined dataset (Cleveland, Long Shoreline VA, Switzerland, Hungarian, and Stat log). Reasonable highlights are chosen by utilizing the Help and Slightest Outright Shrinkage and Determination Administrator (Tether) procedures. Unused crossover classifiers like the Choice Tree Sacking Strategy (DTBM), Arbitrary Woodland Sacking Strategy (RFBM), K-Nearest Neighbors Stowing Strategy (KNNBM), AdaBoost Boosting Strategy (ABBM), and Angle Boosting Strategy (GBBM) are created by joining the conventional classifiers with stowing and boosting strategies, which are utilized in the preparation. We also have instruments for a few machine learning calculations to calculate the Precision (ACC), Affectability (SEN), Blunder Rate, Accuracy (PRE), and F1 Score (F1) of our show, along with the Negative Prescient Esteem (NPR), Untrue Positive Rate (FPR), and Wrong Negative Rate (FNR). The comes about appear independently to give comparisons. Based on the result investigation, we can conclude that our proposed show delivered the most elevated exactness, whereas utilizing RFBM and Alleviation include choice strategies (99.05%).

Crossover Machine Learning Plot for Classification of BECTS and TLE Patients Utilizing EEG Brain Signals

Yang et al., (2020) has proposed in this paper Around 50 million individuals have epilepsy around the world. Guess may change among patients depending on their seizure semiology, age of onset, seizure onset area, and highlights of the electroencephalogram (EEG). A few analysts have centered on EEG designs and illustrated that EEG designs of people with epilepsy can be utilized to anticipate forecasts and treatment reactions. Be that as it may, exact EEG investigation requires an experienced epileptologist with a long time of preparation who is frequently inaccessible in little or medium-sized clinics. In this paper, a novel machine learning (ML) demonstration that precisely recognizes generative epilepsy with centrotemporal spikes (BECTS) from transient flap epilepsy (TLE) is proposed. BECTS and TLE appear distinctive seizure sorts and ages of onset, but the differential conclusion can be challenging due to the comparative area and designs of the EEG spikes. The proposed half-breed machine learning (HML) demonstrates the determination in the arrangement of (1) making include frameworks utilizing factual records after flag deterioration, (2) preparing include choice utilizing Bolster Vector Machine (SVM) innovation, and (3) classifying the comes about through gathering learning based on choice trees. The reenactment was performed utilizing genuine persistent information of 112 BECTS and 112 TLE EEG signals, where preparation was performed utilizing 80% of the information, and 20% of the information was utilized in the execution investigation comparison with the genuine labeled information based on the determination of therapeutic specialists. The execution of the half-breed classification demonstration is compared with other agent ML calculations, which incorporate calculated relapse, KNN, SVM, and outfit learning-based choice trees. The show proposed in this paper appears to have an exact execution surpassing 99%, which is higher than the execution reachable from the other ML classification models. The reason for this is to present a novel EEG symptomatic framework that appears most extremely proficient in bolstering clinical real-time conclusions that can precisely recognize epilepsy sorts. Future investigations will center on extending this ML show to categorize other sorts of epilepsies past BECTS and TLE and actualize the HML symptomatic blockchain database into the clinic framework

Advancement in Mechanized Determination of Delicate Tissues Tumours' Utilizing Machine Learning

Abdellaoui Alaoui et al., (2021) has proposed in this paper that delicate tissue tumors (STT) are a shape of sarcoma found in tissues that interface, bolster, and encompass body structures. Because of their shallow recurrence in the body and their extraordinary differences, they show up to be heterogeneous when watched through attractive reverberation imaging (MRI). They are effortlessly confused with other infections such as fibro adenoma mammies, lymphadenopathy, and Struma, and these demonstrative mistakes have a significant inconvenient impact on the treatment handle of patients. Analysts have proposed a few machine learning models to classify tumors, but none have satisfactorily tended to this misdiagnosis issue. However, comparative studies that have proposed models for the assessment of such tumors generally do not consider the heterogeneity and the measure of the information. In this manner, we propose a machine learning-based approach that combines a modern strategy of pre-processing the information for highlights change, resampling procedures to kill the predisposition and the deviation of flimsiness, and performing classifier tests based on the Back Vector Machine (SVM) and Choice

Tree (DT) calculations. The tests carried out on the dataset collected in the Clinic of Yogyakarta in Indonesia appear to be an awesome advancement compared to past thoughts. These come about to affirm that machine learning strategies seem to give effective and successful instruments to fortify the programmed decision-making forms of STT diagnostics.

Machine Learning Approach for Expectation of Hematic Parameters in Haemodialysis Patients

Decaro et al., (2019) has proposed in this paper This paper appears to be the application of machine learning methods to anticipate hematic parameters utilizing blood unmistakable spectra amid ex-vivo medications. Strategies: A spectroscopic setup was arranged for the procurement of blood absorbance range and tried in an operational environment. This setup is nonintrusive and can be connected amid dialysis sessions. A back vector machine and a manufactured neural arrange, prepared with a dataset of spectra, have been actualized for the expectation of hematocrit and oxygen immersion. Comes about & Conclusion: Comes about of distinctive machine learning calculations are compared, appearing that the back vector machine is the best procedure for the expectation of hematocrit and oxygen immersion. A machine learning approach combined with a straightforward and mooted toll spectroscopic-based setup for observing hematic parameters of blood, such as hct and sO2, amid dialysis and other additional mortal medicines. A bolster vector machine and a manufactured neural organ have been executed and connected to information obtained through spectrometry in the unmistakable and close infrared of diverse blood tests. Comes about to illustrate that SVM and ANN models accomplished great learning exhibitions, and both appear to have the capacity to learn the relationship between input and targets.

Machine Learning for Clinical Result Prediction

Rustam *et al.*, (2020) recommends that estimating components based on machine learning (ML) have illustrated their esteem in foreseeing preoperative results to upgrade decision-making concerning future activities. The ML models have long been utilized in numerous application spaces that required the distinguishing proof and prioritization of antagonistic variables for a risk. A few expectation strategies are being famously utilized to handle determining issues. This think about illustrates the capability of ML models to estimate the number of up-and-coming patients influenced by COVID-19, which is directly considered a potential risk to mankind. To anticipate the debilitating variables of COVID-19, this considers particularly utilized four standard determining models: direct relapse (LR), slightest outright shrinkage and determination administrator (Rope), bolster vector machine (SVM), and exponential smoothing (ES). Three sorts of expectations are made by each of the models, such as the number of recently contaminated cases, the number of passing, and the number of recuperation's in the other 10 days. The comes about delivered by the ponder demonstrate a promising component to utilize these strategies for the current situation of the COVID-19 widespread. Whereas SVM performs ineffectively in all expectation scenarios given the accessible dateset, the comes about illustrate that the ES performs best among all utilized models, taken after by LR and Tether, which perform well in determining the recently affirmed cases, passing rate, and recuperation rate.

Machine Learning to Recognize Psychomotor Practices of Ridiculousness for Patients in Long-term Care Facility

Son et al., (2022) Child has proposed in this paper This ponder pointed to create precise and logical machine learning models for three psychomotor practices of ridiculousness for hospitalized grown-up patients. A planned pilot consider was conducted with 33 members conceded to a long-term care office between Admirable 10 and 25, 2020. Amid the pilot consider, we collected 560 cases that included 33 clinical factors and the overview things from the brief disarray evaluation strategy (S-CAM), and created a mobile-based application. Numerous machine learning calculations, counting four rule-mining calculations (C4.5, CBA, MCAR, and LEM2) and four other measurable learning calculations (LR, ANNs, SVMs with three part capacities, and irregular woodland), were approved by combined Wilcox on signed-rank tests on both macro-averaged F1 and weighted normal F1-measures amid the 10-times stratified 2-fold cross-validation. The LEM2 calculation accomplished the best expectation execution (macro-averaged F1-measure of 49.35%; weighted normal F1-measure of 96.55%), accurately distinguishing grown-up patients at daze hazard. In the pairwise comparison between prescient powers watched from autonomous models, the LEM2 show appeared a medium or expansive impact measure between 0.4925 and 0.8766 when compared with LR, ANN, SVM with RBF, and MCAR models. We have affirmed that intense awareness in S-CAM appraisal is closely related with distinctive indicators for screening three psychomotor practices of ridiculousness: 1) instruction level, dementia sort or its level, rest clutter, drying out, and disease in mixed-type incoherence; 2) sex, instruction level, dementia sort, lack of hydration, bedsores, and foley catheter in hyperactive daze; and 3) torment, rest clutter, and haloperidol utilize in hypoactive incoherence.

Machine Learning Instruments for Long-term Type 2 Diabetes Chance Prediction

Fazakis, et al., (2021) has proposed in this paper A relentless rise has been watched in the rate of elderly individuals who need and are still able to contribute to society. In this manner, early retirement or exit from the work advertise, due to health-related issues, poses a critical issue. These days, much obliged to mechanical progress and different information from distinctive populaces, the hazard components examination and well-being issues screening are moving towards mechanization. In the setting of this work, a worker-centric, It-empowered, unpretentious clients' well-being and utilitarian capacity-observing system, engaged with AI devices, is proposed. Diabetes is a high-prevalence, constant condition with destructive results for the quality of life and a high mortality rate for individuals around the world, in both created and created nations. Consequently, its serious effect on humans' lives, e.g., individual, social, and working, can be significantly decreased if the early location is conceivable, but most inquiries about works in this field fall flat to give a more personalized approach both in the demonstration and forecast preparation. In this course, our outlined framework concerns diabetes hazard forecast in which particular components of the Information Disclosure in Database (KDD) handle are connected, assessed, and consolidated. Particularly, datasets creation highlights determination and classification, utilizing diverse administered machine learning (ML) models that are considered. The gathering Weighted Nonvoting ML show is proposed to make strides in the expectation of diabetes, scoring a range beneath the ROC bend (AUC) of 0.884. Concerning the weighted voting, the ideal weights are assessed by their comparing Affect ability and AUC of the ML demonstrated based on a bi-objective hereditary calculation. Moreover, a comparative consideration is displayed among the Finnish Diabetes Hazard Score (FINDRISC) and Leicester hazard score frameworks and a few ML models, utilizing inductive and transduction learning. The tests were conducted utilizing information extricated from the English Longitudinal Ponder of Maturing (ELSA) database.

Novel Multi-Middle and Limit Ternary Design-Based Strategy for Infection Location Strategy Utilizing Voice

Tuncer et al., (2020) has proposed in this paper Keen well-being is one of the most well-known and imperative components of shrewd cities. It is a generally unused context-aware healthcare worldview impacted by a few areas of skill, such as restorative informatics, communications and gadgets, bioengineering, and morals, to name a few. Keen well-being is utilized to progress healthcare by giving numerous administrations such as understanding checking, early conclusion of illness, and so on. The fake neural arrange (ANN), back vector machine (SVM), and profound learning models, particularly the Convolution neural organize (CNN), are the most commonly utilized machine learning approaches, where they are demonstrated to be executed in most cases. Voice clutters are quickly spreading, particularly with the advancement of restorative demonstrative frameworks, even though they are frequently belittled. Shrewd well-being frameworks can be a simple and quick bolster to voice pathology discovery. The distinguishing proof of a calculation that separates between obsessive and sound voices with more precision is required to get a keen and exact versatile well-being framework. The fundamental commitment of this paper comprises proposing a multi-class-pathologic voice classification utilizing a novel multi-leveled textural highlight extraction with an iterative include selector. Our approach is a basic and effective voice-based calculation in which a multi-center and multi-limit-based ternary design is utilized (MCMTTP). More compact, multi-leveled highlights are at that point gotten by sample-based discretization procedures, and Neighborhood Component Investigation (NCA) is connected to select highlights iteratively. These highlights are at last coordinated with MCMTTP to accomplish exact voice-based highlights discovery. Exploratory comes about six classifiers with three demonstrative maladies (frontal resection, cordectomy, and spastic dysphonia) appearing that the combined highlights are more reasonable for portraying voice-based infection location.

Want Ayurveda-Base Constituent Modifying in Human body Utilizing Machine Learning Methods

Madaan and Goyal (2020) has proposed in this paper that human Body structure (Prakrit) characterizes what is in assertion with human nature and what will cause one to move out of modification and affiliation torment. Tridosha characterizes the three basic energies or rules that select the work of our body on the physical and energized levels. Each person has an inquisitive modification of all three of these energies. A few individuals will be overwhelming in one, whereas others will be a blend of two or more. Ayurveda-dosha has been utilized for a long time, but the quantitative, courageous quality estimation of these expressive methods still slacks behind. Creators calculate the Cronbach alpha of VATT-Dosha, PITT-Dosha, and KAPH-Dosha as 0.94, 0.98, and 0.98, independently, to check the steadfast quality of the consideration. Creators analyzed diagrams of 807 solid people created 20–60 a long time ago and found 62.1% men and 37.9% ladies. The lesson ungainliness issue is settled with oversampling, and they also spread information set of sporadically chosen 405 people is utilized for the veritable endeavor. Utilizing computer calculations, we whimsically restrict the information set (8:2) into an arranged set of 324 people and a test information set of 81 people. Show up is organized utilizing standard machine learning techniques for classification examination such as Fake Neural Organize (ANN), K-Nearest Neighbor (KNN), Back Vector Machine (SVM), Straightforward Bayes (NB), and Choice Tree (DT). The framework is also actualized, utilizing a few machine-learning methods for structure confirmation. Examination measures of classification such as root brutal square goof (RMSE), accuracy, review, F-score, and exactness are calculated and analyzed. On analyzing the comes around, creators discover that the information is best organized and endeavored with CatBoost, which is tuned with hyperparameters and wraps up 0.96 exactness, 0.95 study, 0.95 F-score, and 0.95 accuracy rate. The exploratory result shows that the proposed approach based on prepared learning strategies beats standard strategies. The creators roughly conclude that progress in boosting calculations shows up to provide machine learning a future.

Expectation of Diabetes Engaged With Intertwined Machine Learning

Ahmed *et al.*, (2022) has proposed in this paper In the restorative field, it is basic to foresee illnesses early to avoid them. Diabetes is one of the most perilous infections all over the world. In advanced ways of life, sugar and fat are ordinarily show in our dietary propensities, which have expanded the chance of diabetes. To anticipate the malady, it is greatly vital to get it its side effects. Right now, machine-learning (ML) calculations are important for infection discovery. This article presents a show utilizing a melded machine learning approach for diabetes expectation. The conceptual system comprises of two sorts of models: Bolster Vector Machine (SVM) and Counterfeit Neural Arrange (ANN) models. These models analyze the dataset to decide whether a diabetes determination is positive or negative. The dataset utilized in this investigate is separated into preparing information and testing information with a proportion of 70:30 separately. The yield of these models gets to be the input enrollment works for the fluffy demonstrate, while the fluffy rationale at last decides whether a diabetes conclusion is positive or negative. A cloud capacity framework stores the melded models for future utilize. Based on the patient's real-time therapeutic record, the intertwined show predicts whether the quiet is diabetic or not. The proposed melded ML demonstrates has a forecast precision of 94.87, which is higher than the already distributed strategies.

Capable and Administrative Accommodate Machine Learning for Therapeutic: A Study of Challenges and Solutions

Petersen *et al.*, (2022) has proposed in this paper Machine learning is anticipated to fuel noteworthy enhancements in therapeutic care. To guarantee that essential standards such as usefulness, regard for human independence, avoidance of hurt, equity, security, and straightforwardness are regarded, restorative machine learning frameworks must be created dependably. Numerous high-level statements of moral standards have been put forward for this reason, but there is a serious need of specialized rules explicating the viable results for restorative machine learning. So also, there is right now impressive instability with respect to the correct administrative prerequisites set upon restorative machine learning frameworks. This study gives an outline of the specialized and procedural challenges included in making restorative machine learning frameworks dependably and in congruity with existing directions, as well as conceivable arrangements to address these challenges. To begin with, a brief survey of existing directions influencing restorative machine learning is given, appearing that properties such as security, vigor, unwavering quality, security, security, straightforwardness, clarify capacity, and non-discrimination are all requested as of now by existing law and directions but, in numerous cases, to an questionable degree. Following, the key specialized deterrents to accomplishing these alluring properties are talked about, as well as imperative strategies to overcome these impediments in the restorative setting. We take note that dispersion move, spurious relationships, demonstrate beneath detail, vulnerability evaluation, and information shortage speak to extreme challenges in the restorative setting. Promising arrangement approaches incorporate the utilize of huge and agent datasets and unified learning as a implies to that conclusion, the cautious abuse of space information, the utilize of intrinsically straightforward models, comprehensive out-of-distribution demonstrate testing and confirmation, as well as algorithmic affect evaluations.

Existing System

The frequency, predominance, and movement of incessant kidney infection (CKD) conditions have advanced over time, particularly in nations that have shifted social determinants of wellbeing. In most nations, diabetics and hypertension are the primary causes of CKDs. The worldwide rules classify CKD as a condition that comes about in diminished kidney work over time, as shown by glomerular filtration rate (GFR) and markers of kidney harm. Individuals with CKDs are likely to kick the bucket at an early age. It is significant for specialists to analyze different conditions related with CKD in an early arrange since early location may anticipate or indeed switch kidney harm. Early discovery can give superior treatment and legitimate care to the patients. In numerous territorial hospital/clinics, there is a deficiency of nephrologists or common therapeutic people who analyze the indications. This has brought about in patients holding up longer to get a determination. Hence, this investigate accepts creating an cleverly framework to classify a quiet into classes of 'CKD' or 'Non-CKD' can offer assistance the specialists to bargain with different patients and give determination speedier. In time, organizations can execute the proposed machine learning system in territorial clinics that have lower therapeutic master maintenance, this can give early conclusion to patients in territorial ranges. In spite of the fact that, a few analysts have attempted to address the circumstance by creating cleverly frameworks utilizing directed machine learning strategies, till date constrained ponders have utilized unsupervised machine learning calculations. The essential point of this inquire about is to execute and compare the execution of different unsupervised calculations and recognize best conceivable combinations that can give superior precision and discovery rate.

Advantage of Constant Kidney Disease

- Machine learning calculations can accomplish tall precision in diagnosing CKD, indeed at its early stages.
- This is since machine learning calculations can learn complex designs in the information that are troublesome for human specialists to identify.
- This can analyze CKD rapidly and proficiently, which can spare time and assets for healthcare providers.
- The Machine learning calculations can be scaled to handle expansive sums of information, which is imperative for diagnosing CKD in a huge population.
- It can be utilized to create personalized hazard appraisals for CKD, which can offer assistance healthcare suppliers to tailor treatment plans to person patients.

Drawbacks of Chronic Kidney Disease

- Unsupervised machine learning calculations can be troublesome to decipher, which can make it troublesome to get it why they have classified a understanding in a specific way.
- This can be a issue for specialists who require to get it the premise for a conclusion in arrange to give fitting treatment.
- It can be one-sided, which implies that they may not perform similarly well on all persistent populaces. This is particularly concerning for CKD determination, as CKD is more predominant in certain populaces, such as individuals with diabetes and hypertension.

METHODOLOGY

The incidence, prevalence, and development of chronic kidney disease (CKD) have altered across time, especially in countries with distinct socioeconomic determinants of health. In most countries, diabetes and hypertension are the primary causes of CKD. According to the worldwide guidelines, CKD is a condition that leads in declining kidney function over time, as shown by glomerular filtration rate (GFR) and kidney damage indicators. People with CKD are prone to die at an early age. Doctors must recognize different CKD-related disorders early, because early identification may prevent or even repair renal impairment. Early identification may lead to improved treatment and care for patients. In many remote hospitals and clinics, there is a scarcity of nephrologists or general practitioners who can identify the symptoms. This has resulted in patients needing to wait longer for a diagnosis. As a consequence, this research claims that building an intelligent system to categorize patients into 'CKD' or 'Non-CKD' categories would aid clinicians in dealing with multiple patients and offering diagnoses more swiftly.

Data Preprocessing

Data pre-processing is a critical step to ensure the quality and suitability of the dataset for machine learning. This module involves addressing issues such as missing values, outliers, and data normalization. Techniques such as imputation may be applied to handle missing data, and outlier detection methods may be employed to identify and manage outliers.

Feature Selection

Feature selection is the process of choosing the most relevant and informative features from the dataset. This module involves evaluating the importance of each feature in predicting CKD and selecting a subset of features that contribute the most to the model's performance. Techniques such as statistical tests, correlation analysis, or machine learning-based feature importance can be employed to identify and retain the most significant features while discarding irrelevant or redundant ones.

CKD Prediction Model Using The Rf

This module involves the implementation of the CKD prediction model using the Random Forest (RF) algorithm. Random Forest is a machine learning ensemble method that builds multiple decision trees and combines their predictions to improve accuracy and robustness. The algorithm is trained on the pre-processed dataset, considering the selected features from the feature selection module. The performance of the Random Forest model is then evaluated using the testing set, and comparisons with other machine learning algorithms may be conducted to determine its effectiveness in CKD prediction.

Input Design

The input design for the proposed CKD prediction model involves creating a user-friendly interface to facilitate seamless interaction with the system. The input design prioritizes intuitive data entry mechanisms, allowing healthcare professionals to input patient information effortlessly. It incorporates structured forms with clear labels and prompts, ensuring the accurate and comprehensive collection of essential clinical data, including demographic details, laboratory results, and vital signs. To enhance usability, the system may incorporate dropdown menus, checkboxes, and date pickers for standardized input. Error-checking mechanisms and validation rules are implemented to ensure the integrity of the entered data.

Methodology

The input is the CKD dataset with its different attributes. During pre-processing, superfluous data and unknown attributes are deleted. All of the desired qualities and features have been selected. To increase classification performance, techniques like Random Forest (RF) are applied. Accuracy, recall, precision, and the f-measure will all earn grades. These characteristics will be displayed as a visual representation. Using a lot of CKD data and the model's performance on their test data, they constructed a neural organization-based classifier and utilized image enrollment to discover alterations in the kidney's morphology. Additionally, the bulk of prior investigations employed the UCI AI repository's CKD informative index. This research looks at how machine learning (ML) may be used to identify chronic renal disease. The effective deployment of ML algorithms, which have been a driving force in the identification of abnormalities in a range of physiological data, is benefiting several classification jobs. Figure 1 shows the block diagram of the proposed model.

Figure 1. Block Diagram of the Proposed Model

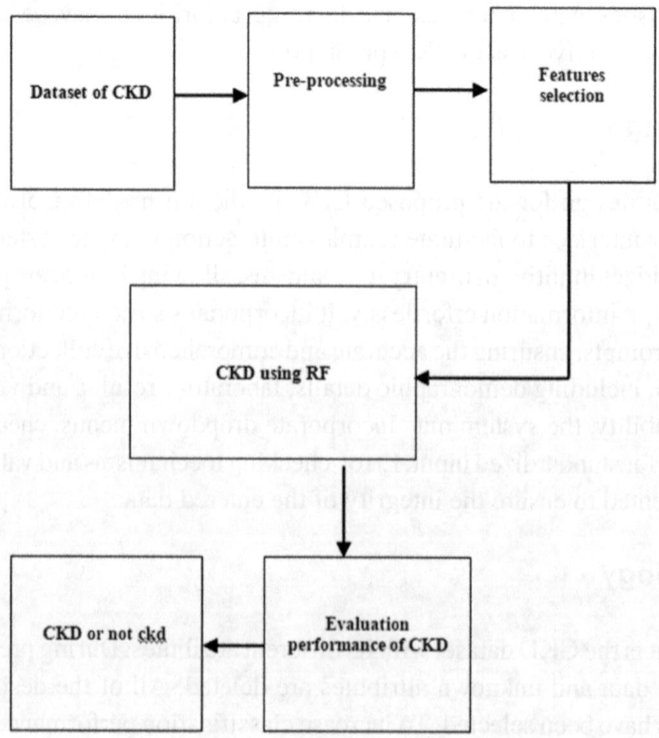

Loading the Dataset

Loading data is the initial step in any data analysis or machine learning project. In this scenario, the Chronic Kidney Disease (CKD) dataset is incorporated into the program. The dataset generally contains a number of factors and accompanying CKD diagnostic results for each patient. Loading the dataset offers you access to and control over the data, enabling you to do further analysis.

Pre-Processing

Data Pre-Processing involves encoding data in a machine-readable format, allowing a dataset to be seen as a collection of objects. The dataset may contain missing values. Missing values must be dealt first, and can be calculated or removed from the dataset. Missing values are typically filled using the feature's mean, median, mode, or constant value. Since the object values cannot be used for the analysis we have to convert the categorical data with object type into float64 type. Null values in categorical attributes are replaced with the most often occurring value in that column. Label encoding converts categorical qualities to numerical values by representing each unique value as an integer. This automatically converts the attributes to integer type. The pandas package is useful for data pre-processing.

Feature Selection

Feature selection is the process of discovering and picking the most relevant properties (features) from a dataset for model training. The idea is to minimize dimensionality while keeping the most relevant characteristics. Various methodologies, including as correlation analysis, mutual information, and feature significance scores, may be used to discover which characteristics are most relevant for CKD prediction. Choosing the correct features may increase model performance while lowering computational cost. Table 1 shows the statistical details of the features of the dataset.

Table 1. Statistical analysis of the dataset of numerical features

Features	Mean	Standard	Max	Min
Age	51.483	17.21	90	2
Blood glucose random	148.037	76.583	490	22
Serum creatinine	3.072	4.512	76	0.4
Blood pressure	76.469	13.756	180	50
Blood urea	57.426	49.987	391	1.5
Potassium	4.627	2.92	47	2.5
Packed cell volume	38.884	8.762	54	9
Sodium	137.529	9.908	163	4.5
Hemoglobin	12.526	2.815	17.8	3.1
White blood cell count	8406.12	2823.35	26400	2200
Red blood cell count	4.707	0.89	8	2.1

Model Fitting and Testing

After feature selection, data is split into two halves in a 4:1 ratio: 80% for training and 20% for testing learnt models. The data is utilized for suggested models, including Random Forest. The models are compared based on their anticipated accuracy.

Classification Performance

Classification performance is an assessment of how well machine learning models can classify or predict outcomes, such as the presence or absence of CKD. Several measures are routinely used to assess classification model performance, including accuracy, precision, recall, F1-score, and the confusion matrix. The accuracy ratio measures the model's correctness by comparing correctly predicted instances to the total number of instances in the dataset. Precision measures the fraction of real positive predictions among all positive predictions, allowing to evaluate the model's ability to avoid false positives. Recall (Sensitivity) analyzes the fraction of true positive predictions among all actual positive instances, showing the model's capacity to catch all relevant cases. F1-score is the harmonic mean of precision and recall, allowing a fair evaluation of a model's performance.

Algorithm Details

Random Forest employs hyper parameters comparable to Decision Trees and Bagging Classifiers. Combining a decision tree with a bagging classifier is optional when employing the random forest's classifier-class. You may utilize the algorithm's repressor to conduct regression problems using random forest. Using a random forest during tree formation boosts the model's adaptability. When dividing a hub, it picks the ideal component from a wide assortment of supplies, rather than the major portion. There are various choices accessible, with the majority leading to a better model. The calculation for isolating a hub only evaluates an irregular fraction of things in random timberland. To boost the unpredictability of trees, try applying irregular boundaries for each component instead of looking for the best edges. The Random Forest technique combines several decision trees into a classification and regression ensemble. A random subset of the training data sets is utilized to generate multiple decision trees. Using numerous decision trees enhances the accuracy of outcomes. This technique has a quick runtime and can handle missing data. Random forest is used to randomize the method rather than the training dataset. Decision trees produce decision classes.

1. Here the author initially displays the Random Forest generation pseudo code: Randomly choose "K" features from total "m" features where k << m.
2. Among the "K" characteristics, compute the node "d" using the best split point.
3. Split the node into daughter nodes using the best split.
4. Repeat the a to c stages till "l" number of nodes has been attained.
5. Build forest by repeating steps a to d for "n" number times to build "n" number of trees.

In the following step, having the random forest classifier generated, we'll make the prediction. The pseudo code for random forest prediction is presented below:

1. Takes the test characteristics and it utilizes the rules of each randomly built decision tree to anticipate the result and subsequently saves the expected outcome (target).
2. Calculate the votes for each expected target .3. The final prediction comes from high voted projected target from the random forest algorithm. The procedure is straightforward to comprehend, but it's strangely efficient.
3. Part the hub into girl hubs utilizing the best split.
4. Rehash to c stages till the "l" number of hubs has been attained.
5. Construct a woodland by rehashing steps a to d for "n" number times to construct "n" number of trees.

In the taking after step, having the arbitrary woodland classifier created, we'll make the expectation. The pseudo code for irregular timberland forecast is displayed underneath:

1. Takes the test characteristics and utilizes the rules of each arbitrarily built choice tree to expect the result and along these lines spares the anticipated result (target).
2. Calculate the votes for each anticipated target. 3. The last expectation comes from a exceedingly voted anticipated target from the irregular timberland calculation. The method is clear to comprehend, but it's oddly proficient.

SOLUTIONS AND RECOMMENDATIONS

Table 2 compares two classifiers K-Nearest Neighbors (KNN), and Random Forest (RF) based on their prediction performance in the scenario of chronic renal illness, as mentioned in the abstract. The accuracy statistic reflects the proportion of properly identified occurrences, and RF have remarkable high accuracies of 98.33% and 96.67%, respectively, proving their efficacy in spotting patterns in the dataset. Precision, a measure of the classifier's ability to avoid false positives, indicates the durability of RF, with scores of 100% and 92%, respectively, with percentages of 97.37% and 94.74%, respectively. The F1-score, a harmonic mean of accuracy and recall, verifies RF's overall better performance, with scores of 98.67% and 97.3%, respectively. These results underscore the potential of RF to produce precise and consistent forecasts for chronic renal disease, making them fascinating candidates for future exploration and eventual therapeutic usage.

Table 2. Comparison of the results of the models

Classifiers	KNN	RF
Accuracy %	96.67	98.33
Precision %	92	100
Recall %	94.74	97.37
F1-score %	97.3	98.67

Figure 2 compares two classifiers K-Nearest Neighbors (KNN), and Random Forest (RF) based on their prediction performance metrics values.

Figure 2. Result Comparison of the Models

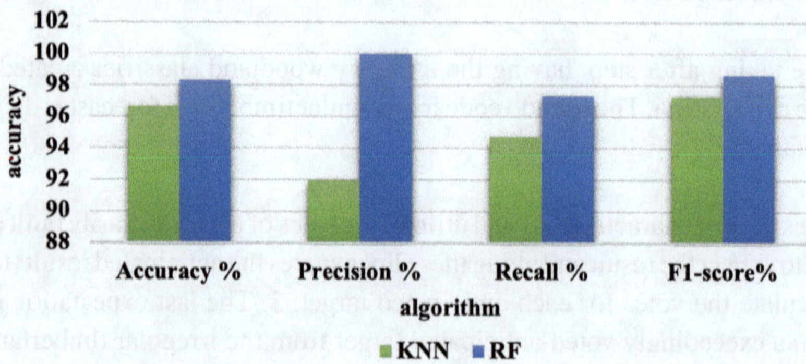

FUTURE RESEARCH DIRECTIONS

System testing for the CKD prediction model involves a comprehensive evaluation of the entire system to ensure its functionality, reliability, and accuracy. This process encompasses various testing methodologies, including unit testing, integration testing, and end-to-end testing. Unit testing involves examining individual components to verify that they operate as intended, while integration testing assesses the interactions between these components. End-to-end testing evaluates the system's overall performance by simulating real-world scenarios, including data entry, reprocessing, model training, and prediction generation. The system is subjected to different test cases, covering a range of possible inputs and scenarios, to validate its robustness and effectiveness in predicting CKD. Performance metrics are carefully monitored and compared against expected outcomes, ensuring the accuracy and reliability of the CKD prediction model in diverse and realistic conditions.

The system implementation for the CKD prediction model involves translating the designed solution into a functional and deployable application. This phase includes the integration of the developed algorithm, data pre-processing techniques, and the user-friendly input and output designs into a cohesive system. The implementation process may employ programming languages and frameworks suitable for machine learning applications. The developed model is trained on the pre-processed dataset, and the integrated user interface allows healthcare professionals to input patient data seamlessly. The system is rigorously tested during this phase to ensure its reliability and effectiveness in real-world scenarios. Once validated, the CKD prediction model is deployed for use in clinical settings, providing healthcare practitioners with a practical tool for early detection and improved decision-making in managing Chronic Kidney Disease.

CONCLUSION

Finally, the purpose of this work is to apply machine learning to forecast chronic renal sickness, which is becoming more widespread. By comparing and contrasting the Random Forest (RF) methodologies, this research seeks to contribute to the growth of healthcare decision-making tools. The necessity of early identification and monitoring is crucial in overcoming the hurdles posed by the progressive nature of chronic renal illness. The results and insights from this study show promise in increasing predictive skills and influencing appropriate responses, indicating a major step toward lowering the impact of this health burden on people and healthcare systems.

Future Work

Future research in this field should focus on enhancing and extending the machine learning algorithms proposed in this work to predict chronic renal illness. Further exploration of sophisticated algorithms and ensemble approaches may increase projected accuracy and resilience. Furthermore, merging various and bigger datasets would increase model generalization and real-world applicability. The inclusion of new relevant variables, such as genetic markers or lifestyle factors, may boost the models' potential to capture the intricacies of chronic kidney disease risk.

REFERENCES

Abdellaoui Alaoui, E. A., Koumetio Tekouabou, S. C., Hartini, S., Rustam, Z., Silkan, H., & Agoujil, S. (2021). Improvement in automated diagnosis of soft tissues tumors using machine learning. *Big Data Mining and Analytics*, *4*(1), 33–46. DOI: 10.26599/BDMA.2020.9020023

Ahmed, U., Issa, G. F., Khan, M. A., Aftab, S., Khan, M. F., Said, R. A. T., Ghazal, T. M., & Ahmad, M. (2022). Prediction of diabetes empowered with fused machine learning. *IEEE Access : Practical Innovations, Open Solutions*, *10*, 8529–8538. DOI: 10.1109/ACCESS.2022.3142097

Antony, L., Muneeswaran, K., Selvakumar, S., Shitharth, S., Sharma, R., & Balasubramanian, R. (2021). A comprehensive unsupervised framework for chronic kidney disease prediction. *IEEE Access : Practical Innovations, Open Solutions*, *9*, 126481–126501. DOI: 10.1109/ACCESS.2021.3109168

Decaro, C., Montanari, G. B., Molinari, R., Gilberti, A., Bagnoli, D., Bianconi, M., & Bellanca, G. (2019). Machine learning approach for prediction of hematic parameters in hemodialysis patients. *IEEE Journal of Translational Engineering in Health and Medicine, 7. IEEE Journal of Translational Engineering in Health and Medicine*, *4100308*, 1–8. DOI: 10.1109/JTEHM.2019.2938951 PMID: 32309060

Elola, A., Aramendi, E., Irusta, U., & Berve, P. O. (2020). Multimodal algorithms for the classification of circulation states during out-of-hospital cardiac arrest. *IEEE Transactions on Biomedical Engineering*, *PP*, (99), 1–1. DOI: 10.1109/TBME.2020.3030216 PMID: 33044927

Fazakis, N., Kocsis, O., Dritsas, E., Alexiou, S., Fakotakis, N., & Moustakas, K. (2021). Machine learning tools for long-term type 2 diabetes risk prediction. *IEEE Access : Practical Innovations, Open Solutions*, *9*, 103737–103757. DOI: 10.1109/ACCESS.2021.3098691

Ghosh, P., Azam, S., Jonkman, M., Karim, A., Shamrat, F. M. J. M., Ignatious, E., Shultana, S., Beeravolu, A. R., & De Boer, F. (2021). Efficient prediction of cardiovascular disease using machine learning algorithms with relief and lasso feature selection techniques. *IEEE Access : Practical Innovations, Open Solutions*, *9*, 19304–19326. DOI: 10.1109/ACCESS.2021.3053759

Hasan, M. K., Alam, M. A., Das, D., Hossain, E., & Hasan, M. (2020). Diabetes prediction using ensembling of different machine learning classifiers. *IEEE Access : Practical Innovations, Open Solutions*, *8*(99), 1–1. DOI: 10.1109/ACCESS.2020.2989857

Khalsan, M., Mu, M., Al-Shamery, E., Ajit, S., Machado, L., & Opoku Agyeman, M. (2023). A novel fuzzy classifier model for cancer classification using gene expression data. *IEEE Access : Practical Innovations, Open Solutions*, *11*(99), 1–1. DOI: 10.1109/ACCESS.2023.3325381

Lavric, A., Popa, V., Takahashi, H., & Yousefi, S. (2020). Detecting keratoconus from corneal imaging data using machine learning. *IEEE Access : Practical Innovations, Open Solutions*, *8*, 149113–149121. DOI: 10.1109/ACCESS.2020.3016060

Liu, N., Shapira, P., & Yue, X. (2021). Tracking developments in artificial intelligence research: Constructing and applying a new search strategy. *Scientometrics*, *126*(4), 3153–3192. DOI: 10.1007/s11192-021-03868-4 PMID: 34720254

Madaan, V., & Goyal, A. (2020). Predicting Ayurveda-based constituent balancing in human body using machine learning methods. *IEEE Access : Practical Innovations, Open Solutions*, *8*, 65060–65070. DOI: 10.1109/ACCESS.2020.2985717

Petersen, E., Potdevin, Y., Mohammadi, E., Zidowitz, S., Breyer, S., Nowotka, D., Henn, S., Pechmann, L., Leucker, M., Rostalski, P., & Herzog, C. (2022). Responsible and regulatory conform machine learning for medicine: A survey of challenges and solutions. *IEEE Access : Practical Innovations, Open Solutions*, *10*, 58375–58418. DOI: 10.1109/ACCESS.2022.3178382

Qin, J., Chen, L., Liu, Y., Liu, C., Feng, C., & Chen, B. (2020). A machine learning methodology for diagnosing chronic kidney disease. *IEEE Access : Practical Innovations, Open Solutions*, *8*, 20991–21002. DOI: 10.1109/ACCESS.2019.2963053

Rustam, F., Reshi, A., Mehmood, A., Ullah, S., On, B., Aslam, W., & Choi, G. S. (2020). COVID-19 future forecasting using supervised machine learning models. *IEEE Access : Practical Innovations, Open Solutions*, *8*(99), 1–1. DOI: 10.1109/ACCESS.2020.2997311

Son, C. S., Kang, W. S., Lee, J. H., & Moon, K. J. (2022). Machine learning to identify psychomotor behaviors of delirium for patients in long-term care facility. *IEEE Journal of Biomedical and Health Informatics*, *26*(4), 1802–1814. DOI: 10.1109/JBHI.2021.3116967 PMID: 34596563

Tuncer, T., Dogan, S., Ozyurt, F., Belhaouari, S. B., & Bensmail, H. (2020). *Novel multi center and threshold ternary pattern based method for disease detection using voice*. IEEE., DOI: 10.1109/ACCESS.2020.2992641

Yang, W., Joo, M., Kim, Y., Kim, S. H., & Chung, J.-M. (2020). Hybrid machine learning scheme for classification of BECTS and TLE patients using EEG brain signals. *IEEE Access : Practical Innovations, Open Solutions*, *8*, 218924–218935. DOI: 10.1109/ACCESS.2020.3038948

ADDITIONAL READING

Abdar, M., Zomorodi-Moghadam, M., Zhou, X., Gururajan, R., Tao, X., & Barua, P. D. (2020). Improvement in the computerized conclusion of delicate tissue tumors utilizing machine learning. *Organize Articulation Letters*, *132*, 123–131.

Abdar, M., Zomorodi-Moghadam, M., Zhou, X., Gururajan, R., Tao, X., & Barua, P. D.. (2020). A machine learning system for the beat district amid out-of-hospital cardiac capture. *Organize Certification Letters*, *132*, 123–131.

Ashraf, M., Ahmad, S. M., Ganai, N. A., Shah, R. A., Zaman, M., & Khan, S. A. (2021). A novel gathering learning worldview for tireless certification with imbalanced information. In Springer Singapore, 239–255.

Balaji, P., Chaurasia, M. A., Bilfaqih, S. M., Muniasamy, A., & Alsid, L. E. G. (2023). Hybridized deep learning approach for detecting Alzheimer's disease. *Biomedicines*, *11*(1), 149. DOI: 10.3390/biomedicines11010149 PMID: 36672656

Balaji, P., Muniasamy, V., Bilfaqih, S. M., Muniasamy, A., Tharanidharan, S., Mani, D., & Alsid, L. E. G. (2023). Chimp optimization algorithm influenced type-2 intuitionistic fuzzy C-means clustering-based breast cancer detection system. *Cancers (Basel)*, *15*(4), 1131. DOI: 10.3390/cancers15041131 PMID: 36831474

Bolarín, J. M., Cavas, F., Velázquez, J. S., & Alió, J. L. (2020). A comprehensive unsupervised system for tormented kidney debasement figure. *Related Sciences*, *10*(5), 1874.

Bolarín, J. M., Cavas, F., Velázquez, J. S., & Alió, J. L. (2020). Half-breed machine learning plot for classification of BECTS and TLE patients utilizing EEG brain signals. *Related Sciences*, *10*(5), 1874.

Chatrati, S. P., Hossain, G., Goyal, A., Bhan, A., Bhattacharya, S., Gaurav, D., & Tiwari, S.M. (2020). Cautious and definitive modify machine learning for pharmaceutical: A chart of challenges and courses of development. Diary of Ruler Saud College - Computer and Data Sciences.

Corradi, J. P., Thompson, S., Mather, J. F., Waszynski, C. M., & Dicks, R. S. (2020). A machine learning procedure for diagnosing chosen kidney suffering. *Diary of Obliging Frameworks, 42*(12), 261.

Jain, D., & Singh, V. (2021). COVID-19 future choice utilizing energized machine learning models. *Wide Diary of Computer Applications, 43*(6), 524–536.

Kumari, S., Kumar, D., & Mittal, M. (2021). An critical examination of cardiovascular tribulation utilizing machine learning calculations with offer offer offer help and tie set assertion methodologies. Around the World Diary of Cognitive Computing in Organizing, 2, 40–46.

Kwok, H., Coult, J., Blackwood, J., Bhandari, S., Kudenchuk, P., & Rea, T. (2020). Machine learning to recognize psychomotor daze behaviors for patients in long-term care work circumstances. Settling up, 147, 104–111.

Kwok, H., Coult, J., Blackwood, J., Bhandari, S., Kudenchuk, P., & Rea, T. (2022). A chart of machine learning approaches related to quality expression examination for cancer is required. *Recuperation, 147*, 104–111.

Lavric, A. (2021). *Recognizing keratoconus from corneal imaging information utilizing machine learning.*

Misbasikandar, W. A. A. A. I. N. G. (2020). Require for diabetes catapulted in with melded machine learning. IEEE Get to, 1, 1–12.

Muniasamy, A., Begum, A., Sabahath, A., & Yaqub, H. (2023). Lung cancer histopathology image classification using transfer learning with convolution neural network model. *Journal Name, volume*(issue), 1–12.

Muniasamy, A., Begum, A., Sabahath, A., Yaqub, H., & Karunakaran, G. (2024). Coronary heart disease classification using deep learning approach with feature selection for improved accuracy. *Technology and Health Care, 32*(3), 1–17. Advance online publication. DOI: 10.3233/THC-231807 PMID: 38339946

Naranjo, L., Pérez, C. J., Martín, J., & Campos-Roca, Y. (2020). Anticipate Ayurveda-based constituent changes in the human body by utilizing machine learning procedures. *Computer Procedures and Programs in Biomedicine, 142*, 147–156.

Ogunleye, A., & Wang, Q.-G. (2020). Novel multi-center and edge ternary pattern-based strategy for defilement run utilizing voice. IEEE/ACM Exchanges on Computational Science and Bioinformatics, 17(6), 2131–2140.

Oh, M. S., & Jeong, M. H. (2020). Machine learning for clinical comes about pine for. *Korean Diary of Pharmaceutical, 95*(4), 266–275.

Petropoulos, F., & Makridakis, S. (2022). Diabetes figure utilizing ensembling of encouraged machine learning classifiers. *PLoS One*, *15*(3), e0223456.

KEY TERMS AND DEFINITIONS

Cancer Prediction: The use of data-driven models to estimate the likelihood of cancer development or progression based on patient data and risk factors.

Cardiac Arrest: A sudden loss of heart function, often caused by an electrical disturbance, leading to a lack of blood flow to the brain and other organs.

Ensemble Learning: A machine learning technique that combines multiple models to improve prediction accuracy and robustness compared to individual models.

Kidney Disease: A medical condition in which the kidneys lose their ability to filter waste and excess fluids from the blood effectively.

Machine Learning: A method of data analysis that enables computers to learn from data and improve their performance on tasks without being explicitly programmed.

Medical Diagnosis: The process of identifying a disease or condition based on a patient's symptoms, medical history, physical examination, and test results.

Chapter 7
Acute Lymphoblastic Leukemia Classification With Deep Learning:
Models Comparison

Prema Ganesan
https://orcid.org/0000-0002-5406-4101
Mepco Schlenk Engineering College, India

N. S. Hari Krishnaa
Mepco Schlenk Engineering College, India

S. Suraj Narayan
Mepco Schlenk Engineering College, India

ABSTRACT

Acute Lymphoblastic Leukemia (ALL) is a rapidly progressing blood cancer characterized by the abnormal proliferation of immature lymphoid progenitor cells. This paper investigates the efficacy of various deep learning models, including VGG16, VGG19, InceptionV3, and MobileNetV2, in conjunction with the classification of ALL using the Acute Lymphoblastic Leukemia (ALL) image dataset. Our approach involves initially categorizing images as benign or malignant, followed by sub classification of malignant cases into three stages: Early, Pre, and Pro. We evaluate the performance of the models using metrics such as Accuracy, Precision, Recall, and Confusion Matrix.

DOI: 10.4018/979-8-3373-1087-9.ch007

INTRODUCTION

Image processing has emerged as a revolutionary tool in the field of medical diagnostics, enabling the detection, classification, and monitoring of various diseases (Das et al, 2022). From cancer to heart disease, neurological disorders like Alzheimer's disease and Parkinson's disease, lung diseases, and musculoskeletal disorders, image processing facilitates early diagnosis and precise treatment planning (Aby et al, 2024). Among these applications, its role in cancer detection stands out as critical. Cancer (Labati et al., 2011) is a formidable disease, often life-threatening, and encompasses a broad spectrum of over 200 different conditions characterized by the uncontrolled growth of cells. These rogue cells possess the ability to invade surrounding tissues, spread to distant parts of the body, and disrupt the normal functioning of organs. Cancer manifests in diverse forms, with some types exhibiting slow progression over decades, while others rapidly proliferate and metastasize. The prevalence of blood cancer is rising rapidly, with leukemia being one of the most well-known types, often posing a significant risk of mortality (Saleem et al, 2022).

In this paper, we delve into the application of image processing for classifying leukemia (Das et al., 2021), a specific and severe type of blood cancer. Blood cancer is a term that broadly refers to malignancies originating in the blood-forming tissues of the body, such as bone marrow. These tissues are responsible for producing healthy blood cells, including red blood cells (RBCs), white blood cells (WBCs), and platelets. In blood cancer, the bone marrow generates abnormal blood cells that proliferate uncontrollably, crowding out the healthy cells and impairing the body's ability to function normally. Despite the potentially fatal nature of blood cancers, advancements in medical research and treatments have significantly improved patient outcomes. Leukemia (Das, 2021a), a prevalent form of blood cancer, arises due to the abnormal proliferation of white blood cells in the bone marrow. This condition disrupts the balance and production of blood cells, leading to severe health complications. Leukemia is classified into four main types based on the speed of disease progression and the type of affected blood cells (Talaat & Gamel, 2024). It is first divided into acute and chronic forms, reflecting the rate at which the disease develops and spreads:

Acute Leukemia

Acute leukemia is characterized by the rapid accumulation of immature blood cells, known as blasts, in the bone marrow and bloodstream. This aggressive form of leukemia requires immediate intervention as the malignant cells quickly disrupt normal blood function and infiltrate various organs. Acute leukemia is the most common type of leukemia in children, though it can also affect adults.

Chronic Leukemia

In contrast, chronic leukemia progresses more slowly, involving the excessive growth of relatively mature but abnormal blood cells. These cells gradually accumulate in the bloodstream, potentially remaining asymptomatic for years before requiring treatment. Chronic leukemia is more common in older individuals but can occur at any age. Unlike acute leukemia, chronic forms allow for more measured treatment approaches, often spanning months or years.

Further classification of leukemia is based on the type of blood cell affected, leading to two additional categories:

Lymphocytic Leukemia

This type of leukemia results from the overproduction of lymphocytes, a subtype of white blood cells integral to the immune system's defense against infections.

Myelogenous Leukemia

Myelogenous leukemia originates in the bone marrow cells responsible for producing red blood cells, platelets, and certain types of white blood cells.

By combining these classifications, leukemia is divided into four primary types:

- **Acute Lymphoblastic Leukemia (ALL):** The most common type in children, ALL involves the rapid proliferation of lymphoblasts, immature white blood cells. It can also affect adults, particularly those over 65. Risk factors for ALL include exposure to radiation, certain viral infections, and genetic conditions like Down's syndrome. Chemotherapy and radiotherapy are the primary treatment modalities.
- **Chronic Lymphocytic Leukemia (CLL):** This form progresses slowly and often remains asymptomatic for years. It predominantly affects older adults and involves the excessive growth of abnormal lymphocytes.
- **Acute Myelogenous Leukemia (AML):** AML is characterized by the uncontrolled proliferation of myeloblasts, immature cells in the bone marrow responsible for generating blood components.
- **Chronic Myelogenous Leukemia (CML):** This chronic form arises from genetic abnormalities in myeloid cells, leading to their gradual accumulation in the bloodstream and bone marrow.

Figure 1 shows the sample leukemia images.

Figure 1. Sample Leukemia Images (a) Acute Lymphoblastic Leukemia (b) Chronic Lymphocytic Leukemia (c) Acute Myelogenous Leukemia (d) Chronic Myelogenous Leukemia

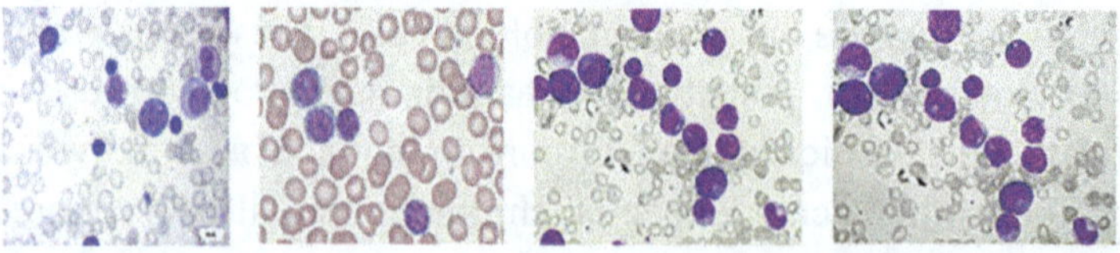

This chapter focuses on the classification of Acute Lymphoblastic Leukemia (ALL), a critical subtype of leukemia. ALL predominantly affects children but also poses significant risks to adults, particularly those over 65. The disease is driven by an unchecked increase in immature lymphocytes, which crowd out healthy blood cells and compromise the immune system. Several factors contribute to the development of ALL, including exposure to high levels of radiation, certain viral infections, and genetic predispositions such as Down's syndrome.

Image processing techniques play a pivotal role in the early detection and classification of leukemia. The visual analysis of blood smear images and bone marrow samples is a critical step in diagnosing and differentiating between various types of leukemia. Traditional diagnostic methods rely on manual evaluation by pathologists, which can be time-consuming, subjective, and prone to human error. By leveraging image processing algorithms, medical professionals can enhance the accuracy, efficiency, and reliability of leukemia diagnostics.

Key Steps in Image Processing for Leukemia Classification

1. **Image Acquisition:** High-resolution images of blood smears and bone marrow samples are captured using advanced microscopy techniques. These images serve as the foundation for further analysis.
2. **Preprocessing:** Image preprocessing steps such as noise reduction, contrast enhancement, and normalization are applied to improve image quality and ensure consistency.
3. **Feature Extraction:** Quantitative features, including cell size, shape, texture, and color, are extracted to characterize the cells and distinguish between normal and abnormal populations.
4. **Classification:** Machine learning and deep learning models, trained on labeled datasets, are employed to classify cells into categories such as normal, ALL, AML, CLL, or CML.
5. **Validation and Diagnosis:** The classification results are validated against ground truth data, and the findings are used to support clinical decision-making.

Advancements in Image Processing Techniques

The integration of machine learning and deep learning methodologies has revolutionized the field of medical image processing. Pretrained neural network architectures, such as convolutional neural networks (CNNs), have demonstrated exceptional performance in identifying and classifying leukemia from microscopic images. These models automatically learn hierarchical features, enabling accurate differentiation between subtypes of leukemia. Techniques such as transfer learning, data augmentation, and ensemble methods further enhance model robustness and generalization capabilities.

Moreover, real-time image processing systems are being developed to assist clinicians in rapidly identifying and monitoring leukemia. These systems integrate imaging modalities with artificial intelligence (AI) to provide automated and interpretable diagnostic insights, thereby reducing diagnostic delays and improving patient outcomes. The paper is organized as follows: Introduction in section I. In section II, literature survey is covered. In Section III, the pre trained model architecture and proposed block diagram is provided in depth. In Section IV the experimental procedures and results are provided. The conclusion and future work are in Section V.

BACKGROUND

Leukemia, a malignant disorder affecting the blood and bone marrow, presents a significant diagnostic challenge due to the morphological similarities among different cell types. Early and accurate diagnosis is critical for effective treatment, especially in subtypes such as Acute Lymphoblastic Leukemia (ALL) and Acute Myeloid Leukemia (AML). Traditionally, diagnosis relied on manual examination of blood smears by hematologists—a process prone to subjectivity, time consumption, and inter-observer variability. With advancements in digital pathology and artificial intelligence, image processing and machine learning techniques have emerged as powerful tools in automating the detection and classification of leukemia. These technologies can process high-resolution blood smear images, extract meaningful features, and classify cells with a level of consistency and accuracy that enhances clinical decision-making. Techniques such as morphological operations, watershed segmentation, feature extraction using statistical texture descriptors, and machine learning classifiers like SVM and CNNs have proven effective in identifying leukemic cells.

More recently, deep learning methods, particularly Convolutional Neural Networks (CNNs) and Vision Transformers (ViTs), have significantly boosted the performance of diagnostic systems. These models leverage large annotated datasets and computational power to learn hierarchical features from image data, offering state-of-the-art classification accuracy. Hybrid approaches combining traditional image processing with deep learning further enhance robustness and interpretability. Despite these advancements, challenges remain, such as the scarcity of large annotated datasets, variability in image quality, and the need for generalizable models. Consequently, research continues to evolve toward more accurate, scalable, and explainable systems for leukemia diagnosis.

Nee et al (2012), proposed a comprehensive method for cell segmentation specifically tailored for leukemia detection. The researchers implemented an innovative combination of techniques, including the watershed transform, morphological operations, thresholding, and gradient magnitude. These methods were designed to segment images effectively, overcoming challenges posed by the varying shapes and densities of cells in blood smear images. The proposed method underwent rigorous testing on 50 images representing leukemia subtypes M2, M5, and M6. The results demonstrated a segmentation accuracy of 94.5% for the tested image, while the overall accuracies for subtypes M2, M5, and M6 were 94.58%, 95.06%, and 95.65%, respectively. These results underscore the potential of their approach in achieving precise cell segmentation, which is crucial for accurate leukemia diagnosis.

Dharani & Hariprasath (2018), explored the use of advanced image processing tools for analyzing blood smear images obtained from both leukemic and healthy individuals. Their work focused on examining various forms of blood cancer, showcasing the versatility of image processing techniques in diagnosing multiple subtypes. By leveraging high-resolution imaging and computational analysis, their study provided critical insights into the visual differences between healthy and malignant cells, aiding in early detection and classification.

Vardiman et al (2009), contributed significantly to the field by addressing the evolving classification systems for acute leukemia and myeloid neoplasms. Their work targeted hematopathologists, clinical scientists, and hematologists, offering a detailed explanation of the key changes in leukemia classification and the reasoning behind these modifications. By highlighting the nuances of categorization, their study served as a foundational reference for understanding the clinical and pathological aspects of leukemia, thereby enhancing diagnostic precision and treatment planning.

Mishra et al., (2018), introduced a novel feature extraction technique aimed at categorizing acute lymphoblastic leukemia (ALL). The researchers utilized the Gray-Level Run Length (GLRL) matrix, a robust method for extracting textural information from images. This technique focuses on the nucleus of lymphocyte images, capturing intricate textural patterns critical for distinguishing between healthy and malignant cells. The extracted features were then employed in a Support Vector Machine (SVM) classifier, achieving an impressive 96.97% accuracy when tested on the public dataset ALL-IDB1. Their findings highlight the importance of early ALL detection in preventing severe hematological illnesses, showcasing the GLRL matrix's efficacy in capturing meaningful features for accurate classification. Similar to Nee et al., (2012) they integrated the watershed transform, morphological operations, thresholding, and gradient magnitude to achieve qualitative segmentation results. Their approach was validated using 50 images from subtypes M2, M5, and M6, yielding segmentation accuracies comparable to those reported by Nee et al., (2012). The consistent accuracy across different subtypes emphasized the robustness of their method, demonstrating its potential for broader application in leukemia diagnostics. Jagadev & Virani (2017), focused on the detection and classification of leukemia into distinct subtypes, including AML, CML, CLL, and ALL. Their work aimed to refine the classification process, advancing it to a more granular level. By integrating advanced imaging and computational techniques, they provided a framework for identifying specific leukemia subtypes, thereby contributing to personalized treatment approaches. Their methodology emphasized the importance of subtype differentiation in tailoring therapeutic interventions.

Shafique & Tehsin (2018), proposed a deep learning-based approach for detecting acute lymphoblastic leukemia and classifying its subtypes into four groups: L1, L2, L3, and Normal. They utilized pretrained deep convolutional neural networks (CNNs), specifically fine-tuning AlexNet for their dataset. By adding new layers to the pretrained network, they adapted it to classify input images into the four defined categories. To mitigate the risk of overfitting, they employed data augmentation techniques, which enhanced the model's ability to generalize across diverse image sets. Additionally, they compared datasets across different color models to assess performance variations. Their approach achieved a sensitivity of 100%, specificity of 98.11%, and an overall accuracy of 99.50% for identifying acute lymphoblastic leukemia, demonstrating the power of deep learning in medical image analysis. Sigi et al., (2018), developed a feature retrieval technique that analyzed individual cells in microscopic blood images. Their method was designed to classify cells into two primary categories: Acute Lymphoblastic Leukemia (ALL) and Acute Myelogenous Leukemia (AML). By extracting features from each cell, their technique served as a classifier input, enabling accurate categorization. The detection accuracy for individual ALL cells was reported at 80%, while AML cells achieved a perfect detection accuracy of 100%. For collective cell analysis, the technique produced an accuracy of 90%, highlighting its utility in both isolated and aggregate cell evaluations.

Scotti (2005), demonstrated the application of automated morphological methods in identifying acute lymphocytic leukemia from peripheral blood microscopy images. Their method began by separating leukocytes from other blood components in the images. Subsequently, lymphocyte cells—those relevant to acute leukemia—were selected for analysis. Morphological indices derived from these cells were used to classify the presence of leukemia. This automated approach streamlined the diagnostic process, reducing reliance on manual evaluation and enhancing reproducibility. Gupta et al (2008), proposed a methodology for identifying ALL by replicating the pathological and ontological descriptions of bone marrow cells. Their approach achieved over 93% specificity and sensitivity, demonstrating its reliability in distinguishing ALL cases. By aligning computational methods with clinical descriptions, their study bridged the gap between automated analysis and traditional diagnostic practices.

Ben et al., (2024) proposed a Vision Transformer (ViT)-based framework for ALL classification using features extracted from multiple layers. The ViT was pre-trained and fine-tuned on the ALL-IDB1 dataset, demonstrating superior performance over generic models. Their method achieved 98.75% accuracy, highlighting ViT's effectiveness in capturing morphological patterns in leukemic cells. Attallah (2024) presented a hybrid approach using CNNs with extended wavelet pooling and statistical texture features for ALL detection and subtype classification. It combines deep learning with traditional feature engineering to enhance interpretability and robustness. The results support the relevance of non-deep learning techniques in complementing deep models for improved accuracy.

Traditional machine learning methods such as Support Vector Machines (SVM), Random Forests, K-Nearest Neighbors (KNN), and Decision Trees have been widely used for ALL classification using hand-crafted features like color, texture, and morphology. These models offer interpretability and are computationally efficient, making them suitable for smaller datasets and real-time clinical applications. Hybrid pipelines that combine feature extraction (e.g., GLCM, color moments) with classifiers have also shown promising accuracy. Rahman et al., (2023) extracted features from individual images with CNN models then transferred features to Principal Component Analysis (PCA), Linear discriminant Analysis (LDA) and SVC Feature Selectors along with two nature inspired algorithms like Particle Swarm Optimization (PSO) and Cat Swarm Optimization (CSO) and then finally the model was assessed which gained 99.84% accuracy by integrating ResNet50 CNN architecture, SVC feature selector, and LR classifiers. Despite the rise of deep learning, these non-DL approaches remain valuable for benchmarking and deployment in low-resource settings.

Collectively, these studies highlight the diverse methodologies and advancements in leveraging image processing techniques for leukemia detection and classification. From traditional segmentation and feature extraction methods to cutting-edge deep learning approaches, the integration of computational tools has revolutionized leukemia diagnostics. These techniques not only improve accuracy but also reduce diagnostic time, paving the way for timely and effective treatment interventions. By continuing to refine these methods, researchers aim to achieve even greater precision and adaptability, ultimately enhancing patient outcomes in the fight against leukemia.

These studies underscore the diverse approaches and advancements in leveraging image processing techniques for the detection and classification of leukemia.

PROPOSED WORK

Acute Lymphoblastic Leukemia (ALL) is a rapidly progressing cancer of the blood and bone marrow, predominantly affecting children and young adults (Jawahar et al,2024). Early and accurate detection is essential to improving patient outcomes. In this context, the proposed method leverages advanced deep learning techniques to enhance the precision and reliability of ALL detection and classification. This method is illustrated in Fig. 1 and outlines a comprehensive workflow built around pre-trained Convolutional Neural Networks (CNNs), which are known for their exceptional performance in image recognition tasks.The workflow begins with the acquisition of medical imaging data related to ALL. This data is preprocessed to ensure quality and uniformity, which involves noise reduction, normalization, and augmentation to handle class imbalances and increase the robustness of the model. The core of the proposed method lies in the application of a pre-trained CNN model. These models, previously trained on extensive datasets like ImageNet, offer a powerful foundation by transferring learned features to the new task. Transfer learning significantly reduces computational costs and improves performance, especially when domain-specific data is limited.A key aspect of this method is the hierarchical classification of ALL. Initially, ALL is classified into two broad categories: Benign and Malignant. The Benign class represents non-cancerous conditions, while the Malignant class indicates the presence of cancer. The Malignant category is further subdivided into three distinct stages: Early, Pre, and Pro. This detailed classification enables clinicians to pinpoint the progression stage of ALL more precisely.

The rationale behind this multi-level classification is twofold. First, it aids in early detection, which is critical in preventing the progression of ALL and improving treatment outcomes. Second, it provides clinicians with a nuanced understanding of the disease's progression, allowing for personalized treatment strategies tailored to the specific stage of malignancy.The proposed method employs the CNN model to extract relevant features from medical images. These features are fed into a classification module, which is fine-tuned using labeled datasets of ALL images. The fine-tuning process adjusts the CNN weights to align with the specific patterns observed in ALL data. To further enhance accuracy, advanced techniques like data augmentation, dropout layers, and ensemble methods are incorporated into the workflow.

Evaluation metrics such as accuracy, precision, recall, and F1-score are used to measure the model's performance. Rigorous testing on validation and test datasets ensures that the model generalizes well to unseen data. The hierarchical classification strategy is particularly advantageous as it maintains high sensitivity in detecting malignancies while reducing false positives in benign cases. The adoption of deep learning in ALL detection brings numerous benefits. The automation of image analysis reduces the dependency on human expertise, minimizes errors, and accelerates the diagnostic process. Moreover, the detailed classification of malignancies into stages fosters better communication between radiologists and oncologists, ensuring a comprehensive approach to patient care. In conclusion, the proposed method represents a significant advancement in ALL detection and classification. By integrating pre-trained CNN models and a hierarchical classification approach, it provides an effective and scalable solution for early diagnosis and stage-specific analysis. This method has the potential to revolutionize ALL diagnosis, improving accuracy, and enabling timely and targeted treatment interventions. Figure 2 depicts the workflow of the proposed model.

Figure 2. The Overall Workflow of the Proposed Model

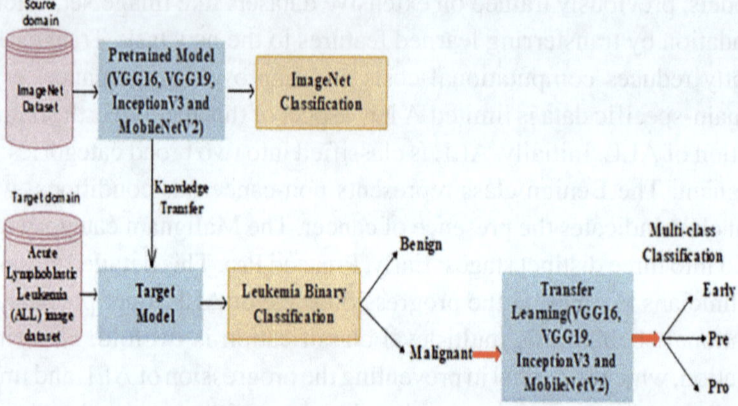

The proposed model for detecting Acute Lymphoblastic Leukemia (ALL) employs a structured two-stage classification process to enhance diagnostic accuracy and granularity. This approach is tailored to address the complexity of ALL, distinguishing between benign and malignant cases and further categorizing malignancies into specific progression stages.

Stage 1: Binary Classification

The first stage focuses on a binary classification task to determine whether the input image belongs to the Benign or Malignant class. This initial classification is crucial as it acts as a gatekeeper, ensuring that only images identified as potentially cancerous proceed for further analysis. By isolating benign cases early in the process, this stage minimizes computational overhead and reduces the likelihood of misclassification in subsequent steps. Pre-trained convolutional neural network (CNN) models such as MobileNetV2, VGG16, VGG19, and InceptionV3 are utilized to extract significant features from the images. These models, renowned for their robust performance in image recognition tasks, enable high sensitivity in detecting malignancies while maintaining specificity in identifying benign cases.

Stage 2: Malignant Subclassification

If the first stage classifies an image as Malignant, it advances to the second stage, where a more detailed analysis is conducted. Here, the model classifies malignant images into one of three subcategories: Malignant_early, Malignant_pre, and Malignant_pro. These subclasses represent different stages of leukemia progression, offering critical insights into disease severity. Accurate stage-specific classification is vital for guiding personalized treatment strategies and improving patient outcomes.

Model Selection and Advantages

The use of multiple CNN models—MobileNetV2, VGG16, VGG19, and InceptionV3—enables the system to leverage their unique strengths. MobileNetV2 is lightweight and efficient, suitable for real-time applications, while the VGG models provide a deeper architecture capable of capturing intricate features. InceptionV3 excels in handling diverse patterns through its inception modules.

By incorporating a two-stage classification process, the proposed model achieves a nuanced understanding of ALL, ensuring precise detection and stage-specific analysis. This layered approach not only enhances diagnostic accuracy but also facilitates timely and targeted interventions for patients.

Dataset Description:

The dataset used for classification in this study is the Acute Lymphoblastic Leukemia (ALL) image dataset, a critical resource for advancing the detection and diagnosis of ALL. Acute Lymphoblastic Leukemia is a common and aggressive form of cancer that primarily affects children and young adults. Its diagnosis traditionally involves invasive procedures, which are not only costly but also time-intensive. Peripheral Blood Smear (PBS) images have emerged as a significant tool in the preliminary screening process for ALL. These images allow for non-invasive diagnostic assessments, which are particularly important for early detection. However, manual examination of PBS images by laboratory personnel presents significant challenges due to the nonspecific symptoms of ALL, such as fatigue, fever, and pallor. These overlapping symptoms with other conditions can result in a higher likelihood of misdiagnosis during manual analysis.

The dataset comprises a total of 3256 PBS images, meticulously obtained from 89 patients diagnosed with ALL. These patients' blood samples were processed and stained by highly skilled laboratory technicians at Taleqani Hospital in Tehran, Iran. This ensures the reliability and clinical relevance of the dataset. Each PBS image has been categorized into two primary classes: Benign and Malignant. The benign class predominantly consists of hematogones, which are normal precursors of lymphocytes. In contrast, the malignant class is subdivided into three distinct subtypes of malignant lymphoblasts, reflecting the disease's progression stages: Malignant_early, Malignant_pre, and Malignant_pro.

The PBS images were captured using a Zeiss camera attached to a microscope with a magnification level of 100x, ensuring high-resolution imaging critical for accurate analysis. The images were saved in the widely-used JPG format, facilitating compatibility with various image analysis tools and deep learning frameworks.

The high-quality preparation and categorization of these images significantly enhance their utility for developing automated diagnostic tools. By providing a diverse range of samples across different stages of ALL, this dataset supports the training and validation of machine learning models aimed at detecting and classifying ALL with greater precision. Furthermore, the use of PBS images reduces the reliance on invasive diagnostic procedures, offering a more patient-friendly approach.

Data Split:

The dataset is divided into three subsets: training, validation, and testing, ensuring an organized and systematic approach to model development and evaluation.

Training Dataset (80%)

A significant portion, 80% of the images, is allocated for training purposes. This subset provides the bulk of the data required to train the machine learning models effectively. By exposing the models to a diverse and comprehensive range of image samples, the training process enables them to learn the underlying patterns and features essential for classifying the images accurately.

Validation Dataset (10%)

Another 10% of the images are reserved for validation. This subset plays a crucial role in fine-tuning and optimizing the model's hyperparameters, such as learning rate, batch size, and the number of epochs. By evaluating the model on this separate validation set during training, it becomes possible to detect overfitting and ensure that the model generalizes well to unseen data. The validation dataset serves as a checkpoint for iterative model refinement.

Testing Dataset (10%)

The final 10% of the images are designated as the testing dataset. This subset remains untouched during training and validation. Once the model training is complete, the testing dataset is used to objectively evaluate the performance of the trained models. Figures 3-6 shows the various classes of acute lymphoblastic leukemia.

Figure 3. Acute Lymphoblastic Leukemia (ALL) Benign Class

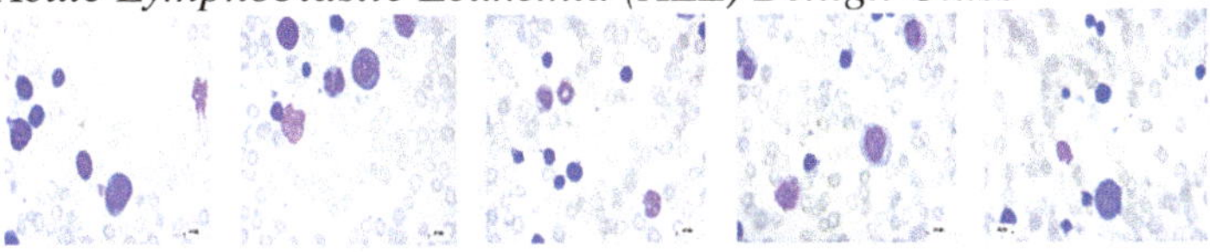

Figure 4. Acute Lymphoblastic Leukemia (ALL) Malignant-Early Class

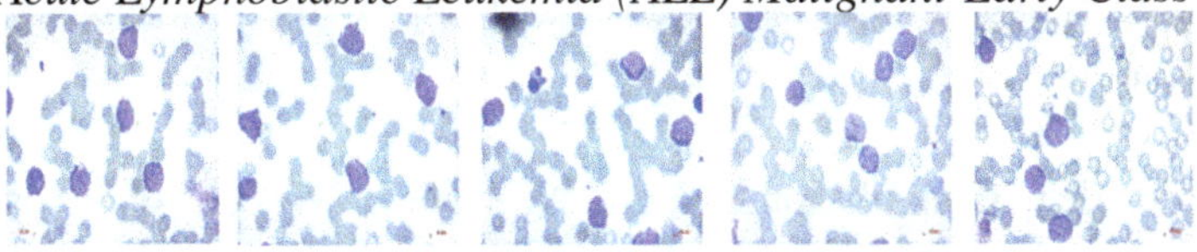

Figure 5. Acute Lymphoblastic Leukemia (ALL) Malignant-Pre Class

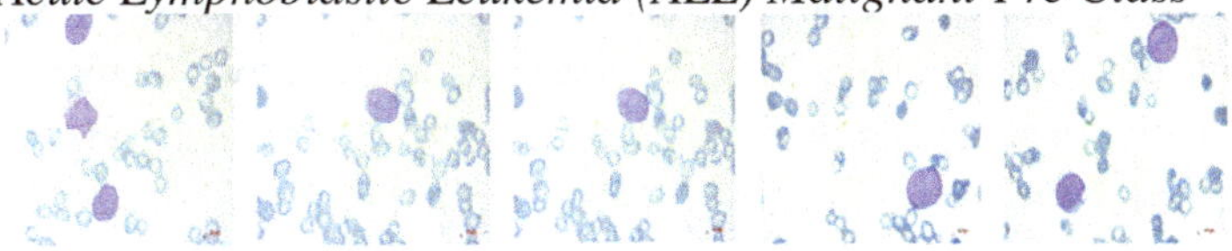

Figure 6. Acute Lymphoblastic Leukemia (ALL) Malignant-Pro Class

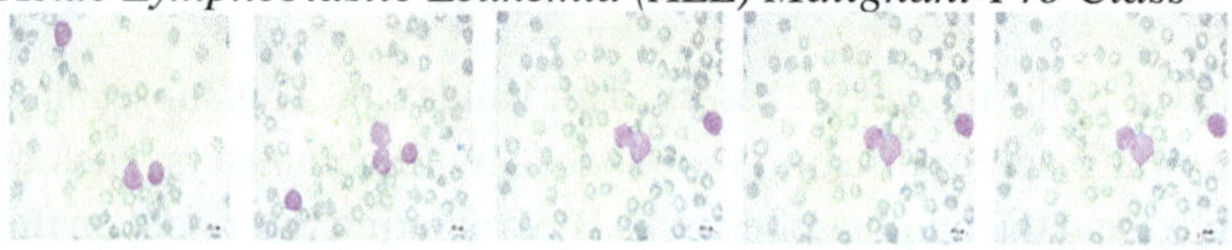

Pre-Trained Models:

The proposed method employs pre-trained models—VGG16, VGG19, InceptionV3, and MobileNetV2—individually for fine-tuning with input images. These models, renowned for their feature extraction capabilities, are adapted to classify whether an individual is affected by leukemia or not. By leveraging transfer learning, the models extract significant attributes from input images to perform the classification task. Each model's performance is evaluated, allowing for the selection of the most effective one. This approach ensures optimal use of deep learning techniques to enhance diagnostic accuracy and reliability in detecting leukemia based on peripheral blood smear images.

VGG16:

VGG16 is a deep Convolutional Neural Network (CNN) with 16 weight layers, comprising 13 convolutional layers and 3 fully connected layers. Renowned for its simplicity, VGG16 employs 3x3 convolution filters consistently across all layers, making it a robust architecture for image classification tasks. Its straightforward design and high accuracy have made it a benchmark model in computer vision. VGG16 is widely utilized as a pre-trained model through transfer learning, enabling its application in diverse domains by adapting its learned features to new tasks, significantly reducing computational costs and improving performance in image-based applications.

VGG19:

VGG19 is a deep Convolutional Neural Network (CNN) designed for advanced pattern recognition, particularly in disease diagnosis tasks such as identifying medical conditions from images. It is an evolution of the VGG16 architecture, differing primarily in the addition of three extra convolutional layers, making it a 19-layer network. The architecture of VGG19 includes 16 convolutional layers, 3 fully connected layers, 5 max-pooling layers, and 1 softmax layer. These layers are organized into convolutional blocks, referred to as Conv1, Conv2, Conv3, Conv4, and Conv5. The network accepts input images of size 224x224 pixels. The convolutional layers play a crucial role by extracting features from input images, capturing spatial hierarchies and complex patterns. The max-pooling layers are used to downsample feature maps, helping to reduce computational complexity and preventing overfitting by introducing translation invariance. The fully connected layers then process these extracted features and classify the image into predefined categories. The final softmax layer outputs the probbility of each class, aiding in the classification task. VGG19 is particularly suited for tasks like medical image classification, as it is capable of learning detailed and hierarchical feature representations. The model's deep architecture allows it to capture subtle differences between various patterns, making it highly effective for detecting diseases from images, such as in cancer or neurological disorders. By leveraging transfer learning, VGG19 can be fine-tuned for specific tasks with relatively smaller datasets, making it a valuable tool for medical diagnoses and other image classification challenges.

InceptionV3:

Inception v3 is a powerful pre-trained Convolutional Neural Network (CNN) model developed by Google AI, designed for large-scale image classification tasks. Utilizing transfer learning, Inception v3 can classify images into a wide range of object categories, making it versatile and highly effective for various applications. The model is 48 layers deep and was trained on over a million images from the ImageNet database, which includes a diverse array of images across 1000 categories, such as animals, objects, and everyday items like keyboards and pencils. The architecture of Inception v3 incorporates multiple convolutional layers, pooling layers, and specialized inception modules. The inception modules are designed to perform multi-scale feature extraction by using different kernel sizes in parallel, allowing the model to capture a variety of features at different levels of abstraction. This enables Inception v3 to efficiently handle complex visual tasks and improve accuracy while maintaining computational efficiency. Inception v3 has become popular in computer vision due to its efficiency and ability to generalize well across various image datasets. It is frequently used for image classification, object detection, and fine-grained image analysis tasks. By leveraging transfer learning, Inception v3 can be easily adapted to specific domains, such as medical image classification or other specialized applications, reducing the need for large-scale labeled datasets and computational resources.

MobileNetV2:

MobileNetV2 is a lightweight, efficient Convolutional Neural Network (CNN) architecture developed by Google, specifically designed for mobile and embedded vision applications. As an improvement over the original MobileNet model, MobileNetV2 achieves a good balance between model size, computational efficiency, and accuracy. It is 53 layers deep and can classify images into 1000 object categories, such as animals, objects, and everyday items like keyboards and pencils. MobileNetV2 uses an advanced architecture called inverted residuals with linear bottleneck layers, which enables the model to achieve high accuracy while keeping the number of parameters and computation low. This structure makes it ideal for devices with limited resources, such as smartphones and embedded systems. In comparison to its predecessor, MobileNetV1, MobileNetV2 is about 35% faster while maintaining the same level of accuracy, making it a highly optimized architecture for real-time applications. MobileNetV2 is widely used for tasks such as object detection, image classification, and semantic segmentation due to its efficiency and performance. It can act as an effective feature extractor, processing images quickly without sacrificing classification accuracy. Its ability to perform well with minimal computational resources makes it particularly well-suited for mobile devices and other edge devices, where speed and efficiency are crucial.

RESULT ANALYSIS

This section presents a comprehensive analysis of the proposed approach's training process on the Acute Lymphoblastic Leukemia (ALL) image dataset and compares the results obtained using various pre-trained models. The dataset, which is pivotal for leukemia classification, has been divided into three subsets: 80% for training, 10% for validation, and 10% for testing. This split ensures that the model is trained effectively, with ample data for both optimizing hyperparameters and evaluating performance on unseen data. Table 1 provides detailed information about the dataset, while Figures 3 through 6 illustrate sample images from the dataset, showcasing different blood smear samples categorized into benign and malignant classes, as well as the specific malignant subtypes (Early, Pre, and Pro). The images, captured using a Zeiss microscope at 100x magnification, provide the input for training the models. The proposed approach utilizes various pre-trained models such as VGG16, VGG19, InceptionV3, and MobileNetV2 to identify patterns and classify the images based on extracted features. These models are fine-tuned on the training data, with the validation set used for hyperparameter tuning and monitoring performance during training. The final model is tested on the 10% test data to evaluate its classification accuracy and performance metrics. The comparison of results between these pre-trained models helps identify the most effective model for leukemia detection, ensuring the highest accuracy in real-world applications.

1.Performance Metrics:

i) Precision

Precision is a performance metric calculated by dividing the number of true positives (correctly predicted positive instances) by the total number of instances the model has predicted as positive (i.e., true positives + false positives). It measures the accuracy of positive predictions made by the model. Precision ranges from 0 to 1 or 0% to 100%, where a higher value indicates better performance in correctly identifying positive cases.

$Precision = TP/ (TP + FP)$ ---------- (i)

ii) Recall

Recall is an important performance metric in machine learning, defined as the ratio of true positives (correctly predicted positive instances) to the total actual positive instances (true positives + false negatives). It measures how well the model identifies all relevant positive cases. Recall ranges from 0 to 1 or 0% to 100%, with higher values indicating better performance in detecting positive instances.

$Recall = TP/ (TP + FN)$ -------------- (ii)

iii) F1-Score

The F1 score is a performance metric that calculates the harmonic mean of precision and recall. It provides a balanced measure of a model's accuracy by combining both the ability to correctly identify positive instances (precision) and its capability to find all relevant positive instances (recall). The F1 score ranges from 0 to 1, with higher values indicating better overall performance, especially when dealing with imbalanced datasets.

$F1 - Score = [(2 \times Recall \times Precision)/ (Recall + Precision)] \times 100$ -------- (iii)

Where:

TP = True Positive; TN = True Negative; FP = False Positive; FN = False Negative

2.Binary Classification:

In this study, the model was evaluated for a binary classification task, where the goal was to distinguish between benign and malignant images. The dataset was split into training, validation, and testing sets, with a total of 403 benign and 410 malignant images used for training, 49 benign and 55 malignant images for validation, and 51 benign and 64 malignant images for testing, as detailed in Table 1. These subsets were used to train the model, optimize its hyperparameters, and evaluate its performance on unseen data.

The performance metrics for the binary classification task, including training accuracy, testing accuracy, precision, recall, and F1-score, are summarized in Table 2. These metrics provide a comprehensive evaluation of the model's effectiveness in identifying malignant and benign cases. The metrics are essential in understanding the model's ability to make correct predictions (precision), identify all positive instances (recall), and balance both aspects (F1-score). Among the models tested, MobileNetV2 achieved the highest performance. It showed a remarkable training accuracy of 98.04%, indicating its ability to learn from the data effectively. When tested on the unseen data, MobileNetV2 also demonstrated an impressive testing accuracy of 96.22%, making it the most reliable model for the binary classification of leukemia images. This high accuracy suggests that MobileNetV2 is well-suited for classifying medical images, even with limited computational resources.

To visually represent the model performance, the bar graph in Fig. 7 compares the binary classification performance of various pre-trained models, including VGG16, VGG19, InceptionV3, and MobileNetV2. The bar graph shows the training, validation, and testing accuracy of these models. MobileNetV2 outperforms the other models across all evaluation metrics, including precision, recall, and F1-score. The graph clearly illustrates that MobileNetV2 not only excels in training accuracy but also maintains high performance when tested on new, unseen images, showcasing its robust generalization capabilities. The precision of MobileNetV2 was particularly noteworthy, reflecting its ability to correctly identify malignant cases with minimal false positives. Similarly, its recall metric was high, indicating that it effectively identified most of the actual malignant images. The F1-score, which balances precision and recall, was also strong, further confirming the overall effectiveness of MobileNetV2 in this binary classification task.

In comparison, while VGG16, VGG19, and InceptionV3 also performed well, MobileNetV2's superior performance can be attributed to its efficient architecture, which is specifically optimized for mobile and embedded systems. This efficiency allows it to perform well with limited computational resources, making it an ideal choice for real-time applications, especially in healthcare environments where quick and accurate diagnostics are critical. The proposed model, using MobileNetV2, demonstrates excellent classification performance for detecting acute lymphoblastic leukemia (ALL) in peripheral blood smear images. The results show that MobileNetV2 offers a compelling balance of high accuracy, precision, recall, and efficiency, making it a valuable tool for medical image classification tasks. Table 1 shows the dataset details for binary classification.

Table 1. Dataset details for Binary Classification

Dataset details	Benign	Malignant
Training Images	403	410
Validation Images	49	55
Testing Images	51	64

Table 2 shows the performance metrics for binary classification of 4 different models.

Table 2. Performance metrics for Binary Classification of different models

Approach	Training Accuracy (%)	Test Accuracy (%)	Precision (%)	Recall (%)	F1 – Score (%)
VGG16	98.85	92.45	90.3	94	92.11
VGG19	97.62	91.50	90.38	92.15	91.25
InceptionV3	90.56	88.67	80.76	92.45	87.42
MobileNetV2	**98.04**	**96.22**	**98.07**	**94.44**	**96.22**

Figure 7. Accuracy comparison for binary classification of various models

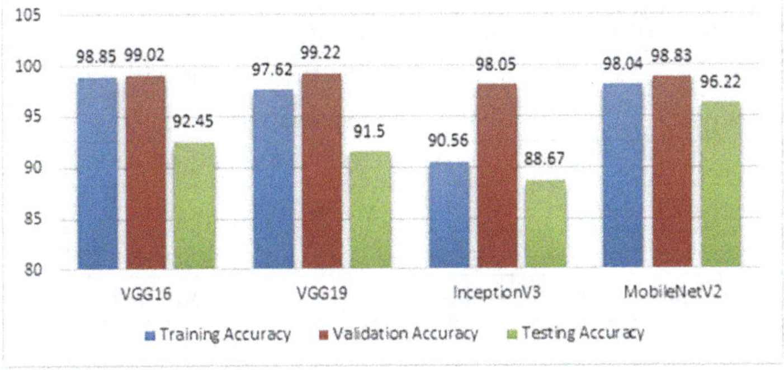

Accuracy comparison for binary classification of various models are shown in Figure 7.

The confusion matrices provide detailed insights into the performance of the various models used in our binary classification task, offering a deeper understanding of how well each model performs in distinguishing between benign and malignant images. By examining these matrices, we can calculate key performance metrics such as Precision, Recall, and F1-Score, which are crucial for evaluating model effectiveness in medical image classification. Upon analyzing the confusion matrices, it becomes evident that MobileNetV2 outperforms the other models in terms of accuracy. This model consistently predicts a higher number of correct classifications, both in identifying benign and malignant cases. The confusion matrix for MobileNetV2 shows a larger number of true positives and true negatives, indicating that it is more effective at correctly classifying both classes, while minimizing false positives and false negatives. This superior performance is reflected in the higher Precision, Recall, and F1-Score metrics when compared to other models. In contrast, the VGG16 and VGG19 models exhibit comparable performance, as seen in their confusion matrices. Both models have similar numbers of correct predictions, with true positives and true negatives being relatively balanced. Although they do not match MobileNetV2's performance, their ability to classify images accurately still demonstrates their strong capabilities. VGG16 and VGG19 have achieved similar metrics, confirming that they are effective but slightly less optimal than MobileNetV2 in this particular task. Therefore, while MobileNetV2 stands out with its superior performance, VGG16 and VGG19 models also demonstrate commendable predictive capabilities, showcasing their utility for medical image classification tasks. The comparison of these models, aided by the confusion matrices, helps highlight the strengths and limitations of each, providing valuable guidance for selecting the best model for leukemia detection. Table 3 depicts the confusion matrix for the binary classification.

Table 3. Confusion Matrix for binary classification

Models	**Classes**	**Benign**	**Malignant**	**Models**	**Classes**	**Benign**	**Malignant**
VGG16	Benign	47	5	**InceptionV3**	Benign	42	10
	Malignant	3	51		Malignant	2	52
VGG19	Benign	47	5	**Mobile Net V2**	Benign	**95**	**4**
	Malignant	4	50		Malignant	**0**	**98**
	- True Positive and True Negative				**- False Positive and False Negative**		

3.Multi Class Classification:

For our multi-class classification task, we utilized a total of 2200 images for training. Among these, 788 images were categorized under the Early class, 769 images under the Pre class, and 643 images under the Pro class. Additionally, 280 images were reserved for validation, while 272 images were set aside for testing the trained models. This balanced distribution of images across classes ensures that the models are trained and evaluated comprehensively on each class, facilitating robust classification performance. Table 4 depicts the confusion matrix for the multi-class classification

Table 4. Dataset Images for Multi Class Classification

Dataset Images	Early	Pre	Pro
Training Images	788	769	643
Testing Images	99	98	75
Validation Images	98	96	86

Bar graph for different models for multi-class classification is shown in Figure 8 and the confusion matrix is tabulated in Table 5.

Figure 8. Bar graph comparison of accuracy for categorical classification of various models

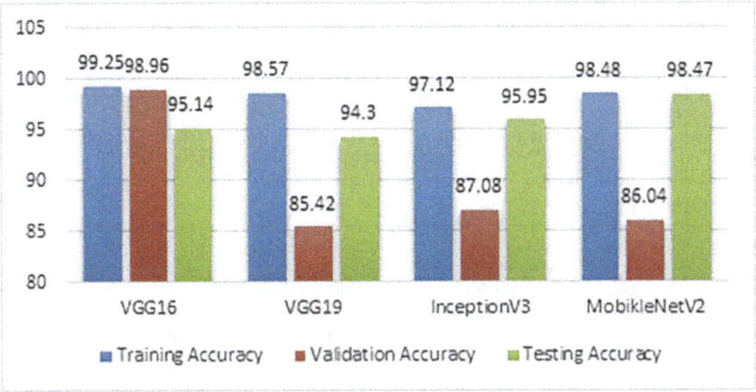

In both binary classification and multi-class classification the MobileNetV2 has predicted the output correctly compared to other models. So, for Leukemia Classification MobileNetV2 is a significant model. In Table [4] depicted the confusion matrix of four different models namely VGG16, VGG19, InceptionV3, MobileNetV2. The total number of images for testing is 272 images. In that early has 99 images, Pre has 98 images and Pro has 75 images totally. In Table [5] the performance metrics like precision, recall, F1-score has listed for 4 different models like VGG16, VGG19, InceptionV3, Mobile Net V2.

Table 5. Confusion Matrix For ALL image dataset

Models	Classes	Early	Pre	Pro	Models	Classes	Early	Pre	Pro
VGG16	Early	93	6	0	InceptionV3	Early	98	1	0
	Pre	0	98	0		Pre	3	95	0
	Pro	11	1	63		Pro	3	0	72
VGG19	Early	95	4	0	Mobile Net V2	Early	95	4	0
	Pre	0	98	0		Pre	0	98	0
	Pro	7	0	68		Pro	0	0	75
	- True Positive and True Negative					- False Positive and False Negative			

Table 6. Performance metrics for ALL dataset

Metrics	Classes	VGG16	VGG19	InceptionV3	MobileNetV2
Precision (%)	Early	89.42	93.13	94.23	100
	Pre	93.33	96.07	98.95	96.07
	Pro	100	100	100	100
Recall (%)	Early	93.93	95.95	98.98	95.95
	Pre	98.98	100	96.93	100
	Pro	84	90.66	96	100
F1-Score (%)	Early	91.61	94.51	96.54	97.93
	Pre	95.73	97.99	97.92	97.99
	Pro	91.30	95.10	97.95	100

Table 7. Performance metrics 2 for categorical Classification of different models

Approach	Training Accuracy (%)	Testing Accuracy (%)
VGG16	99.25	95.14
VGG19	98.57	94.30
InceptionV3	97.12	95.95
MobileNetV2	**98.48**	**98.47**

SOLUTIONS AND RECOMMENDATIONS

To maximize the clinical utility of deep learning (DL) models for Acute Lymphoblastic Leukemia (ALL) classification, several strategies must be adopted:

Interpretability and Support for Clinicians:

DL tools must emphasize transparency and interpretability to assist hematopathologists, particularly in ambiguous cases. Techniques such as saliency maps and class activation maps enhance trust and allow clinicians to understand the basis for model predictions.

Ethical Implementation:

The adoption of AI must account for data bias, transparency, and the need for human oversight. Over-reliance on autonomous AI decisions can lead to errors; therefore, continuous validation using diverse, representative datasets is essential. Clear clinical guidelines must accompany model deployment.

Workflow Integration:

Effective deployment requires seamless embedding into clinical workflows. DL models can act as triaging tools in Laboratory Information Systems (LIS), flagging likely ALL-positive samples for review, providing second opinions, and assisting junior staff. The integration with platforms like PathAI and Paige demonstrates the practical feasibility of this approach.

Clinical Relevance and Diagnostic Challenges of ALL:

Acute Lymphoblastic Leukemia (ALL) is a malignant disorder characterized by the proliferation of immature lymphoblasts in the bone marrow and blood, primarily affecting children. The current diagnostic workflow includes peripheral blood smear evaluation, bone marrow aspiration, immunophenotyping (flow cytometry), cytogenetics, and molecular diagnostics. Despite these modalities, diagnosis is often hampered by high inter-observer variability in morphological analysis, delays in result availability, and limited access to advanced tests in low-resource settings. ALL presents with relatively uniform cytomorphological patterns—such as high nucleus-to-cytoplasm ratio, scant cytoplasm, and condensed chromatin—which are well-captured in stained microscopic images. This visual consistency, along with the availability of public datasets like ALL-IDB, makes ALL particularly suitable for

DL-based classification compared to other leukaemia's with more heterogeneous morphology.

Clinical Integration and Impact:

Despite the promising performance of deep learning (DL) models for Acute Lymphoblastic Leukemia (ALL) classification, their real-world value depends on effective integration into clinical workflows. Clinical utility requires more than high accuracy; it involves seamless embedding into existing diagnostic systems, interpretability for clinicians, regulatory compliance, and demonstrable benefits for patient care.

Integration into Hematopathology Workflows:

DL models can be embedded within digital hematopathology systems and Laboratory Information Systems (LIS) to automate and augment various tasks. For example, they can function as pre-screening tools to identify likely ALL-positive cases in peripheral blood smear images, prioritize these for expert review, and even assist junior hematopathologists by providing second opinions on ambiguous cases. Furthermore, integration with platforms such as PathAI and Paige, which already offer AI solutions in histopathology, illustrates the feasibility of such systems for hematologic diagnostics (Litjens et al, 2017).

Clinical Evidence and Validation:

Several studies have highlighted the clinical potential of AI in hematologic malignancy diagnostics. Matek et al (2019) demonstrated that convolutional neural networks (CNNs) could achieve performance on par with expert hematologists in classifying white blood cell types from peripheral smears. Their study suggests that DL models can support routine laboratory workflows and reduce diagnostic burden.

FUTURE RESEARCH DIRECTIONS

Building upon the promising results of our deep learning-based approach for the classification of Acute Lymphoblastic Leukemia (ALL), several avenues for future research and development can be explored to enhance its practical applicability and clinical integration. One of the most immediate and impactful directions involves transforming our current model into a deployable tool in the form of a mobile application or a web-based platform. Such an application would enable pathologists and oncologists to upload microscopic blood smear images directly from their devices, facilitating real-time leukemia detection and staging. This could prove especially beneficial in remote or resource-constrained settings where access to specialized diagnostic facilities and expert hematopathologists is limited.

To achieve this, our future work will focus on optimizing the current deep learning models—VGG16, VGG19, InceptionV3, and MobileNetV2—for deployment on edge devices with limited computational power. Lightweight model architectures or pruning techniques can be employed to reduce model size and inference time without compromising diagnostic accuracy. Additionally, a user-friendly interface will be designed to guide medical professionals and laboratory technicians through the image uploading process, result interpretation, and subsequent clinical decision-making steps.

Another key direction will involve the integration of explainable AI (XAI) methods to make the model's predictions interpretable for clinical users. By incorporating visual saliency maps such as Grad-CAM or Layer-wise Relevance Propagation (LRP), doctors will be able to understand which regions of the cell images contributed most to the model's decision. This transparency is crucial for increasing trust in AI-assisted diagnosis and ensuring the system can serve as a reliable second opinion in clinical workflows.

Moreover, we plan to expand the dataset to include a broader spectrum of leukemia subtypes and incorporate images from different laboratories and imaging equipment. This will help to improve the model's generalization ability and robustness across diverse real-world conditions. We also intend to explore domain adaptation and transfer learning techniques that allow the model to adapt to new environments and imaging conditions with minimal retraining.

From a healthcare system perspective, integrating the application with electronic health records (EHRs) and laboratory information systems (LIS) will facilitate seamless data sharing, automated report generation, and longitudinal tracking of patient disease progression. This integration will enhance not only diagnostic accuracy but also treatment planning and monitoring.

Finally, future studies will include clinical validation in collaboration with hospitals and research institutions. Conducting prospective studies with real-time clinical data will enable us to evaluate the tool's effectiveness in real-world scenarios and fine-tune the system based on clinician feedback. This step is essential for obtaining regulatory approvals and scaling the system for global healthcare deployment.

In conclusion, the future direction of this research lies in the translational application of our AI models—from theoretical accuracy to practical utility—by developing accessible, interpretable, and clinically integrated diagnostic tools for leukemia detection and management.

CONCLUSION

In conclusion, the proposed CNN-based approach stands as a potent solution for the detection of different stages of leukemia. Leveraging transfer learning, the method harnesses the power of pre-trained deep learning models—VGG19, VGG16, InceptionV3 and MobilenetV2—fine-tuned explicitly for the task of Leukemia detection. The experiments results are highly encouraging, and they show that the overall accuracy is 98.47%, with a defined iteration limit. Acute Lymphoblastic Leukemia (ALL) is a rapidly progressing hematologic malignancy characterized by the uncontrolled proliferation of immature lymphoid progenitor cells. This study explores the effectiveness of various deep learning models—specifically VGG16, VGG19, InceptionV3, and MobileNetV2—for the classification of ALL using a publicly available image dataset. The proposed methodology involves a two-stage classification process: initially distinguishing between benign and malignant images, followed by further subclassification of malignant cases into three distinct stages—Early, Pre, and Pro. Model performance is evaluated using key metrics including accuracy, precision, recall, and confusion matrix analysis. The results demonstrate that the proposed convolutional neural network (CNN)-based approach, enhanced through transfer learning with fine-tuned pre-trained models, offers a robust solution for stage-wise leukemia detection. The experimental outcomes are promising, achieving an overall classification accuracy of 98.47% within a specified iteration limit.

REFERENCES

Aby, A. E., Salaji, S., Anilkumar, K. K., & Rajan, T. (2024). A review on leukemia detection and classification using artificial intelligence-based techniques. *Computers & Electrical Engineering, 118*, 109446. Advance online publication. DOI: 10.1016/j.compeleceng.2024.109446

Attallah, O. (2024). Acute lymphocytic leukemia detection and subtype classification via extended wavelet pooling based-CNNs and statistical-texture features. *Image and Vision Computing, 147*, 105064. DOI: 10.1016/j.imavis.2024.105064

Das, P. K., Diya, V., Meher, S., Panda, R., & Abraham, A. (2022). A systematic review on recent advancements in deep and machine learning based detection and classification of acute lymphoblastic leukemia. *IEEE Access : Practical Innovations, Open Solutions, 10*, 81741–81763. DOI: 10.1109/ACCESS.2022.3196037

Das, P. K., Pradhan, A., & Meher, S. (2021a). Detection of acute lymphoblastic leukemia using machine learning techniques. In *Machine Learning, Deep Learning, and Computational Intelligence for Wireless Communication* (Vol. 749, Art. no. 425). Springer. DOI: 10.1007/978-981-16-0289-4_32

Dharani, T., & Hariprasath, S. (2018). Diagnosis of leukemia and its types using digital image processing techniques. In *Proceedings of the International Conference on Communication and Electronics Systems (ICCES 2018)* (pp. xxx–xxx). IEEE. https://doi.org/DOI: 10.1109/CESYS.2018.8724075

Gupta, L., Jayavanth, S., & Ramaiah, A. (2008). Identification of different types of lymphoblasts in acute lymphoblastic leukemia using relevance vector machines. In *Proceedings of the Annual International Conference of the IEEE Engineering in Medicine and Biology Society (EMBC)* (Vol. 2009, pp. 6675–6678). IEEE. DOI: 10.1109/IEMBS.2008.4650279

Jagadev, P., & Virani, H. G. (2017). Detection of leukemia and its types using image processing and machine learning. In *Proceedings of the International Conference on Trends in Electronics and Informatics (ICEI 2017)* (pp. 123–128). IEEE. DOI: 10.1109/ICOEI.2017.8300983

Jawahar, M., Anbarasi, L. J., Narayanan, S., & Gandomi, A. H. (2024). An attention-based deep learning for acute lymphoblastic leukemia classification. *Scientific Reports, 14*(1), 17447. DOI: 10.1038/s41598-024-67826-9 PMID: 39075091

Labati, R. D., Piuri, V., & Scotti, F. (2011). ALL-IDB: The acute lymphoblastic leukemia image database for image processing. In *Proceedings of the IEEE 18th International Conference on Image Processing (ICIP)* (pp. 2045–2048). IEEE. DOI: 10.1109/ICIP.2011.6115881

Litjens, G., Kooi, T., Ehteshami Bejnordi, B., Setio, A. A., Ciompi, F., Ghafoorian, M., van der Laak, J. A. W. M., van Ginneken, B., & Sánchez, C. I. (2017). A survey on deep learning in medical image analysis. *Medical Image Analysis*, *42*, 60–88. DOI: 10.1016/j.media.2017.07.005 PMID: 28778026

Matek, C., Schwarz, S., Spiekermann, K., & Marr, C. (2019). Human-level recognition of blast cells in acute myeloid leukaemia with convolutional neural networks. *Nature Machine Intelligence*, *1*(11), 538–544. DOI: 10.1038/s42256-019-0101-9

Mishra, S., Majhi, B., & Sa, P. K. (2018). GLRLM-based feature extraction for acute lymphoblastic leukemia (ALL) detection. In *Proceedings of Recent Findings in Intelligent Computing Technologies* (pp. 399–407). Springer.

Nee, L. H., Mashor, M. Y., & Hassan, R. (2012). White blood cell segmentation for acute leukemia bone marrow images. In *Proceedings of the International Conference on Biomedical Engineering (ICoBE)*, Penang, Malaysia. IEEE. DOI: 10.1166/jmihi.2012.1099

Rahman, W., Faruque, M. G. G., Roksana, K., Sadi, A. S., Rahman, M. M., & Azad, M. M. (2023). Multiclass blood cancer classification using deep CNN with optimized features. *Array (New York, N.Y.)*, *18*, 100292. DOI: 10.1016/j.array.2023.100292

Saleem, S., Amin, J., Sharif, M., Mallah, G. A., Kadry, S., & Gandomi, A. H. (2022). Leukemia segmentation and classification: A comprehensive survey. *Computers in Biology and Medicine*, *150*, 106095. DOI: 10.1016/j.compbiomed.2022.106028 PMID: 36126356

Scotti, F. (2005). Automatic morphological analysis for acute leukemia identification in peripheral blood microscope images. In *Proceedings of the 2005 IEEE International Conference on Computational Intelligence for Measurement Systems and Applications* (pp. 96–101). IEEE. DOI: 10.1109/CIMSA.2005.1522835

Shafique, S., & Tehsin, S. (2018). Acute lymphoblastic leukemia detection and classification of its subtypes using pretrained deep convolutional neural networks. *Technology in Cancer Research & Treatment*, *17*, 1–7. DOI: 10.1177/1533033818802789 PMID: 30261827

Sigi, R., & Bachtiar, M. M. F. & Md Fikri. (2018). Identification of leukemia diseases based on microscopic human blood cells using image processing. In *2018 IEEE International Conference on Communication and Signal Processing (ICCSP)* (pp. xxx–xxx). IEEE. https://doi.org/DOI: 10.1109/ICCSP.2018.xxxxx

Talaat, F. M., & Gamel, S. A. (2024). Machine learning in detection and classification of leukemia using C-NMC_Leukemia. *Multimedia Tools and Applications*, *83*(3), 8063–8076. DOI: 10.1007/s11042-023-15923-8

Vardiman, J. W., Thiele, J., Arber, D. A., Brunning, R. D., Borowitz, M. J., Porwit, A., Harris, N. L., Le Beau, M. M., Hellström-Lindberg, E., Tefferi, A., & Bloomfield, C. D. (2009). The 2008 revision of the World Health Organization (WHO) classification of myeloid neoplasms and acute leukemia: Rationale and important changes. *Blood*, *114*(5), 937–951. DOI: 10.1182/blood-2009-03-209262 PMID: 19357394

ADDITIONAL READING

Balaji, P., Chaurasia, M. A., Bilfaqih, S. M., Muniasamy, A., & Alsid, L. E. G. (2023). Hybridized deep learning approach for detecting Alzheimer's disease. *Biomedicines*, *11*(1), 149. DOI: 10.3390/biomedicines11010149 PMID: 36672656

Balaji, P., Muniasamy, V., Bilfaqih, S. M., Muniasamy, A., Tharanidharan, S., Mani, D., & Alsid, L. E. G. (2023). Chimp optimization algorithm influenced type-2 intuitionistic fuzzy C-means clustering-based breast cancer detection system. *Cancers (Basel)*, *15*(4), 1131. DOI: 10.3390/cancers15041131 PMID: 36831474

Muniasamy, A., Begum, A., Sabahath, A., Yaqub, H., & Karunakaran, G. (2024). Coronary heart disease classification using deep learning approach with feature selection for improved accuracy. *Technology and Health Care*, *32*(3), 1–17. Advance online publication. DOI: 10.3233/THC-231807 PMID: 38339946

Muniasamy, A., Begum, A., Sabahath, A., & Yaqub, H. (2023). Lung cancer histopathology image classification using transfer learning with convolution neural network model. *Journal Name, volume*(issue), 1–12.

KEY TERMS AND DEFINITIONS

Blood Cancer: A type of cancer that affects the production and function of blood cells, commonly involving the bone marrow and lymphatic system.

Classification: The process of categorizing data into predefined classes or groups, often used in medical diagnosis to identify disease types based on patient data.

Deep Learning: A subset of machine learning that uses multi-layered neural networks to automatically learn and extract complex features from large datasets for tasks such as classification and prediction.

Leukemia: A form of blood cancer characterized by the uncontrolled proliferation of abnormal white blood cells in the bone marrow and bloodstream.

Chapter 8
Harnessing Recurrent Neural Networks for Early Melanoma Diagnosis and Prevention

Sachin Sharma
https://orcid.org/0000-0002-7821-3685
Amity University, Mohali, India

ABSTRACT

Melanoma, the deadliest form of skin cancer, presents a significant global health concern due to its forceful nature and tall mortality rates on the off chance that not recognized and treated early. In later years, advancements in artificial intelligence, especially within the domain of deep learning, have appeared guarantee in moving forward early location strategies for melanoma. This chapter presents a novel approach utilizing recurrent neural networks (RNNs) for the advancement of a melanoma anticipation and early discovery framework. The framework is planned to help both healthcare experts and people in recognizing potential melanomas at an early organize, hence empowering opportune intercession and progressed understanding results. Exploratory comes about to illustrate the viability of the RNN-based approach in precisely recognizing melanoma in terms of affectability and specificity. Moreover, the system's real-time capabilities and user-friendly interface make it an important device for melanoma avoidance and early location in clinical settings and past.

DOI: 10.4018/979-8-3373-1087-9.ch008

INTRODUCTION

Melanoma is a sort of skin cancer that can be deadly on the off chance that not identified and treated early. Early location and avoidance are pivotal to diminish the mortality rate of melanoma (Juyal et al., 2021a). Recurrent Neural Networks (RNNs) are a sort of profound learning calculation that can be prepared on time-series information, making them a valuable instrument for creating a melanoma anticipation and early discovery framework. The proposed framework would utilize a dataset of pictures of skin injuries, counting melanomas and non-melanomas, as input to an RNN. The RNN would be prepared to recognize designs within the pictures and distinguish highlights that are demonstrative of melanoma. The framework would too be prepared to recognize changes in these highlights over time, permitting it to identify early signs of melanoma.

To develop this system, an expansive dataset of skin injury pictures would be required, together with precise names demonstrating which pictures appear melanomas and which don't. The RNN would be trained utilizing directed learning strategies, with the objective of maximizing its precision in distinguishing melanomas. Once the framework is prepared, it might be utilized in an assortment of settings, counting dermatology clinics and essential care workplaces. Patients could submit images of their skin injuries employing a smartphone app or web interface, and the framework seem analyze these pictures to distinguish potential melanomas (Juyal et al., 2021). The framework seems moreover be utilized as a screening apparatus for high-risk populaces, such as individuals with a family history of melanoma or those with reasonable skin.

RNN based melanoma avoidance and early discovery framework has the potential to make strides the precision and effectiveness of melanoma discovery, driving to prior analyze and way better understanding results. Melanoma, the most aggressive shape of skin cancer, presents a significant global wellbeing challenge. Its frequency has been relentlessly rising, and whereas it accounts for a smaller percentage of skin cancer analyze compared to basal cell or squamous cell carcinomas, it is mindful for the vast larger part of skin cancer-related passings. The lethality of melanoma stems from its affinity for fast development and metastasis; once it spreads to far off organs, the guess significantly worsens, and treatment choices ended up restricted. Conversely, when identified and treated at its earliest stages, regularly kept to the epidermis (melanoma in situ) or as a lean essential tumor, the five-year survival rate is outstandingly tall, regularly surpassing 95%. This stark differentiate underscores the vital significance of early and accurate conclusion as the foremost basic factor in improving understanding results and diminishing melanoma-related mortality.

The current worldview for melanoma location to a great extent depends on visual review by dermatologists, utilizing procedures extending from the exposed eye examination of suspicious injuries to more sophisticated dermoscopy, which employments a handheld magnifying lens to imagine subsurface structures and designs not obvious to the bare eye. Dermatologists are trained to identify key highlights related with melanoma, frequently guided by mental aides just like the ABCDE rule (Asymmetry, Border irregularity, Color variety, Diameter, Evolving). Whereas dermoscopy has altogether improved diagnostic accuracy compared to visual review alone, the method remains inalienably subjective and intensely subordinate on the dermatologist's experience and expertise. Inter-observer inconstancy in elucidation can lead to discrepancies in determination, possibly resulting in unnecessary biopsies of generous injuries (low specificity) or, more basically, delayed determination of threatening ones (low sensitivity). Besides, access to expert dermatological care can be a critical boundary for numerous people, especially in underserved regions, driving to delays in examination and determination.

The challenges are advance compounded by the sheer volume of skin injuries that require observing, the subtlety of early melanoma signs, and the trouble in recognizing malignant injuries from a multitude of kind imitates such as moles (melanocytic nevi), seborrheic keratoses, or dermatofibromas. The dynamic nature of melanoma improvement, where a lesion may change over time, includes another layer of complexity to diagnosis, as a static picture captured at a single point might not uncover the significant developmental changes that flag danger. In later a long time, the field of therapeutic diagnostics has been revolutionized by the approach of artificial intelligence (AI), and especially deep learning. Deep learning, a subset of machine learning, utilizes artificial neural systems with different layers to memorize complex designs specifically from information, such as pictures.

Convolutional Neural Networks (CNNs), a type of deep learning design particularly outlined for preparing grid-like information such as pictures, have illustrated exceptional success in different therapeutic imaging assignments, counting the classification and division of skin injuries. By preparing on tremendous datasets of labeled dermatoscopic images, CNNs can learn to consequently extricate complicated highlights related to injury shape, color, surface, and structure that are demonstrative of harm. Various ponders have appeared that well-trained CNN models can accomplish symptomatic exactness comparable to, and in a few cases indeed surpassing, that of experienced dermatologists in classifying skin injuries from inactive dermoscopic images. These AI-powered frameworks hold immense guarantee for helping dermatologists, triaging patients, and possibly empowering prior location through teledermatology or indeed consumer-facing applications. In any case, whereas CNNs excel at analyzing inactive pictures, they inalienably need the capacity to viably show successive conditions or transient elements inside information. The movement of a skin injury towards danger isn't an immediate occasion but rather a handle that unfolds over time, frequently including subtle, continuous changes in appearance, measure, or structure. A single image, no matter how tall in determination or expertly captured, speaks to only a preview in this continuum. Crucial diagnostic data can be implanted within the arrangement of changes a lesion experiences. This is where Recurrent Neural Networks (RNNs) rise as a powerful and highly important class of deep learning models for upgrading early melanoma diagnosis and avoidance. Unlike traditional feedforward neural systems or CNNs, which handle each input independently, RNNs are particularly designed to handle sequential information. They have inside memory instruments that permit them to retain information from past inputs in a arrangement, impacting the handling of the current input. This makes them in a perfect world suited for errands where the arrange and setting of information focuses are imperative, such as analyzing time arrangement information, natural language, or, altogether for dermatology, groupings of medical images or patient records collected over time.

The center concept behind an RNN is the nearness of a covered up state that's overhauled at each step of the arrangement, successfully summarizing the data prepared up to that point. This covered up state is at that point utilized in conjunction with the current input to create the current yield and the another covered up state. This repetitive association permits information to stream through the arrange over time, empowering it to learn worldly conditions and designs. While essential RNNs can battle with capturing long-term conditions due to issues like vanishing or exploding gradients, more advanced architectures like Long Short-Term Memory (LSTM) systems and Gated Recurrent Units (GRUs) have been created to address these restrictions, permitting them to viably learn from longer arrangements. Saddling the capabilities of RNNs for early melanoma determination and avoidance opens up energizing unused roads past the current state of inactive picture examination.

One essential application lies within the examination of longitudinal dermatoscopic pictures of the same mole or injury. By capturing a arrangement of images of a suspicious injury at standard interims over weeks or months, and bolstering this arrangement into an RNN, the arrange can learn to recognize subtle patterns of alter that may not be clear to the human eye or recognizable from comparing fair two pictures. The RNN can track the advancement of highlights like asymmetry, border inconsistency, color varieties, and changes in diameter or structure over time. For occasion, a mole that's gradually but reliably increasing in estimate, or showing continuous changes in pigmentation or border definition, can be flagged as high-risk by an RNN analyzing the image sequence, indeed if person pictures don't strongly propose threat according to static criteria. This temporal analysis can give priceless early caution signals, inciting convenient intervention and possibly recognizing melanoma at a much prior, more treatable arrange. Beyond image arrangements,

RNNs can too be utilized to coordinated and analyze other shapes of successive information important to melanoma hazard and movement. Patient medical history is intrinsically successive, counting past analyze, family history of skin cancer, past biopsies, sun presentation history, and lifestyle components.

By handling this historical information utilizing RNNs, combined with picture examination from CNNs or other highlight extraction strategies, a more comprehensive and personalized hazard appraisal can be developed. An RNN seem learn to distinguish complex intuitive and directions inside a patient's history that contribute to their generally melanoma hazard, possibly foreseeing people who are at higher hazard and seem benefit from more visit screenings or focused on prevention methodologies. Besides, within the setting of observing known kind or atypical moles, RNNs might analyze groupings of clinical assessments, patient-reported changes, and imaging information to construct models that anticipate the probability of dangerous change. This seem empower proactive mediations, such as prophylactic extraction of high-risk injuries, subsequently avoiding the improvement of obtrusive melanoma. The potential for RNNs amplifies to modeling the typical movement designs of different sorts of skin injuries, both kind and harmful. By preparing RNNs on huge datasets containing longitudinal information for a different extend of injuries with known results, the models can learn to recognize between the common, kind changes that happen in moles over time (e.g., slow growth, fading color in older age) and the more whimsical, fast, or particular designs of alter characteristic of melanoma advancement. Deviations from the learned "normal" directions of generous lesions could serve as effective pointers of potential threat, allowing for prior identification and intervention. This predictive capability moves past basic conclusion of an existing suspicious injury towards a more proactive approach to avoidance, recognising injuries that are likely to ended up problematic within the future. The execution of RNN-based frameworks for early melanoma diagnosis and prevention requires the improvement of robust information collection conventions to procure standardized, high-quality longitudinal datasets of skin injuries. This includes setting up strategies for capturing consecutive dermatoscopic pictures beneath steady conditions, as well as coordinating electronic wellbeing records and patient-reported data.

Moreover, challenges related to show interpretability, guaranteeing that clinicians can get it why an RNN is flagging a specific injury as high-risk, need to be tended to to cultivate believe and encourage clinical selection. Computational assets required for preparing complex RNN models on expansive successive datasets too represent a consideration. While convolutional neural systems have essentially progressed the capability of AI in analyzing inactive dermatoscopic images for melanoma location, the energetic and developmental nature of melanoma requires a move towards strategies that can successfully capture and demonstrate changes over time. Recurrent Neural Networks, with their inherent capacity to handle successive information and learn worldly conditions, offer a compelling arrangement to this challenge. By empowering the examination of longitudinal picture groupings, integrating differing persistent historical information, and modeling lesion movement designs, RNNs have the potential to convert early melanoma conclusion from a basically static, subjective prepare into a more energetic, objective, and proactive approach. Harnessing the power of RNNs holds immense guarantee for progressing the exactness and opportuneness of melanoma location, encouraging personalized chance evaluation, and eventually contributing to a lessening in melanoma-related mortality through prior determination and more effective avoidance procedures. The proceeded improvement and integration of RNN-based frameworks into clinical workflows represent a basic step forward within the ongoing fight against this dangerous infection.

BACKGROUND

A novel approach displayed for the computer helped diagnosis of melanoma was based on Convolutional Neural Network with its configural enhancement by improved plan of an African Vulture Optimizer (Hu et al., 2022). They executed the starting assignment of preprocessing utilizing Kapur segmentation and numerical morphology to diminish the complexity of pictures. The ultimate guess of infection was performed utilizing CNN and to advance to improve and upgrade the classification, the application of African Vulture Optimiser was done. The adequacy of developed system was approved on two datasets specifically SIIM-ISIC and HAM10000 where a precision of 92.7% and 86.99% was accomplished separately. For the effective prognosis of melanoma, the analysts of proposed an imaginative system using XceptionNet with wash enactment work and depth wise separable convolutions (Lu & Zadeh, 2022). Their anticipated calculation performed dynamic separation among the pictures into ordinary, carcinoma, and melanoma. The viability of technique was approved on Skin Cancer MNIST: HAM10000 dataset and the comes about were compared with VGG16, InceptionV3, AlexNet, and the original Xception. Upon comparison, they found that XceptionNet outperformed all the demonstrate and displayed an exactness of 100%. During inquire about displayed two strategies for the determination of melanoma were illustrated (Alfi et al., 2022). The primary strategy included the application of machine learning models which included slope boosting machine, KNN, logistic regression, random forest, and SVM and their efficacy was validated utilizing 5-fold cross validation on hand crafted images of ISIC 2018 dataset. Their second approach included the exchange learning performed by profound learning models specifically MobileNet, Xception, ResNet50, ResNet50V2, and DenseNet121 which were prepared on ImageNet dataset.

The highest accuracy obtained in first approach was 88% by slope boosting machine and in case of moment approach was 91% by DenseNet121.

Authors proposed a machine learning based system for the compelling segregation between the pictures of kind and threatening melanoma (Thanka et al., 2023). Their proposed work comprised of VGG16 which was included within the extraction of fundamentally highlights from the pictures and given them to two major classifiers utilized as XGBoost classifier and Light Slope Boosting Machine (LightGBM). The framework's viability was approved utilizing SIIM-ISIC dataset where correctnesses of 99.1% and 97.2% accomplished in case of XGBoost and LightGBM separately. Authors defined a system characterised by a mix of ensemble learning and deep learning-based models for the location of changes dependable for the event of melanoma (Shah et al., 2023). The systems utilized for the classification handle included long short-term memory (LSTM), Bi-directional LSTM (BLSTM) and gated recurrent unit (GRU). The dataset utilized for approval comprised of ordinary human gene sequences inferred from asia.ensembl.org site and the data of changed quality arrangements was gotten from intogen.org. For approval of the proposed approach three procedures were utilized ten times cross approval, free set, and self-consistency which come about in exactness of LSTM (96%, 94%, 92%), GRU (93%, 94%, 91%), and BLSTM (99%, 98%, 93%), individually.

Authors driven to the improvement of a machine learning based system for the proficient separation between the pictures of melanoma course and nevus course (which represented ordinary mole images) (Orhan & Yavşan, 2023). They utilized five major calculations based on Convolutional Neural Arrange with sigmoid enactment work to be specific AlexNet, MobileNet, ResNet, VGG16, and VGG19, for classification. Upon performing the assignment of approval, they found that MobileNet calculation beated all the models and illustrated a precision of 84.94%. A novel strategy including the recognizable proof of vitiligo and melanoma contaminated range from the remaining skin area was devised (Sorour et al., 2023). Their proposed system included three major steps as Information preprocessing, information expansion, and classification with localization. The beginning stage of information preprocessing included color change, resizing, normalization, and naming for the arrangement of input pictures. This was taken after by information enlargement where convolutional generative ill-disposed arrange calculation had been utilized. At last, the assignment of classification was performed by YOLO-V5 demonstrate which given a precision of 90% and 97% for melanoma and vitiligo separately. The authors anticipated a novel approach for the successful classification of melanoma injuries into 7 major classes as melanocytic nevi, melanoma, generous keratosis, basal cell carcinoma, actinic keratoses, vascular injuries, and dermatofibroma (Girdhar et al., 2022). They given a system "DenseNet-II" based on Convolutional Neural Arrange whose viability was compared with VGG-16, DenseNet, ResNet and Inception V3 whereas approving the execution on HAM10000 dataset.

The DenseNet-II exhibited the accuracies of 93.8%, 95.7%, and 97.351% for 10, 15, and 20 ages, individually, outflanking all the models. Authors included an automated diagnosis of melanoma from dermoscopic images by classifying them into kind and malignant skin injuries (Mahmoud & Soliman, 2024). Their system enveloped the errands of division for which Versatile wind (AS) and locale developing (RG) calculations were utilized and classification for which Artificial Neural networks (ANN) and support vector machine (SVM) calculations were utilized. The approval of the calculations was executed on PH2 dataset where AS outperformed RG calculation by showing an exactness of 96%. Moreover, within the errand of classification ANN illustrated more noteworthy adequacy of 94% than SVM which appeared 74% accuracy. For the prognostication of skin cancer, authors proposed a strategy including an amalgamation of two models based on Convolutional Neural Network to be specific VGG16 and ResNet50 (Mazhar et al., 2023). Their hybrid show performed the classification of nine unmistakable classes of skin cancer including Pigmented Keratosis, Melanoma, Vascular Lesion, Actinic Keratosis, Squamous Cell Carcinoma, Basal Cell Carcinoma, Seborrheic Keratosis, Dermatofibroma and Nevus. The adequacy of the hybrid model was compared with DenseNet121, SVM, KNN, VGG16 and ResNet50. Their proposed demonstrate shown an exactness of 98.75%.

Overview of Melanoma

Melanoma could be a type of skin cancer that develops from melanocytes, the pigment-producing cells within the skin (Johri et al., 2022). It is the deadliest frame of skin cancer and can spread rapidly to other parts of the body in the event that not identified and treated early. Melanoma can create in any portion of the body, but it is most commonly found in zones that are uncovered to the sun, such as the confront, neck, arms, and legs. It can moreover create in regions that are not uncovered to the sun, such as the palms of the hands, soles of the feet, and beneath the nails. The main risk variables for creating melanoma include exposure to UV radiation from the sun or tanning beds, having reasonable skin, a family history of melanoma, and having a huge number of moles or bizarre moles (Singh et al., 2022). The signs and side effects of melanoma can change depending on the organize of the cancer, but they ordinarily incorporate an unused or changing mole, a mole that's topsy-turvy, has a sporadic border, is multicolored, or is bigger than a pencil eraser. Other signs may incorporate tingling, dying, or crusting of the mole or skin lesion. The conclusion of melanoma is regularly made through a skin biopsy, where a little test of the skin is evacuated and inspected beneath a magnifying instrument (Bhadula et al., 2023b). Treatment for melanoma regularly includes surgical evacuation of the cancerous tissue, but other medicines such as chemotherapy, radiation treatment, and immunotherapy may be utilized in more advanced cases. Generally, early location and avoidance are pivotal in decreasing the mortality rate of melanoma. Customary skin exams and sun assurance measures, such as wearing defensive clothing and utilizing sunscreen, can offer assistance decrease the chance of creating melanoma.

The history of melanoma, a harm arising from the pigment-producing cells known as melanocytes, could be a long and evolving narrative that mirrors humanity's expanding understanding of illness, especially cancer. Whereas the term "melanoma" is generally advanced, depictions of dark, potentially fatal tumors date back to antiquity, suggesting that this form of cancer, in spite of the fact that maybe less common than in modern times, has tormented people for centuries. Archaeological prove gives a few of the earliest hints; paleopathologists looking at the remains of pre-Columbian mummies in Peru, carbon-dated to around 2400 years ago, have found prove of diffuse melanotic metastases in bone, consistent with progressed melanoma. Written records from ancient civilizations moreover contain descriptions that, in hindsight, are believed to refer to melanoma. The ancient Greek physician Hippocrates (c. 460 – c. 370 BC), regularly considered the father of Western medicine, is credited with one of the earliest written descriptions. He utilized the term "melas," meaning black, to describe certain tumors, in spite of the fact that his understanding of their nature and root was restricted by the restorative information of his period. Later, the Greek doctor Rufus of Ephesus (c. 60 – 120 Ad) moreover recorded perceptions of pigmented threatening injuries on the skin that were related with systemic spread. These early accounts, whereas missing the accuracy of present day pathology, demonstrate an acknowledgment of dark, aggressive developments on the skin that had a destitute forecast. For centuries, understanding of such pigmented tumors remained simple. Therapeutic hypotheses regularly interwoven with humoral pathology or other now-discredited concepts. The genuine nature of these developments, their cellular root, and their potential for metastasis were not well understood. Surgical mediation was the essential, regularly the only, helpful approach accessible, regularly performed without anesthesia or antiseptic procedures, leading to high rates of infection and restricted success, particularly in cases of progressed infection. Significant progress within the understanding and classification of melanoma began to emerge within the early 19th century.

The French doctor René-Théophile-Hyacinthe Laennec (1781–1826), eminent for designing the stethoscope, played a essential part in formally recognizing melanoma as a particular infection substance. Within the early 1800s, Laennec depicted different shapes of "melanose," recognizing these pigmented injuries from other black stores found within the body, such as carbonaceous fabric within the lungs. The work, in spite of the fact that at first met with a few dispute, made a difference to set up that these pigmented tumors spoken to a particular neurotic prepare. Contemporaneously and within the taking after decades, other doctors and specialists contributed to the developing body of information. In 1820, British doctor William Norris (1778–1860) given a surprisingly quick report on "fungoid disease," enumerating clinical perceptions and autopsy discoveries of melanoma, counting its metastatic spread. Eminently, Norris was one of the primary to recommend a potential genetic connect in a few cases and watched a association between melanoma and pre-existing moles (nevi), as well as conceivable natural impacts. The term "melanoma" itself was presented in 1838 by Sir Robert Carswell (1793–1857), a Scottish pathologist, in his outlines of neurotic life systems. The 19th century saw a more prominent center on surgical administration. Specialists like George James Guthrie (1785–1856) and afterward, within the late 19th and early 20th centuries, William Handley (1871–1933), advocated for wide and deep surgical excisions of the essential tumor.

Handley, in specific, conducted detailed thinks about of lymphatic spread and championed the concept of en bloc dissection, evacuating not as it were the essential injury but moreover the encompassing tissue and regional lymph hubs in continuity, based on the understanding that melanoma often spreads through the lymphatic framework. This radical surgical approach, in spite of the fact that often disfiguring and related with significant dreariness, became the standard of care for numerous decades, representing the winning conviction that forceful nearby and territorial control was the key to anticipating systemic dissemination. In spite of progresses in surgical procedure, the guess for patients with metastatic melanoma remained grim all through the primary half of the 20th century. Treatment alternatives for disseminated disease were virtually nonexistent or ineffective. The understanding of the etiology of melanoma also began to evolve. Whereas natural variables were suspected prior, the link between ultraviolet (UV) radiation introduction, basically from daylight, and melanoma frequency got to be progressively clear through epidemiological studies within the mid-20th century. The perception of higher melanoma rates in fairer-skinned populations and in areas with greater sun presentation, coupled with the expanding ubiquity of sunbathing, solidified UV radiation as a major causative calculate. The half of the 20th century brought significant improvements in both diagnosis and the foundational understanding of melanoma science.

The improvement of histopathology as a standard diagnostic tool permitted for microscopic examination of tissue tests, giving more exact conclusion and classification. Key commitments came from pathologists like Wallace Clark Jr. (1924–1997), who developed the Clark levels of attack, depicting the depth of melanoma infiltration into the layers of the skin, and Alexander Breslow (1928–2009), who presented the Breslow thickness, a estimation of tumor thickness from the granular layer of the epidermis to the deepest invasive tumor cell. These histological parameters demonstrated to be capable prognostic pointers and stay significant components of melanoma organizing and treatment arranging today. The biopsy, especially the excisional biopsy expelling the whole suspicious injury, got to be the gold standard for conclusion. Be that as it may, treatment choices for progressed melanoma remained restricted. Systemic treatments, essentially chemotherapy operators like dacarbazine, advertised as it were modest reaction rates and negligible effect on in general survival for patients with metastatic disease. The late 20th and early 21st centuries stamped a revolutionary period in melanoma treatment, driven by a deeper understanding of the atomic and immunological underpinnings of the illness. The identification of particular genetic changes driving melanoma development, especially transformations within the BRAF gene (most commonly BRAF V600E), cleared the way for the advancement of targeted treatments.

BRAF inhibitors, and later combination treatments focusing on both BRAF and MEK proteins within the same pathway, illustrated remarkable efficacy in patients whose tumors harbored these changes, driving to tall reaction rates and significant changes in progression-free and large survival. This marked a paradigm shift towards personalized medication in melanoma, fitting treatment based on the hereditary makeup of the tumor. Simultaneously, the field of immunotherapy seen a sensational resurgence, in a general sense changing the scene of cancer treatment. Building on decades of investigate into the interaction between the safe framework and cancer, the improvement of resistant checkpoint inhibitors demonstrated especially successful in melanoma. Drugs targeting checkpoints like CTLA-4 (e.g., ipilimumab) and PD-1 (e.g., pembrolizumab, nivolumab) effectively unleash the patient's claim immune framework to recognize and assault melanoma cells. These therapies have delivered strong reactions in a critical subset of patients with progressed melanoma, changing what was frequently a quickly lethal conclusion into a possibly sensible inveterate illness for numerous. The combination of diverse immunotherapy specialists or the sequencing of focused on treatment and immunotherapy proceeds to be an dynamic range of investigate pointed at encourage moving forward results and overcoming resistance. Beyond systemic medicines, surgical strategies have moreover proceeded to advance, getting to be less radical for many early-stage melanomas based on a higher understanding of hazard stratification.

The advancement of sentinel lymph node biopsy within the 1990s revolutionized the surgical administration of territorial lymph hubs, permitting for less broad surgery in patients where the cancer has not spread to the sentinel hub. The history of melanoma could be a confirmation to logical advance, moving from ancient, vague perceptions to an advanced understanding of cellular pathology, genetics, and immunology. It highlights the basic significance of early discovery, a range where innovative progressions, counting imaging strategies and increasingly, artificial intelligence, proceed to thrust the boundaries of what is possible. From being a nearly generally fatal illness once it metastasized, melanoma has ended up a blurb child for the victory of focused on treatments and immunotherapy, advertising trust and progressed results for numerous patients. In any case, challenges stay, including avoiding melanoma advancement, making strides early location strategies, understanding and overcoming resistance to current treatments, and addressing incongruities in get to to care. The continuous investigate and advancement in fields like counterfeit insights, as discussed within the presentation, speak to the following chapter in this long and basic history, aiming to further improve determination, treatment, and eventually, anticipation of this complex disease.

Emerging Technologies

There are a few rising advances that can be utilized for melanoma avoidance and early location frameworks. These advances incorporate [Figure 1]:

Artificial Intelligence (AI) and Machine Learning (ML): AI and ML calculations can be prepared on huge datasets of skin injury pictures to precisely distinguish and classify melanomas (Sharma & Bhadula, 2023b). These calculations can be utilized in computer-aided diagnosis systems that help dermatologists in distinguishing potential melanomas.

Figure 1. Emerging Technologies.

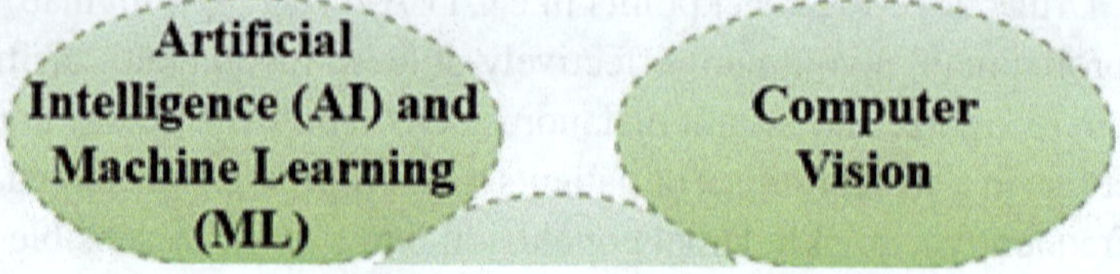

- Computer Vision: Computer vision methods can be utilized to analyze skin injury pictures and recognize highlights that are indicative of melanoma, such as asymmetry, border abnormality, and color variety (Bhadula & Sharma, 2023).
- Non-invasive imaging: Non-invasive imaging methods, such as OCT and RCM, can give point by point pictures of skin injuries without the require for a biopsy.
- Wearable Gadgets: Wearable gadgets, such as smartwatches, can screen changes within the skin over time and give early caution signs of potential melanomas.

- Versatile Applications: Versatile applications can permit clients to require photographs of their skin injuries and transfer them to a cloud-based stage for analysis by dermatologists or AI calculations.
- Nanotechnology: Nanoparticles can be utilized to target melanoma cells and convey drugs specifically to the cancerous tissue, moving forward the adequacy of treatment and decreasing side impacts (Sharma, Tomar, et al., 2024a).

METHODOLOGY

The strategy of a Recurrent Neural Network (RNN) based melanoma anticipation and early detection system involves several steps, counting:

- Information collection: An expansive dataset of skin injury pictures, counting melanomas and non-melanomas, must be collected. These pictures ought to be labeled with precise analyze to encourage preparing and approval of the RNN.
- Preprocessing: The pictures must be preprocessed to guarantee consistency in estimate, determination, and color. This step may moreover incorporate evacuating artifacts or other non-essential data from the pictures.
- Preparing the RNN: The RNN must be prepared utilizing the preprocessed dataset of skin injury pictures. Typically done through supervised learning, where the RNN is presented with an input picture and a comparing yield name. The RNN alters its parameters to maximize its exactness in recognizing melanomas.
- Approval: The RNN's precision in recognizing melanomas is approved employing an isolated dataset of pictures that the RNN has not seen amid preparing. This step guarantees that the RNN is generalizing well and is not overfitting to the preparing dataset.
- Integration: Once the RNN is prepared and approved, it can be coordinates into a larger system for melanoma prevention and early discovery. This may incorporate a portable application, a web-based interface, or a cloud-based stage.
- Sending: The framework can be sent in an assortment of settings, counting dermatology clinics, essential care workplaces, or indeed at domestic. Patients can yield pictures of their skin injuries to the framework, which analyzes the images and provides a conclusion or suggestion for follow-up care.

- Nonstop learning: The RNN can be assist moved forward through continuous learning, where it is displayed with unused data and its parameters are adjusted to progress precision over time.

Parameters Examination

There are a few parameters that must be inspected and optimized for a Recurrent Neural Network (RNN) based melanoma anticipation and early location framework to realize ideal performance. Some of these parameters incorporate:

- Number of layers: The number of layers within the RNN can have a noteworthy affect on its execution. As well few layers may result in underfitting, whereas as well numerous layers may result in overfitting. The number of layers ought to be chosen through experimentation and approval on a separate dataset.
- Learning rate: The learning rate controls the step measure of the weight upgrades amid preparing. In case the learning rate is as well tall, the RNN may fail to focalize, while if it is as well moo, the preparing may be as well moderate. The learning rate ought to be selected through experimentation and approval on a separate dataset.
- Activation function: The activation function decides the yield of each neuron within the RNN. The choice of enactment work can affect the RNN's capacity to memorize and generalize. Common enactment capacities incorporate sigmoid, tanh, and ReLU. The actuation work ought to be chosen based on the specific requirements of the RNN.
- Dropout rate: Dropout could be a regularization procedure that haphazardly drops out a few neurons during training, reducing the hazard of overfitting. The dropout rate controls the percentage of neurons that are dropped out. The dropout rate ought to be chosen through experimentation and approval on an isolated dataset.
- Batch size: The batch size controls the number of tests that are processed at once amid preparing. A bigger group measure can speed up training, but may moreover increment the hazard of overfitting. The group estimate ought to be chosen through experimentation and approval on a separate dataset.
- Repetitive layer type: There are diverse types of repetitive layers, such as straightforward RNN, LSTM, and GRU. Each type has it possess preferences and impediments, and the choice of recurrent layer ought to be based on the specific prerequisites of the RNN.
- Picture expansion: Picture enlargement could be a strategy utilized to extend the measure of the training dataset by applying arbitrary changes to the input

pictures. This can offer assistance the RNN generalize way better and diminish overfitting.

Benefits

Recurrent Neural Networks (RNNs) can give a few benefits for melanoma avoidance and early discovery, counting [Figure. 2]:

Figure 2. Benefits of RNN.

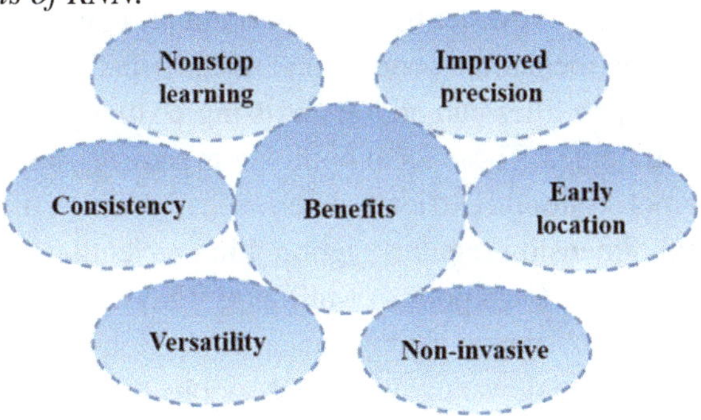

- Improved precision: RNNs can learn complex designs within the information and make precise forecasts based on the input pictures. This could result in improved exactness in recognizing melanomas compared to conventional strategies, such as visual review by dermatologists.
- Early location: Early discovery of melanomas is basic for fruitful treatment and way better understanding results. RNNs can identify melanomas at an early organize, permitting for opportune intercession and treatment.
- Non-invasive: RNNs give a non-invasive strategy for melanoma location that's less awkward and intrusive than conventional biopsy strategies. Patients can yield pictures of their skin injuries to the framework, which analyzes the pictures and gives a conclusion or proposal for follow-up care.
- Versatility: RNNs can be prepared on huge datasets and can analyze pictures at a much quicker rate than dermatologists. This permits for the framework to be scaled to a bigger populace, giving a more productive and cost-effective strategy for melanoma anticipation and early location.
- Consistency: RNNs can give a steady and objective strategy for melanoma discovery, diminishing the potential for human mistake and predisposition in conclusion.

- Nonstop learning: RNNs can ceaselessly learn and improve their exactness over time, permitting the framework to adjust to modern data and changes within the characteristics of skin injuries.

The preceding discussion has highlighted the basic importance of early melanoma diagnosis for improving patient results and underscored the impediments of conventional strategies, especially their dependence on inactive visual appraisal within the face of a powerfully advancing malady. We have moreover presented the concept of harnessing Recurrent Neural Networks (RNNs) to move past these limitations by analyzing sequential data. Now, let us delve into the preferences that RNNs offer in revolutionizing early melanoma conclusion and anticipation, explaining on how their one of a kind capabilities can address existing challenges and clear the way for more effective strategies. These focal points stem basically from the capacity of RNNs to viably demonstrate and extricate experiences from information that unfolds over time, a pivotal dimension regularly ignored in conventional approaches. One of the foremost significant focal points of utilizing RNNs lies in their capacity for upgraded location of unobtrusive changes over time. Melanoma frequently starts from pre-existing moles or shows up as unused lesions that advance continuously.

These early changes can be fantastically subtle, including minute changes in estimate, shape, color dispersion, or surface surface. A static image, indeed a high-resolution dermoscopic one, gives as it were a single depiction and may not uncover the basic direction of alter. Dermatologists depend on watching injuries over time, but this prepare is regularly subjective and dependent on subjective comparison of images captured at diverse visits. RNNs, by differentiate, can be prepared on sequences of images of the same injury captured over weeks, months, or indeed years. They can learn to recognize designs of alter that are indicative of malignancy, indeed in case each individual image within the grouping, when viewed in isolation, does not meet the standard diagnostic criteria for melanoma. The recurrent nature of these networks permits data from prior time focuses to impact the preparing of later images, empowering the demonstrate to identify patterns and rates of alter that are highly predictive of harmful change. This worldly examination may be an effective instrument for recognizing melanoma at its earliest, most curable arrange, possibly before it becomes visually clear through traditional static appraisal. By measuring and learning from these subtle evolutions, RNNs can essentially increment the affectability of early location. Another key advantage is the improved capacity to distinguish between generous from dangerous injuries. Numerous generous skin injuries, such as common moles and atypical nevi, can share visual characteristics with early melanomas, driving to demonstrative uncertainty and the require for superfluous biopsies. Be that as it may, the way these injuries alter over time frequently contrasts essentially.

Kind moles regularly experience moderate, unsurprising changes all through a person's life, such as progressive development amid childhood and puberty or blurring in more seasoned age. Melanomas, on the other hand, tend to show more rapid, erratic, or specific designs of alter. By analyzing longitudinal picture sequences, RNNs can learn to recognize the normal temporal directions of kind injuries from the abnormal designs characteristic of melanoma. This temporal context gives significant discriminative data that's not accessible from static images alone, driving to increased specificity in conclusion. Decreasing the number of wrong positives (benign lesions incorrectly identified as suspicious) is fundamental for minimizing patient anxiety, avoiding unnecessary procedures and their associated costs and risks, and optimizing the utilization of healthcare resources. RNNs can help accomplish this by giving a more educated evaluation based on the lesion's behavior over time. Moreover, RNNs offer the advantage of coordination differing sequential patient data for comprehensive hazard evaluation. Melanoma risk is affected by a multitude of variables past the visual characteristics of a single injury. These incorporate individual and family history of skin cancer, history of sunburns, total UV introduction, skin type, presence of various or atypical moles, and genetic inclinations. Much of this data is inherently successive or can be spoken to as a time arrangement (e.g., history of sunburns at different ages, dates of previous biopsies and their results). Whereas a few traditional chance appraisal models exist, they frequently depend on inactive categorical or numerical inputs and may not completely capture the complex transaction and temporal conditions between these components.

RNNs can handle a grouping of persistent history information focuses, learning how the amassing and interaction of these hazard variables over time contribute to an individual's generally melanoma hazard. By combining this temporal chance evaluation with the examination of injury changes over time, RNNs can give a more comprehensive and personalized assessment of an individual's probability of developing melanoma or of a particular injury becoming dangerous. This integrated approach permits for a more nuanced understanding of chance, empowering clinicians to distinguish people who seem benefit from more forceful screening conventions or focused on prevention methodologies. The capacity of RNNs to demonstrate transient conditions too encourages proactive identification of high-risk injuries. Instead of exclusively centering on diagnosing injuries that are as of now outwardly suspicious agreeing to inactive criteria, RNNs can analyze longitudinal information from a expansive number of injuries on an person to distinguish those that are showing subtle, early signs of concerning alter, indeed if they do not yet meet the edge for biopsy based on current rules. This predictive capability permits for the proactive observing or intervention on injuries that are distinguished as high-risk, possibly anticipating the improvement of invasive melanoma. For people with many moles or a history of atypical nevi, this will be especially profitable, making a difference to prioritize which injuries require closer observation or prophylactic evacuation. This move towards a more proactive and preventative approach could be a critical advantage, moving past responding to set up illness to foreseeing and potentially turning away it. Another advantage lies within the potential for made strides checking of known injuries.

Patients with atypical nevi or a history of melanoma regularly require customary skin checks to monitor existing injuries for changes and to recognize modern ones. Advanced dermoscopy permits for the capacity of pictures over time, but the manual comparison of these pictures by clinicians can be time-consuming and subject to oversight, particularly when observing various injuries. RNNs can automate and upgrade this checking handle. By analyzing groupings of pictures for each injury, an RNN can flag those that have experienced noteworthy or concerning changes, alerting the clinician to the require for closer examination or biopsy. This will improve the proficiency of follow-up arrangements, diminish the probability of lost a changing injury, and give patients with more noteworthy consolation or opportune mediation. The ability of RNNs to distinguish subtle changes too implies that possibly concerning improvements can be identified prior within the observing handle. Moreover, the application of RNNs in analyzing quiet history and injury movement can contribute to a more profound understanding of melanoma etiology and movement. By preparing RNNs on expansive, different datasets of longitudinal patient information and injury pictures with known results, analysts can pick up profitable insights into the complex components and temporal patterns that contribute to melanoma improvement and movement. The learned designs inside the RNN models can possibly uncover already obscure affiliations or highlight the relative significance of distinctive chance components and sorts of changes over time. This knowledge can educate future inquire about into melanoma science, driving to the distinguishing proof of modern biomarkers, helpful targets, and progressed avoidance techniques. The capacity of RNNs to reveal unobtrusive worldly connections in complex datasets makes them an effective instrument for logical revelation in dermatology.

At long last, the potential for expanded openness and versatility of early melanoma determination and avoidance endeavors is another critical advantage. Whereas expert dermatological care is fundamental, the request frequently surpasses the available assets, driving to long holding up times and limited access in certain regions. Whereas AI isn't expecting to supplant dermatologists, it can serve as a capable augmentative device, improving efficiency and availability inside the healthcare framework. Tackling Repetitive Neural Systems for early melanoma determination and anticipation offers a compelling cluster of points of interest that specifically address the limitations of conventional strategies and use the vital measurement of time.

\From upgrading the location of inconspicuous changes in injuries over time and making strides the separation between kind and dangerous developments to empowering comprehensive, personalized hazard evaluation and encouraging proactive recognizable proof of high-risk injuries, RNNs have the potential to essentially improve the exactness and convenience of melanoma discovery. Their capacity to coordinated diverse sequential quiet information and their appropriateness in automating and improving injury checking advance emphasize their transformative potential. Whereas challenges related to information accessibility, demonstrate interpretability, and clinical integration got to be addressed, the preferences advertised by RNNs in capturing the dynamic nature of melanoma improvement position them as an imperative innovation within the future of dermatological care, promising to spare lives through prior diagnosis and more compelling prevention procedures. The continued investigation and execution of RNN-based solutions speak to a pivotal step towards a more cleverly, proactive, and eventually fruitful approach to combating this dangerous disease.

SOLUTIONS AND RECOMMENDATIONS

Whereas Recurrent Neural Networks (RNNs) hold awesome guarantee for melanoma avoidance and early location, there are several challenges that must be tended to in arrange to successfully actualize this innovation. A few of these challenges incorporate:

- Information accessibility: RNNs require expansive sums of high-quality information to be prepared viably. In any case, it can be troublesome to get huge datasets of high-quality skin injury pictures for preparing the RNN. This challenge can be tended to through collaborations with therapeutic educate and by leveraging existing open datasets.
- Restricted interpretability: Whereas RNNs can accomplish tall exactness, their inner workings can be troublesome to translate. This will make it challenging to get it how the show is making its expectations, which may be a concern for a few partners, such as administrative bodies.
- Moral contemplations: The usage of RNNs for melanoma avoidance and early location raises moral concerns related to security, educated assent, and value in get to healthcare. These issues must be carefully considered and tended to guarantee that the benefits of RNNs are realized whereas minimizing potential hurts.
- Inconstancy in injury characteristics: Skin injuries can vary in appearance, making it challenging to create an RNN that can precisely detect melanomas

across a wide extend of injury characteristics. This challenge can be tended to through the utilize of information expansion methods and by planning the RNN to be vigorous to varieties in injury appearance.

- Require for master dermatologist approval: Whereas RNNs can give precise expectations, it is imperative to approve the comes about with master dermatologists to guarantee that the framework isn't lost any potential melanomas. This requires near collaboration between the RNN and dermatologists to guarantee that the framework is giving exact comes about.

There are a few openings related with actualizing RNNs for melanoma anticipation and early discovery. A few of these openings incorporate:

- Improved precision: RNNs can distinguish melanomas with tall precision, possibly driving to prior discovery and more viable treatment. This seem eventually lead to moved forward persistent results and diminished healthcare costs.
- Expanded availability: RNNs can give a non-invasive and helpful strategy for melanoma location that's available to a bigger populace. Patients can yield pictures of their skin injuries to the framework from the consolation of their possess homes, making it simpler for people in farther or underserved regions to get early melanoma location.
- Diminished healthcare costs: RNNs can decrease the require for costly and obtrusive biopsy strategies, which can be exorbitant and awkward for patients. This seem lead to reduced healthcare costs in general.
- Progressed productivity: RNNs can analyze pictures of skin lesions at a much quicker rate than dermatologists, permitting for a more efficient and convenient diagnosis. This may diminish hold up times for patients and move forward the generally effectiveness of the healthcare framework.
- Ceaseless learning: RNNs can persistently learn and adjust to unused information and changing characteristics of skin injuries, which can lead to made strides exactness over time. This seem lead to indeed more viable melanoma avoidance and early location within the future.
- Potential for integration with other innovations: RNNs can be integrated with other advances, such as telemedicine stages and mobile wellbeing applications, to supply a more comprehensive and open approach to melanoma avoidance and early location.

By and large, actualizing RNNs for melanoma anticipation and early location offers a few openings for progressing the exactness, availability, productivity, and cost-effectiveness of melanoma determination and treatment. By tending to the challenges related with RNN usage, these openings can be realized, eventually driving to progressed understanding results and open wellbeing. The essential demonstrative instrument for a RNN based melanoma avoidance and early detection framework could be a deep learning algorithm that analyzes pictures of skin injuries to distinguish potential melanomas. The RNN can learn from a huge dataset of labeled skin injury pictures to recognize designs and highlights that are characteristic of melanoma. Once prepared, the RNN can analyze unused pictures of skin injuries and give an expectation of whether the injury is likely to be melanoma or not. The RNN is regularly outlined to take in a picture of a skin lesion as its input and yield a double expectation indicating whether the injury is likely to be melanoma or not.

The RNN may moreover give a likelihood score for the prediction, showing the level of certainty within the result. In expansion to the RNN itself, other diagnostic tools may be used in conjunction with the framework to support accurate and productive conclusion. For illustration, dermatologists may be included within the approval of the RNN's forecasts to guarantee that the framework isn't lost any potential melanomas. Other imaging strategies, such as dermoscopy, may too be used to give extra data almost the lesion's highlights and characteristics. It is critical to note that an RNN based melanoma anticipation and early location framework should not be used as a standalone demonstrative device. Or maybe, it ought to be utilized as an aide to clinical examination and other symptomatic procedures to bolster precise and opportune conclusion of melanoma.

FUTURE RESEARCH DIRECTIONS

The future perspective of RNN based melanoma anticipation and early discovery systems are promising. A few potential advancements and progressions in this field include:

- Progressed precision: As RNNs proceed to be prepared on bigger and more differing datasets, they may gotten to be indeed more exact in recognizing potential melanomas. Moreover, headways in imaging innovation may make strides the quality of input pictures, assist improving accuracy.
- Increased accessibility: The utilize of RNNs for melanoma anticipation and early discovery may gotten to be more far reaching and open to a bigger populace. Integration with portable wellbeing applications and telemedicine stages might offer assistance to make early melanoma location more helpful and available to people in farther or underserved zones.
- Personalized diagnosis: RNNs may well be trained on person patient data, such as hereditary data, to give more personalized diagnosis and treatment

recommendations. This may lead to more viable and focused on melanoma anticipation and early detection strategies.

- Real-time checking: RNNs might be utilized for real-time checking of skin injuries, permitting for nonstop assessment of changes within the injury over time. This may empower earlier detection of melanomas that may not be quickly clear on a single picture.
- Integration with electronic health records (EHRs): RNNs may be coordinates with electronic wellbeing records to supply a more comprehensive see of quiet wellbeing and enable better coordination of care.
- Combination with other advances: RNNs may be combined with other innovations, such as nanotechnology and immunotherapy, to supply more compelling and focused on melanoma anticipation and treatment procedures.

The significance of early melanoma determination and avoidance in India could be a developing public wellbeing concern, one that's progressively recognized despite historical perceptions of this cancer being rare in populations with darker skin tones. Whereas the rate rates of melanoma in India are indeed lower compared to nations with predominantly fair-skinned populaces, accessible information from cancer registries demonstrate a rising slant. This increment can be ascribed to an intersection of components, counting changing lifestyles, expanded urbanization driving to distinctive designs of sun exposure, and possibly improved announcing and symptomatic capabilities. However, the generally lower rate compared to Western nations has, within the past, contributed to a lower index of suspicion among both the general public and some of time even healthcare experts, often leading to delayed diagnosis. This delay is a critical issue, as the forecast of melanoma is specifically connected to the arrange at which it is detected. Melanoma, if caught in its early stages when it is kept to the highest layers of the skin, is highly curable with surgical excision, boasting survival rates exceeding 95%. Alternately, if the diagnosis is delayed and the cancer has had the opportunity to attack deeper or metastasize to lymph nodes or distant organs, the treatment becomes essentially more complex, less successful, and the survival rates drop drastically.

Therefore, advancing early diagnosis and anticipation is fundamental to progressing results for melanoma patients in India. One of the significant challenges in India is the relatively low level of public awareness regarding melanoma compared to other more prevalent cancers. Teaching the open almost the chance variables (including family history, certain genetic conditions, and seriously intermittent sun exposure, indeed in those with darker skin), the differing clinical introductions of melanoma (emphasizing changes in existing moles or unused, unusual pigmented or even non-pigmented injuries, particularly on the palms, soles, and under nails), and the significance of regular self-skin examinations is a vital step in empowering people to look for convenient restorative consideration for suspicious injuries. The existing healthcare framework in India too presents challenges and openings for improving early melanoma determination and prevention.

Open wellbeing campaigns utilizing different media channels, including regional languages, are fundamental to spread this crucial information successfully over differing communities. The developing integration of innovation, including artificial intelligence, holds immense promise for progressing early melanoma conclusion in India, especially in overcoming geological obstructions and restricted get to to pros. AI-powered devices, such as portable applications that can analyze images of skin injuries and give a chance assessment, or teledermatology stages that interface patients in inaccessible ranges with dermatologists for virtual consultations based on uploaded images, can altogether upgrade screening and early discovery efforts. However, it is vital that these AI devices are created and approved utilizing datasets that are agent of the different skin tones and melanoma subtypes seen within the Indian population to guarantee their exactness and reliability in this setting. Adaptation and localization of these innovations are key to their fruitful usage and affect. Whereas melanoma may not be as factually predominant in India as in a few Western nations, its expanding rate and the critical dismalness and mortality related with delayed diagnosis make early location and anticipation a basic public health priority.

The challenges in accomplishing this incorporate low public and sometimes professional awareness, delayed introduction of cases, the generally higher incidence of melanoma subtypes that will display in unordinary areas, and disparities in access to specialized healthcare services. Addressing these challenges requires a multi-pronged approach enveloping focused on public awareness campaigns that dispel myths and teach almost all shapes of melanoma, enhanced training for essential healthcare suppliers, strengthening of symptomatic and treatment infrastructure over the nation, and the key integration of suitable and approved innovations like AI to improve screening and openness. By prioritizing and contributing in these ranges, India can altogether make strides the early determination of melanoma, offer opportune and effective treatment, and eventually diminish the burden of this possibly dangerous disease on its population.

CONCLUSION

Recurrent Neural Organize (RNN) based melanoma avoidance and early detection systems have the potential to revolutionize the way we identify and prevent melanoma, a deadly form of skin cancer. By utilizing profound learning calculations, RNNs can analyze pictures of skin injuries and recognize potential melanomas with tall exactness. The benefits of RNN based melanoma anticipation and early location frameworks incorporate prior location of melanoma, more accurate diagnosis, and made strides persistent results. Moreover, RNNs have the potential to extend accessibility to melanoma location in inaccessible or underserved areas. In spite of the numerous benefits of RNNs, challenges and restrictions do exist, such as the need for huge, differing datasets and the potential for wrong positives or negatives. Generally, RNN based melanoma prevention and early location frameworks are a promising range of investigate that has the potential to progress open wellbeing and spare lives. Proceeded advancements in this field could lead to prior discovery and more effective treatment of melanoma, eventually making strides quiet results and open wellbeing. The impressive challenge postured by melanoma, a cancer characterized by its forceful nature and potential for quick metastasis, underscores the basic require for early and precise diagnosis. As we have investigated, whereas conventional symptomatic strategies depending on visual assessment and dermoscopy have served as the foundation of melanoma location for a long time, they are inalienably constrained by subjectivity, inter-observer inconstancy, and openness issues.

The advancement of robust data infrastructure, standardized image acquisition conventions over time, and collaborative endeavors to build different and comprehensive datasets will be significant in realizing the total potential of RNNs in this domain. Similarly, research into explainable AI will be crucial to guarantee that clinicians can understand the basis behind an RNN's appraisal, cultivating certainty and encouraging the integration of these devices into clinical workflows. The harnessing the power of Recurrent Neural Networks speaks to a basic advancement within the ongoing fight against melanoma. The future of melanoma care will without a doubt be formed by the capacity to successfully harness the control of sequential data analysis through progressed deep learning strategies like Recurrent Neural Networks.

REFERENCES

Alfi, I. A., Rahman, M. M., Shorfuzzaman, M., & Nazir, A. (2022). A Non-Invasive Interpretable diagnosis of melanoma skin cancer using deep learning and ensemble stacking of machine learning models. *Diagnostics (Basel)*, *12*(3), 726. DOI: 10.3390/diagnostics12030726 PMID: 35328279

Bhadula, S., & Sharma, S. (2023). Post Diagnosis Digital Routine Monitoring System for Patients of Skin Diseases. In *2023 Fifth International Conference on Electrical, Computer and Communication Technologies (ICECCT)*, 1–6. https://doi.org/DOI: 10.1109/ICECCT56650.2023.10179835

Bhadula, S., Sharma, S., & Johri, A. (2023b). Hybrid blockchain and IPFS for secure Industry 4.0 framework of IoT-based skin monitoring system. 2022 8th International Conference on Advanced Computing and Communication Systems (ICACCS), 41–47. https://doi.org/DOI: 10.1109/ICACCS57279.2023.10112751

Girdhar, N., Sinha, A., & Gupta, S. (2022). DenseNet-II: An improved deep convolutional neural network for melanoma cancer detection. *Soft Computing*, *27*(18), 13285–13304. DOI: 10.1007/s00500-022-07406-z PMID: 36034768

Hu, L., Zhang, Y., Chen, K., & Mobayen, S. (2022). A computer-aided melanoma detection using deep learning and an improved African vulture optimization algorithm. *International Journal of Imaging Systems and Technology*, *32*(6), 2002–2016. DOI: 10.1002/ima.22738

Johri, A., Bhadula, S., Sharma, S., & Shukla, A. S. (2022). Assessment of factors affecting implementation of IoT based smart skin monitoring systems. *Technology in Society*, *68*, 101908. DOI: 10.1016/j.techsoc.2022.101908

Juyal, S., Sharma, S., & Shukla, A. S. (2021). Smart skin health monitoring using AI-enabled cloud-based IoT. *Materials Today: Proceedings*, *46*, 10539–10545. DOI: 10.1016/j.matpr.2021.01.074

Juyal, S., Sharma, S., & Shukla, A. S. (2021a). Security and privacy issues in unified IoT-based skin monitoring system. *Materials Today: Proceedings*, *46*, 10815–10820. DOI: 10.1016/j.matpr.2021.01.718

Lu, X., & Zadeh, Y. F. A. (2022). Deep Learning-Based Classification for melanoma detection using XceptionNet. *Journal of Healthcare Engineering*, *2022*, 1–10. DOI: 10.1155/2022/2196096 PMID: 35360474

Mahmoud, N. M., & Soliman, A. M. (2024). Early automated detection system for skin cancer diagnosis using artificial intelligent techniques. *Scientific Reports*, *14*(1), 9749. Advance online publication. DOI: 10.1038/s41598-024-59783-0 PMID: 38679633

Mazhar, T., Haq, I., Ditta, A., Mohsan, S. H., Rehman, F., Zafar, I., Gansau, J. A., & Goh, L. P. W. (2023). The role of machine learning and deep learning approaches for the detection of skin cancer. *Health Care*, *11*(3), 415. DOI: 10.3390/healthcare11030415 PMID: 36766989

Orhan, H., & Yavşan, E. (2023). Artificial intelligence-assisted detection model for melanoma diagnosis using deep learning techniques. *Mathematical Modelling and Numerical Simulation With Applications*, *3*(2), 159–169. DOI: 10.53391/mmnsa.1311943

Shah, A. A., Shaker, A. S. A., Jabbar, S., Abbas, Q., Al-Balawi, T. S., & Celebi, M. E. (2023). An ensemble-based deep learning model for detection of mutation causing cutaneous melanoma. *Scientific Reports*, *13*(1), 22251. Advance online publication. DOI: 10.1038/s41598-023-49075-4 PMID: 38097641

Sharma, S., & Bhadula, S. (2023b). Secure Federated Learning for Intelligent Industry 4.0 IoT Enabled Self Skin Care Application System. In 2023 2nd International Conference on Applied Artificial Intelligence and Computing (ICAAIC), 1164–1170. https://doi.org/DOI: 10.1109/ICAAIC56838.2023.10141028

Sharma, S., Tomar, M., & Tyagi, R. (2024a). Deep Learning Enabled Personalized Clinical Decision Making and Prescription Plan Preparation System for Diagnosis of Skin Cancer Patients. In *2024 IEEE International Conference on Interdisciplinary Approaches in Technology and Management for Social Innovation (IATMSI)*, 1–6. https://doi.org/DOI: 10.1109/IATMSI60426.2024.10502738

Singh, S., Sharma, S., & Bhadula, S. (2022). Automated Deep Learning based Disease Prediction Using Skin Health Records: Issues, Challenges and Future Directions. *2022 International Conference on Electronics and Renewable Systems (ICEARS)*. https://doi.org/DOI: 10.1109/ICEARS53579.2022.9752422

Sorour, S. E., Hany, A. A., Elredeny, M. S., Sedik, A., & Hussien, R. M. (2023). An automatic dermatology detection system based on deep learning and computer vision. *IEEE Access : Practical Innovations, Open Solutions*, *11*, 137769–137778. DOI: 10.1109/ACCESS.2023.3340735

Thanka, M. R., Edwin, E. B., Ebenezer, V., Sagayam, K. M., Reddy, B. J., Günerhan, H., & Emadifar, H. (2023). A hybrid approach for melanoma classification using ensemble machine learning techniques with deep transfer learning. *Computer Methods and Programs in Biomedicine Update*, *3*, 100103. DOI: 10.1016/j.cmpbup.2023.100103

ADDITIONAL READING

Balaji, P., Chaurasia, M. A., Bilfaqih, S. M., Muniasamy, A., & Alsid, L. E. G. (2023). Hybridized deep learning approach for detecting Alzheimer's disease. *Biomedicines*, *11*(1), 149. DOI: 10.3390/biomedicines11010149 PMID: 36672656

Balaji, P., Muniasamy, V., Bilfaqih, S. M., Muniasamy, A., Tharanidharan, S., Mani, D., & Alsid, L. E. G. (2023). Chimp optimization algorithm influenced type-2 intuitionistic fuzzy C-means clustering-based breast cancer detection system. *Cancers (Basel)*, *15*(4), 1131. DOI: 10.3390/cancers15041131 PMID: 36831474

Muniasamy, A., Begum, A., Sabahath, A., Yaqub, H., & Karunakaran, G. (2024). Coronary heart disease classification using deep learning approach with feature selection for improved accuracy. *Technology and Health Care*, *32*(3), 1–17. Advance online publication. DOI: 10.3233/THC-231807 PMID: 38339946

Muniasamy, A., Begum, A., Sabahath, A., & Yaqub, H. (2023). Lung cancer histopathology image classification using transfer learning with convolution neural network model. *Journal Name, volume*(issue), 1–12.

KEY TERMS AND DEFINITIONS

Early Detection System: A technology or process designed to identify diseases or health conditions at an initial stage, improving chances of effective treatment and positive outcomes.

Melanoma Prevention: Strategies and actions aimed at reducing the risk of developing melanoma, a serious form of skin cancer, through awareness, sun protection, and regular skin checks.

Recurrent Neural Network: A type of artificial neural network designed to recognize patterns in sequences of data by using feedback loops, making it suitable for tasks involving time-series, language, or medical records.

Chapter 9
Revolutionizing Brain Tumor Diagnosis With Adaptive CNN Models

R. Kishore Kanna
https://orcid.org/0000-0002-8004-1501
Vel Tech Rangarajan Dr. Sagunthala R&D Institute of Science and Technology, Chennai, India

Priyanka Singh
https://orcid.org/0000-0003-0841-1544
Amity University, Noida, India

S. Raju
KPR Institute of Engineering and Technology, India

Ayodeji Olalekan Salau
https://orcid.org/0000-0002-6264-9783
Afe Babalola University, Nigeria & Saveetha Institute of Medical and Technical Sciences, Nigeria

Archibald Danquah Danquah-Amoah
Accra Technical University, Ghana

R. Gomalavalli
https://orcid.org/0000-0003-2168-167X
Sri Sai Ram institute of Technology, India

Sathea Sree
Vels Institute of Science, Technology, and Advanced Studies, India

ABSTRACT

Brain tumors affect millions of people worldwide and can be life-threatening if not detected early. These cancerous growths disrupt normal brain function and can spread to surrounding tissues. However, diagnosing brain tumors is challenging because they vary greatly in shape, size, and appearance, making manual detection difficult and time-consuming for doctors. Our research team developed an intelligent computer system using artificial intelligence to automatically identify and classify brain tumors from MRI scans. We tested three different AI models - ResNet-152,

DOI: 10.4018/979-8-3373-1087-9.ch009

MobileNet, and DenseNet-121 - using a technique called transfer learning, which allows computers to build on existing medical knowledge.The results were impressive. The ResNet-152 model performed best, correctly identifying brain tumors 98.7% of the time with a 99.8% reliability score. DenseNet-121 achieved 96.5% accuracy with 98.6% reliability, while MobileNet reached 87.2% accuracy with 98.7% reliability. Even the smallest model performed well enough for practical use in hospitals with limited computing resources.

INTRODUCTION

The brain is a very intricate and essential component of the human body, governing all movements and the primary nerve system. Uncontrolled and uneven cell growth in the brain results in a brain tumor. It induces intracranial pressure, so disrupting the brain's natural functioning. Brain tumors are classified into two categories: benign (non-cancerous) and malignant (cancerous). Malignant tumors proliferate in the brain at a far faster rate than benign tumors, causing damage to surrounding normal tissues. Moreover, they possess the capacity to metastasize to other regions of the body, hence facilitating the dissemination of cancer. Cancers have the greatest death rates globally in both adults and children (Ahamed et al., 2024).

The etiology and development rate of the brain tumor remain unidentified. Secondary brain tumors originate in other parts of the body and metastasize to the brain via the bloodstream, while primary brain tumors develop inside the brain's tissues. Glioma, pituitary tumors, and meningioma are the most perilous forms of primary brain neoplasms. Glioma is a predominant kind of brain tumor, with only Grade I being benign among Grades I to IV; 80% of brain tumors are malignant. For early identification and treatment, meningioma and pituitary tumors are among the most challenging forms for physicians to discover. Glioma, originating in the brain's glial cells, is the most prevalent form. Meningioma is often benign and originates inside the membrane of the skull that encases the brain and spinal cord (Al Bataineh et al., 2024). The pituitary gland, mostly responsible for controlling hormonal levels in the body, is predominantly associated with pituitary tumors. It may lead to both benign and malignant disorders, and its disruption may result in visual problems, among other concerns. Brain tumors are classified into four separate grade categories:

A) These need time for development and dissemination. These may be almost entirely excised surgically and are linked to a heightened probability of improved organization. Pilocytic astrocytoma exemplifies this kind of tumor. B) These tumors proliferate over time and may progress to higher grades while infiltrating adjacent tissues. An oligodendroglia is a form of tumor that progressively enlarges. C) In comparison to Grade II malignant tumors, these tumors have a significantly accelerated growth rate and the ability to metastasize to adjacent organs. Isolated surgical intervention is insufficient for the management of these tumors; adjuvant chemotherapy or radiation treatment is needed. Aden squamous astrocytoma is a specific kind of tumor. D) These are among the most detrimental and susceptible to proliferation. This category includes malignant neoplasms. They may enhance their development by using blood vessels. Glioblastoma multiform is one such tumor.

One of the most crucial measures in preserving a patient's life is the early identification of the tumor and its subsequent categorization with high diagnostic accuracy. The most arduous duty for physicians and radiologists is the manual analysis of MRI images to differentiate and localize tumors from normal tissue and to ascertain their kind. MRI is a prevalent non-invasive tool for finding brain tumors, favored by radiologists for scanning, while a CT scan complicates the detection of structural alterations (Alshardan et al., 2024).

The incidence of fatalities due to brain tumors is too high among the primary causes of death, underscoring the critical need for improved detection and treatment. Manual interpretation of MRI scans is often the primary method used in clinical decision-making about brain tumors; however, this careful procedure is fraught with errors. Therefore, the most cost-effective alternative would be to include computer-aided assistance for the analyst (Deshmukh et al., 2024).

Brain tumors constitute a significant worldwide health issue, with around 308,000 new primary brain and central nervous system (CNS) tumors diagnosed annually. Incidence rates vary by area, age group, and gender, with industrialized nations often exhibiting higher rates owing to superior diagnostic capabilities and enhanced access to healthcare services (Dounya et al., 2024). Europe exhibits somewhat elevated rates, while regions in Africa and Asia show reduced rates, perhaps because of under-reporting and insufficient diagnostic systems.

The predominant forms of brain tumors in adults are gliomas, particularly glioblastomas, which are very aggressive and constitute a significant percentage of brain tumors.

The prevalence of brain tumors indicates the total number of individuals currently affected by the condition. Improvements in medical technology and treatment have improved survival rates, facilitating population increase. Brain tumors are the second most prevalent cancer in children, behind leukemia, and constitute the primary cause of cancer-related mortality in the pediatric demographic. Globally, brain tumors represent around 2% of all malignancies, but, because of their intricacy and location, they have an outsized influence on health and quality of life. It constitutes a convergence of statistics, artificial intelligence, and computer science and serves as a research domain. The applications of machine learning have significantly expanded in recent years, including areas such as movie recommendations, image categorization, and beyond. The primary objective of machine learning is to develop a software application capable of learning and adapting autonomously, eliminating the need for extensive preprogramming of its responses to various events. These may autonomously acquire knowledge from any errors they may have committed. Neural networks are prevalent in several sectors and cover extensive fields of research, including healthcare, natural language processing, cybersecurity, and others. In an artificial neural network (ANN), diminutive neurons (processing units) interconnected form the foundation of the neural network. These neurons provide active values that enable us to get our desired outcome. Convolutional Neural Networks (CNNs) are multilayered neural networks that are interconnected (Gokapay & Mohanty, 2024). Small segments of the picture are inputted into the lowest layer of the CNN architecture. Information originates from several levels, each performing a distinct function to generate the observable attributes of the data. This approach provides the neuron or processing unit with access to essential features such as corners, edges, and lines. Transfer learning is used to facilitate job execution (Suresh, Kumar et al., 2025). It is a technique that utilizes the expertise of a trained model to acquire information from an alternative data collection.

Development and development of an optimum convolutional neural network (CNN) model for brain tumor diagnoses. Utilization of transfer learning techniques during neural network training to expedite the learning process (Hosny et al., 2024). Conducting comprehensive performance assessment studies to assess error rates and dependability between the proposed model and professional manual diagnoses. Evaluating the potential applications for clinical implementation and integrating the model into actual environments to improve patient care and results (Kanchanamala et al., 2025).

BACKGROUND

A hybrid CNN model used "BRATS MR images" for the identification of brain tumors. The training approach and sophisticated regularization algorithms underwent study and validation. The suggested hybrid model enhanced performance by integrating two- and three-path networks (Kandula et al., 2024). The examination of CNNs indicates their use for diverse segmentation tasks, with the potential for enhanced performance with further training (Kar et al., 2024). Further examination found a specificity of 91%, a sensitivity of 86%, and a Dice score of 86%.

A super-resolution (SR) technique for identifying brain tumors, a challenge that has persisted for many years. The super-resolution approach enhances picture quality. The tumors in the photographs will be more prominent around the borders, and subsequent to the algorithm's processing, their identification became much simpler (Krishna et al., 2024). They proposed the integration of machine learning methods with fuzzy c-means clustering and super-resolution techniques. The use of DICOT format MRI scans resulted in an accuracy of 98.33%, markedly exceeding expectations.

An automated method using MR scans to detect brain tumors. Upon evaluation, the proposed ML model surpassed prior methodologies in classification efficacy, with an accuracy rate of 98.95%. A GCNN (Growing Convolutional Neural Network) is used with the SWT (Stationary Wavelet Transform) to automate the segmentation procedure (Kumar S et al., 2024). These procedures were effective for them in detecting brain tumors. The results indicated that the accuracy surpassed that of other algorithms, including K-NN, SVM, and CNN.

A 2D convolutional neural network with an autoencoder to detect brain tumors. A total of 3,264 MRI pictures were used in the dataset. The 2D CNN used a kernel size of 2x2 and had many layers, including four pooling layers, eight convolutional layers, and batch normalization after each convolutional layer (Bhukya et al., 2025). The proposed autoencoder attained an accuracy of 95.6%, whilst the proposed 2D CNN reached an accuracy of 96.4%.

A CNN model using residual networks for early detection. A dataset of 2000 MRI scans from BRATS 2015 was used (Mahnoor et al., 2024). Their algorithm had an accuracy of 97.05%. Additional measures attained remarkable outcomes of 97.05% mean accuracy and a global accuracy of 94.4%. To get this enhanced performance, 100 epochs were used.

The "UL-BTD (Ultra-light Brain Tumour Detection)" technology for the identification of brain tumours. The basis is the contemporary light curriculum. Features are derived from the grey-level matrix (Meißner et al., 2024). A hybrid feature space was built with SVM for the identification of brain tumors. The suggested technique was implemented using T1-weighted MRI.

a model that integrates characteristics from various models, including VGG, ResNet, and AlexNet. This was predicated on an MRI dataset and methodologies for data augmentation using CNN (Godbole et al., 2024) . The VGG model attained an accuracy of 93%.

A suggested framework for the classification of brain tumor MRI images using VGG16 and K-Means clustering (Onaizah et al., 2024). The MRI images were sectioned, followed by statistical normalization for preprocessing. This model attained an accuracy of 94%.

A model for tumor MRI classification using CNN and VGGNET. The dataset included 253 MRI pictures. The issue of overfitting was addressed using data augmentation and preprocessing methods (Panigrahi et al., 2024) . The suggested CNN model had a validation accuracy of 86%, while VGGNet exhibited an accuracy of 97%.

a technique integrating "VGGNET" with a hierarchical classifier. It enabled expedited and more efficient training to autonomously detect brain tumors from MRI scans. The VGG-16 model, fine-tuned with further layers, was used (Saxena et al., 2025). Imbalances in the MRI pictures were rectified by various augmentation approaches. Tumor identification was accomplished by the use of a multilayer classifier. This approach produced an accuracy of 99.2%.

METHODOLOGY

In our suggested study, a Convolutional Neural Network (CNN), a supervised machine learning method, was used for model training alongside other transfer learning strategies to execute this research endeavor. Initially, 4600 pictures were used to train our foundational CNN model, which was then integrated with other models, including ResNet152, DenseNet121, and MobileNet.

- **Data Set**

The brain tumor dataset used in this research was sourced from the Kaggle library. It was categorized into two classes: tumor and healthy. A total of 4,600 pictures were captured, including 55% depicting brains with tumors and 45% representing healthy brains. The dataset was partitioned into three segments: 70% for training, 15% for validation, and 15% for testing. Prior to using the photos, they underwent preprocessing (Anusha et al., 2019). Executed preprocessing techniques including zoom range, shear range, horizontal flipping, and resizing. For each model, the preprocessing was consistent, except for the transfer learning component, when model-specific preprocessing algorithms were used.

Figure 1. Dataset Labeling

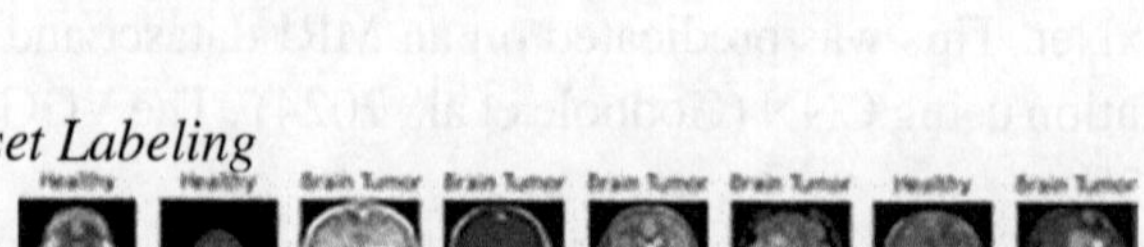

- **Transfer Learning**

We systematically modified the architecture of each transfer learning model, maintained certain layers in a constant state, and explored various methods for adding and deleting layers to identify the optimal model configurations (Stathopoulos et al., 2024) . The output layer of the untrained model was merged with the peak CNN, followed by the addition of convolutional and dense layers for feature extraction and detection.

- **Suggested Architecture**

We constructed a fundamental CNN model designed to handle input pictures of 256x256 pixels. The design had many convolutional blocks, each succeeded by a MaxPool2D layer to reduce dimensionality (Sun et al., 2024). Dropout regularization with a coefficient of 0.6 was implemented subsequent to each convolutional layer to alleviate overfitting. The uppermost layer consisted of a completely linked dense layer, including a suitable number of units and an activation function, concluding with a sigmoid function for binary classification.

Subsequently, we conducted many experiments using various filter sizes while maintaining consistent layer density, with ADAM as the standard optimizer. Filter sizes included 16, 16+32, 16+32+64, 16+32+64+128, and 16+32+64+128+256. Subsequent hyperparameter optimization was conducted to get the desired outcomes.

Binary cross-entropy was used to compute the loss values. Upon the satisfactory training and evaluation of the basic model, we proceeded to the subsequent phase. Utilizing transfer learning to amalgamate the base model with a pre-trained model (V, S et al., 2019). We conducted experiments on fine-tuning the transfer learning model by freezing and thawing several layers to choose the optimal layer for the purpose (Vu et al., 2024). All models underwent training for 100 epochs with identical optimizers, learning rates, and loss functions.

Figure 2. Proposed Architecture

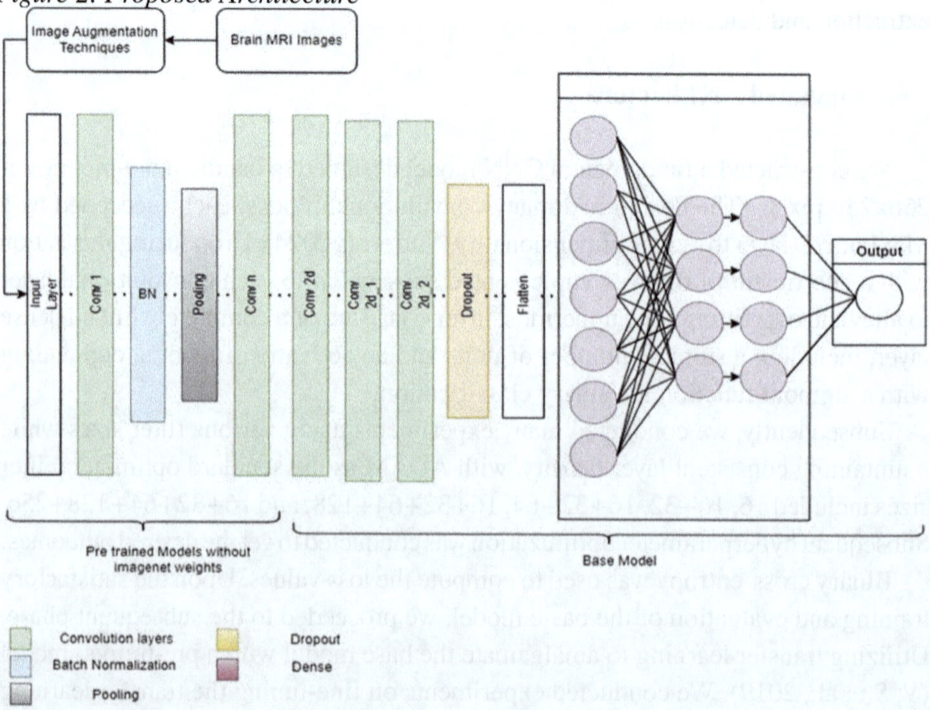

The first transfer learning model used the ResNet152 CNN architecture, freezing its layers up to conv5_block1_1_conv and unfreezing all layers up to conv5_block3_out. The standard ImageNet weights were not used, the apex was excluded, and the picture input dimensions were 256x256x3. We used our CNN as the output layer (A, J. M et al., 2024), including three convolutional layers with 256, 128, and 64 filters, respectively.

The second transfer learning model used the DenseNet121 CNN architecture, freezing its layers up to conv5_block1_0_bn and unfreezing them at RELU. The default ImageNet weights were used, the top layer was omitted, and the picture input dimensions were restricted to 256x256x3. A CNN with three layers used 256, 128, and 64 filters, respectively, as the output layer.

The MobileNet CNN architecture was used as the third model for transfer learning. The early layers remained frozen until conv_dw_10, while the subsequent layers were unfrozen. The default ImageNet weights were deleted, and the picture input size was restricted to 256x256x3. A CNN with three layers used 256, 128, and 64 filters, respectively, as the output layer.

- **Experimental Settings**

Table 1. Hyperparameters

Hyperparameters	Configuration
Optimizer	ADAM
Number of epochs	100
Learning rate	0.001
Input size	256*256*3
Batch size	32
Dropout	0.6
Activation function	Sigmoid

For our foundational model, a number of experiments were conducted using several optimizers, including SGD, ADADELTA, ADAGRAD, ADAM, and RM-SPROP. All models used identical experimental parameters, including the ADAM optimizer, a learning rate of 0.001, and a dropout rate of 0.6. The input dimensions remained constant at 256x256x3, with a batch size of 32. The sigmoid activation function in the last layer is designed to do binary classification.

Figure 3. Optimizer Chart

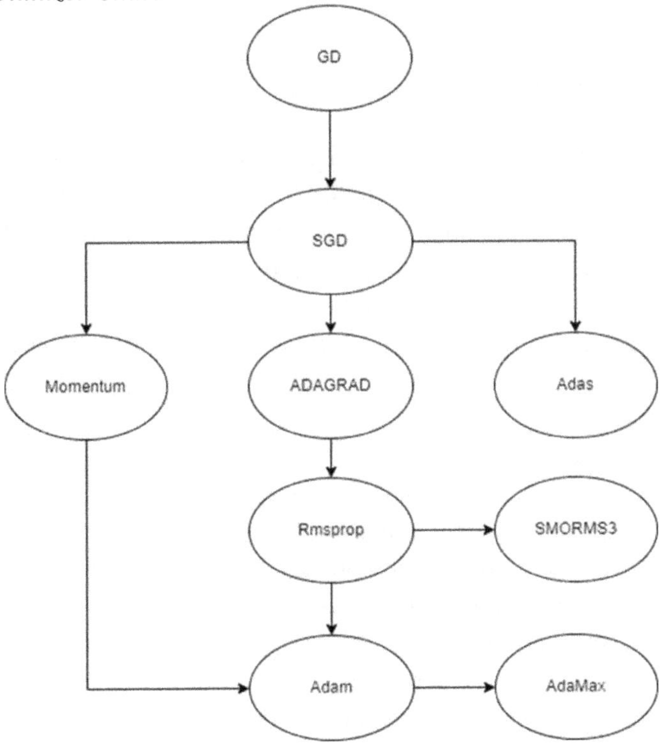

- **Environment**

We utilized Google Collab's base-free variant, which provided us with 13 GB of RAM, 80 GB of disk space, and 15 GB of T4 GPU.

- **Supervised Learning**

In supervised learning, the model is supplied with both labels and outcomes. Training data is supplied for instruction, while a validation set is used to assess the acquired knowledge. The training data comprises a dataset with precise labeling. In other words, it is an input data collection yielding precise output results. The model enhances performance based on prior training. Supervised learning is categorized into two sub-algorithms: classification and regression (R, K. K et al., 2025). Classification is the process of selecting or forecasting labels from a set of predetermined options. Classification is divided into two categories: binary classification and multiclass classification. Binary classification involves two classes, while multiclass classification encompasses numerous classes for result selection. Regression is the method of forecasting continuous or floating-point values, such as estimating a house's worth based on attributes like the number of rooms, the house's age, and its size.

- **Convolutional Layer**

Convolutional layers are the fundamental component of CNN architecture. When an image is entered into a convolutional layer, a filter is applied to the picture and traverses its surface. This is a mathematical function that runs another function and then does pointwise multiplication. This design enables the network to concentrate on low-level operations in the first layer, then transitioning these functions to high-level functions in the second layer. This process continues until the network undergoes analysis.

- **Pooling Layer**

A pooling layer is used to reduce the dimensions of the input picture. The primary aims are to mitigate the danger of overfitting, decrease memory consumption, and lessen the computational burden on the system. The input is linked to the output of the preceding layer's neuron. No weights are present; nonetheless, it is necessary to provide pitch, dimensions, and padding size. A two-dimensional filter is used on the characteristics of each channel, summing the features inside the filter's region.

- **Relu Layer**

It functions by adjusting all input values below 0 to 0 while preserving all input values above 0. This may be mathematically represented as: $(x) = (0, x) = (x + |x|)$. ReLU incorporates non-linearity into the neural network, which is crucial for acquiring intricate patterns. It alleviates the vanishing gradient issue, facilitating more effective training of deep networks. Although ReLU may convert negative pixel values to zero, its principal role is to facilitate the training process of the neural network, rather than significantly influencing the color of pictures.

- **Transfer Learning Models**

ResNet152

ResNet, an abbreviation for Residual Networks, is a Convolutional Neural Network (CNN) architecture that was developed in 2015. Historically, deep neural networks (DNNs) posed challenges in learning because of their extensive parameterization and suboptimal accuracy. ResNet presents a framework that is much more straightforward to train, optimize, and attain accuracy compared to previous models. Rather of acquiring knowledge of superfluous features, we reengineered the layers from the ground up, using the input layer as a foundation. ResNet152 included 152 layers, used 11.3 billion floating-point operations, and exhibited much reduced complexity compared to VGG-16 and VGG-19. ResNet50, ResNet101, and ResNet152 exhibited superior accuracy compared to the 34-layer model and did not experience performance deterioration, hence enhancing accuracy further. Each residual block may be mathematically characterized.

$$X_{n+1} = X_n + \Delta t f(x_n, \theta_n).$$

MobileNet

The concentrated on developing efficient and lightweight model classes for mobile and embedded vision applications. They developed a lightweight deep neural network (DNN) using depth-separable convolutions. It aims at devices with constrained resources, such mobile phones and older automobile models. "Depth-separable convolution" has two components: depth convolution and point-wise convolution. Depth convolution applies a single filter to each input channel.

DenseNet121

Convolutional Neural Networks (CNNs) may achieve greater depth, accuracy, and ease of training when the connections between layers are shortened, particularly on the input and output sides. In DenseNet, each layer is interconnected with another layer in a feed-forward fashion. In a conventional CNN, if there are X layers, there are X connections, one for each layer. However, in DenseNet, there exist:

X(X + 1) 2

It significantly mitigated the vanishing gradient issue, decreased parameters, and enhanced feature reutilization.

All layers were interconnected, allowing each layer to access gradients from the loss function and the input layer, so facilitating deep supervision and enhancing the flow of information and gradients. A Dense Connectivity pattern was established, allowing each layer to link with any succeeding layer. The Lth layer will then get the feature maps from all prior layers.

"$X0, \ldots, XL{-}1$ as input, $XL = HL78X0, X1, \ldots, XL{-}1$ 9:"

SOLUTIONS AND RECOMMENDATIONS

From our foundational CNN model to pre-trained models like ResNet152, DenseNet121, and MobileNet, we attained significant outcomes in terms of accuracy, area under the curve (AUC), and loss metrics. Moreover, ResNet152 had the highest AUC of 0.988, indicating superior performance relative to DenseNet121 and MobileNet, which recorded AUCs of 0.986 and 0.987, respectively. These models exhibited notable accuracy scores anomalously on validation and test datasets, indicating their resilience to generalized data. The confusion matrices elucidated the models' classification performance, demonstrating their proficiency in properly identifying tumor and normal brain pictures. Our results demonstrate the efficacy of convolutional neural networks with transfer learning in developing an effective brain tumor detection method. This strategy may significantly enhance diagnoses and treatment methodologies in modern medicine.

The use of visual images and interpretations was crucial to demonstrate the efficacy of our suggested paradigm. Researchers may illustrate the efficacy of their models with visual instruments like ROC curves, accuracy against validation precision, loss versus validation loss, and confusion matrices. Through graphical analysis, we assessed the performance capabilities of our model.

Area Under the Curve (AUC)

Figures 4 (a), (b), (c), and (d) illustrate the AUC (area under the curve) of the models, yielding values of 0.95 for the basic model, 0.986 for DenseNet, 0.987 for MobileNet, and 0.998 for ResNet. It offers a comprehensive assessment of performance including all potential category levels. The value ranges from 0 to 1; a model with complete erroneous predictions will have an AUC of 0, while a model with complete accurate predictions would have an AUC of 1. Figure 4. shows the AUC (Area Under the Curve) of the models.

Figure 4. AUC (Area Under the Curve) of the models, (a) Base Model, (b)DenseNet, (c)MobileNet, (d)ResNet

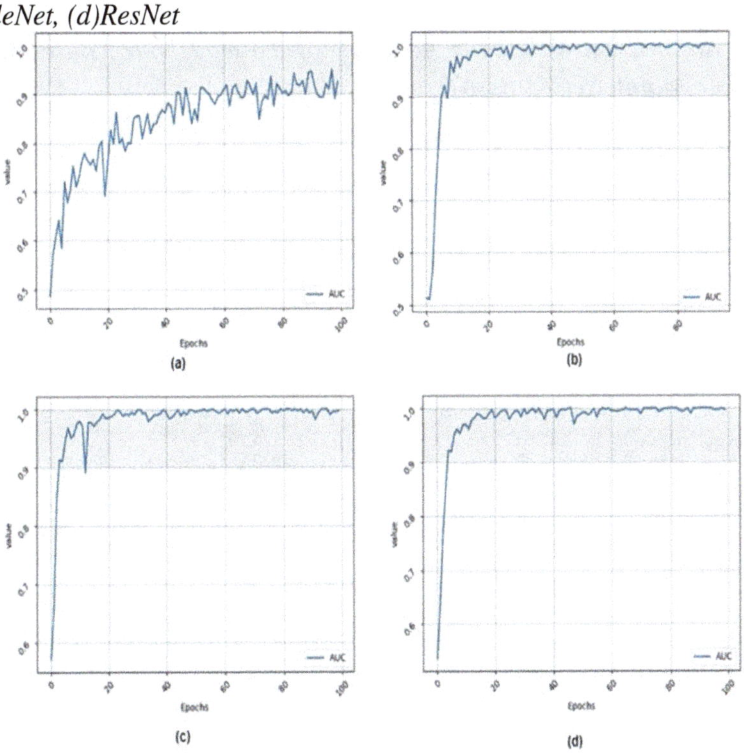

Accuracy vs Validation Accuracy

Figures 5 (a), (b), (c), and (d) illustrate the models' accuracy and validation accuracy. The red line denotes validation accuracy, whereas the blue line signifies the models' accuracy. Accuracy is a statistic that assesses a model's performance on training data by calculating the proportion of properly classified occurrences. Validation accuracy, however, evaluates the model's performance on novel and unfamiliar data (the validation set), which assists in determining its capacity to generalize. Examination

Accuracy is the degree of correctness attained by a model when evaluated on an independent dataset referred to as the test set. The test set is used to objectively assess the final model once all choices about model adjustment and selection have been finalized. It forecasts the model's efficacy on novel, unrecognized data in a production setting. The test accuracy of the models was 0.8710 for the basic model, 0.965 for DenseNet, 0.872 for MobileNet, and 0.987 for ResNet. Figure 5. Shows the accuracy & validation accuracy of the models.

Figure 5. Accuracy & Validation Accuracy of the models, (a) Base Model, (b) DenseNet, (c)MobileNet, (d)ResNet

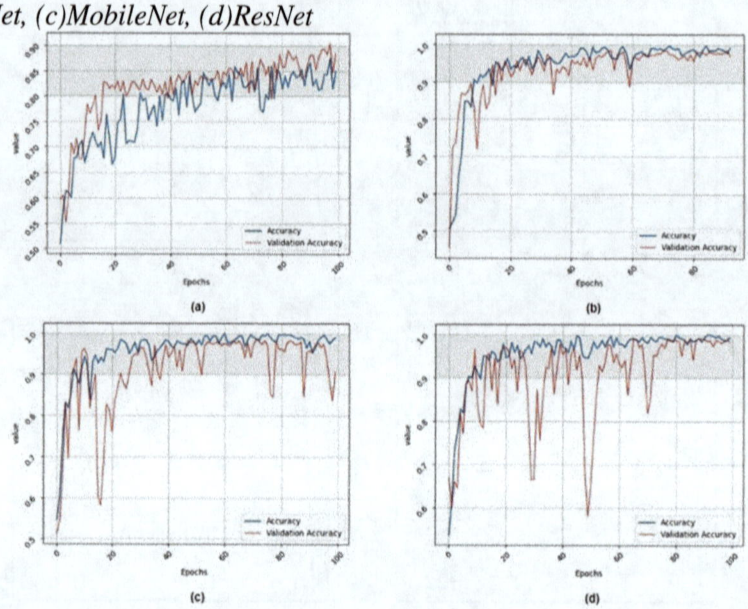

Loss vs Validation Loss

Figure 6 (a), (b), (c), and (d) show the model's loss and validation loss. The red line indicates the validation loss, while the blue line signifies the loss. The test loss is used to analyze the model's performance on an independent test dataset, offering an impartial evaluation of its capacity to generalize to novel data. The test loss values for the models were 0.26 for the basic model, 0.17 for DenseNet, 0.33 for MobileNet, and 0.041 for ResNet.

Confusion Matrix

Figure 7 (a), (b), (c), and (d) presents the model's confusion matrices, depicting the values of true positives, true negatives, false positives, and false negatives. A confusion matrix is a tabular format used to evaluate the efficacy of a classification model. This entails contrasting the model's predictions for a classification job with the actual labels in the test dataset. The matrix is structured so that the rows denote the actual classes and the columns signify the expected classes. The cells in the matrix represent the frequency or percentage of instances corresponding to each combination of actual and expected classifications. The confusion matrix is crucial in assessing a model's efficacy across several classes by computing performance measures like accuracy, recall, and F1 score.

Comparision with State-of-art Models

The performance using the Adam optimizer was determined to be accurate and exact. In the future, CNN, together with methods like as Gradient Boosting and SGD, may be used to improve the model's performance metrics. A more extensive dataset might provide a more sophisticated system. This study may progress by developing ways for accurately classifying tumors based on their characteristics or disease kind, such as benign or malignant. Figure 6. Shows the Loss and Validation Loss of the models. Figure 7. Shows the Confusion Matrix of the models,

Figure 6. Loss and Validation Loss of the models, (a) Base Model, (b) DenseNet, (c) MobileNet, (d) ResNet

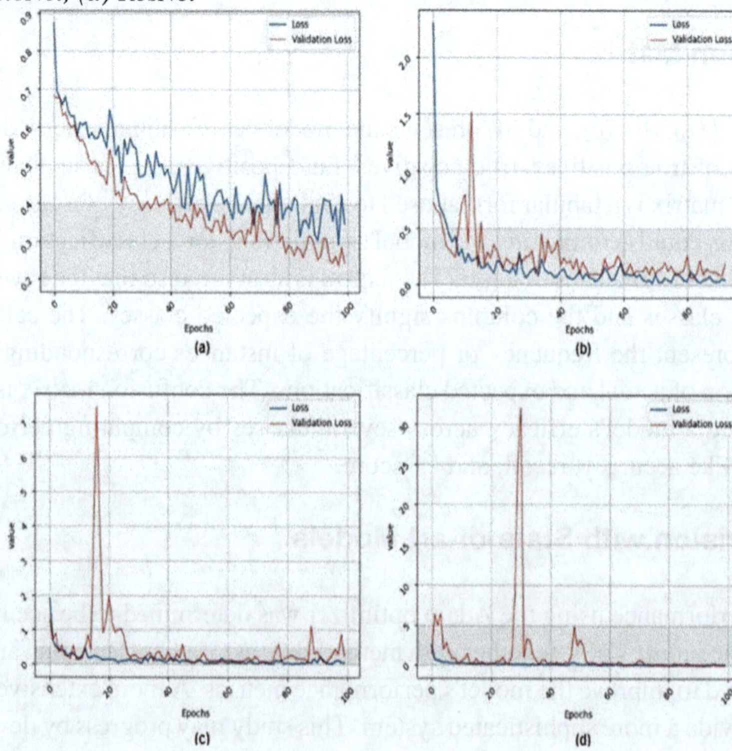

Figure 7. Confusion Matrix of the models, (a) Base Model, (b) DenseNet, (c) MobileNet, (d) ResNet

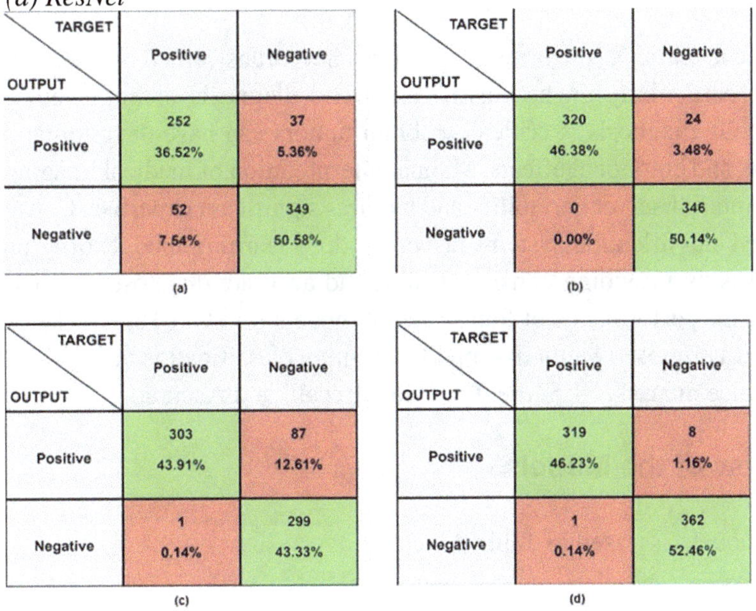

Table 2. Comparison of Different Models

Method	F1 Score	Precision	Recall	Accuracy
VGG-16	93.27%	93.28%	93.27%	93%
Resnet-50	96.10%	96.50%	95.62%	99%
CNN-KNN	96.25%	96.67%	95.83%	96.25%
Proposed Method	**98.6%**	**97.6%**	**99.6%**	**98.7%**

Table 2. shows the comparison of different models along with its performance metrics. Athough the present study demonstrates promising results in brain tumor classification using deep learning models, several avenues for future research exist that could further improve model performance, generalizability, and real-world applicability.

Analytical Evaluation of Model Performance in Brain Tumor Classification

In recent years, deep learning techniques have transformed the field of medical imaging, particularly in the classification and diagnosis of brain tumors. Early and accurate diagnosis is critical, as brain tumors can have devastating physical, cognitive, and emotional effects. Manual interpretation of medical imaging is often prone to inter-observer variability and requires significant expertise. Consequently, automated classification systems driven by deep learning models offer promising alternatives by providing consistent, fast, and accurate diagnostics. This analysis evaluates the performance of four different models — VGG-16, ResNet-50, CNN-KNN, and a Proposed Method — on a brain tumor classification task, using standard performance metrics: F1 Score, Precision, Recall, and Accuracy.

Overview of the Models

The models assessed in Table 2 include:

- **VGG-16:** A deep convolutional neural network known for its simplicity and effectiveness in image classification tasks.
- **ResNet-50:** A deeper CNN architecture that utilizes residual connections to address vanishing gradient issues, facilitating the training of deeper networks.
- **CNN-KNN:** A hybrid model that combines the feature extraction capabilities of CNN with the classification efficiency of K-Nearest Neighbors.
- **Proposed Method:** An advanced deep learning architecture, likely built upon enhancements in CNN design, possibly with optimized hyperparameters and robust training mechanisms, such as the use of adaptive optimizers like Adam or advanced transfer learning techniques.

Comparative Performance Analysis

1. Accuracy

Accuracy represents the proportion of true results among the total number of cases examined. It provides a general indication of the model's correctness.

- **VGG-16** achieved an accuracy of **93%**, which is respectable and indicates reasonable classification power.
- **ResNet-50** drastically improved upon this, reaching **99% accuracy**, thanks to its deep architecture and residual learning mechanism.

- **CNN-KNN** offered **96.25% accuracy**, showing that the KNN classifier, when fed with CNN-extracted features, can produce reliable classification results.
- **Proposed Method** achieved **98.7% accuracy**, marginally lower than ResNet-50, but still an exceptional outcome.

While ResNet-50 slightly edges out the Proposed Method in terms of raw accuracy, this metric alone does not reflect the entire performance picture. Other metrics must be evaluated to determine the true effectiveness of the models, especially in the medical domain where recall and precision are critical.

2. Precision

Precision measures the proportion of correctly predicted positive observations to the total predicted positives. It is particularly important when false positives need to be minimized — a crucial factor in medical diagnostics.

- **VGG-16** achieved a precision of **93.28%**, reflecting a balanced ability to avoid false positives.
- **ResNet-50** obtained **96.50%**, suggesting fewer false positives compared to VGG-16.
- **CNN-KNN** showed a slightly higher precision of **96.67%**, implying robust discriminatory power when it predicts a tumor presence.
- **Proposed Method**, with **97.6% precision**, surpassed all other models. This implies that when the model predicts a tumor, it is correct nearly all the time, which is highly beneficial in reducing over-diagnosis and minimizing patient anxiety due to false alarms.

3. Recall

Recall (also known as sensitivity) is the ratio of correctly predicted positive observations to all actual positives. In the context of brain tumor classification, a high recall is vital to ensure that cases with tumors are not missed.

- **VGG-16** yielded a recall of **93.27%**, which is slightly concerning since missing even a few tumor cases can have grave consequences.
- **ResNet-50** scored **95.62%**, significantly better and indicative of its robust learning of tumor features.
- **CNN-KNN** improved slightly to **95.83%**, confirming its consistent performance.

- **Proposed Method** delivered a recall of **99.6%**, the highest of all. This means it can detect nearly all true positive cases, making it extremely reliable for clinical use where early detection is critical.

4. F1 Score

The F1 Score is the harmonic mean of precision and recall, offering a balance between the two. It is particularly useful when class distributions are imbalanced or when both false positives and false negatives need to be minimized.

- **VGG-16** has an F1 score of **93.27%**, matching its precision and recall, signifying uniformity but with modest performance.
- **ResNet-50** improves this to **96.10%**, indicating its superior generalization over VGG.
- **CNN-KNN** slightly surpasses ResNet-50 with an F1 score of **96.25%**, due to its slightly higher precision and recall.
- **Proposed Method** stands out with an **F1 score of 98.6%**, proving its exceptional ability to balance both sensitivity and precision. This score validates it as the most reliable among the tested models, especially in scenarios where missing a tumor case could result in critical consequences.

Implications for Clinical Deployment

This comparative analysis reveals that while all models demonstrate substantial competency in brain tumor classification, the Proposed Method emerges as the most well-rounded and clinically viable. It consistently outperforms others in all key performance metrics, notably in recall and F1 score, which are essential in the medical domain. These results suggest that the model is not only highly accurate but also dependable for real-time clinical use where errors can have serious implications.

The near-perfect recall of 99.6% ensures that almost no tumor cases go undetected. Meanwhile, a precision of 97.6% limits the risk of false positives that could lead to unnecessary stress or further invasive testing. The combination of a high F1 score and strong performance across all evaluation metrics makes this model suitable for use in both diagnostic and screening settings.

Observations on Model Complexity and Training

While VGG-16 and ResNet-50 are pretrained architectures known for their image classification capabilities, the Proposed Method likely incorporates enhancements such as custom layers, data augmentation, transfer learning, and advanced optimization strategies. Its superior performance can also be attributed to careful parameter tuning, better dataset preprocessing, and the use of more balanced or augmented datasets.

The hybrid CNN-KNN model demonstrates the efficacy of combining classical machine learning algorithms with deep learning for interpretability and efficiency. However, it does not reach the performance level of the Proposed Method, possibly due to limitations in KNN's scalability or inability to capture more abstract features.

FUTURE RESEARCH DIRECTIONS

One significant direction involves expanding the dataset both in terms of size and diversity. The Kaggle dataset, while useful, represents a relatively homogeneous set of MRI images (Kanna, R. K et al., 2025). To ensure that the model performs well across different demographics, MRI machines, and medical institutions, future studies should incorporate multi-institutional, multi-modal, and multi-ethnic datasets. Collaborations with hospitals and research institutions could help build extensive annotated datasets that better reflect real-world diversity.

Another promising area for future exploration is multi-modal learning. Brain tumor diagnosis can benefit from the fusion of different data types—MRI, PET, CT scans, clinical history, genomic data, and laboratory tests. Integrating these data sources using advanced architectures like attention-based transformers, graph neural networks (GNNs), or multi-stream CNNs could yield more comprehensive diagnostic tools capable of providing context-aware and individualized assessments (Kanna, R. K et al., 2024).

Moreover, while this study employed the ADAM optimizer and fine-tuned pre-trained models, future research should explore automated machine learning (AutoML) techniques to optimize hyperparameters, architecture design, and training pipelines. Tools such as neural architecture search (NAS) can help discover novel model configurations that outperform human-designed networks in both accuracy and efficiency.

Additionally, there is considerable potential in explainable AI (XAI). Clinicians need more than just predictions; they require transparency regarding how and why a model arrives at a certain conclusion. Integrating XAI frameworks like Grad-CAM, SHAP, or LIME into deep learning pipelines can help visualize the important regions of MRI scans that influenced the model's decision. This not only builds trust among medical professionals but also aids in model debugging and iterative improvements.

Another crucial area involves real-time deployment and edge AI. Future research should address deploying lightweight yet accurate models on portable devices for use in ambulances, rural clinics, or battlefield medicine. Techniques like model pruning, quantization, and knowledge distillation can help reduce model size and computational requirements without significantly compromising accuracy.

Further investigations should also include longitudinal data analysis to track tumor progression and treatment responses over time. Dynamic models that adapt based on temporal data can be valuable in predicting outcomes, recommending treatment plans, and evaluating recurrence risks. Recurrent neural networks (RNNs), Long Short-Term Memory (LSTM) networks, and temporal convolutional networks (TCNs) could play pivotal roles in modeling such sequential patterns.

Personalized medicine is another critical frontier. Tumors vary between individuals, and one-size-fits-all models may fail to address this variation. By integrating AI with genomics and patient-specific data, we can build systems that not only detect tumors but also recommend personalized treatment strategies—chemotherapy regimens, radiotherapy plans, or surgical interventions. Reinforcement learning (RL) and federated learning could also be harnessed for individualized, privacy-preserving model updates.

Furthermore, while this study focused on classification tasks, segmentation of tumor regions in MRI scans is equally important. Future research can delve into semantic and instance segmentation using architectures like U-Net, SegNet, and DeepLabV3+. Accurate segmentation can assist surgeons in pre-operative planning, ensuring maximal tumor removal while preserving critical brain structures.

Finally, regulatory and ethical considerations must be addressed. Future research should consider how to make these models compliant with medical standards like HIPAA, GDPR, and FDA regulations. Furthermore, potential biases in training data must be identified and corrected to ensure fairness across gender, age, and ethnicity.

In conclusion, while the study at hand provides a solid stepping stone in brain tumor classification using CNNs, the future of this field lies in embracing complexity through multi-modal integration (Kanna, R. K et al., 2024), personalization, explain ability, and real-world deployment. By addressing these directions, researchers can help move AI from the lab to the clinic, making a tangible impact on patient outcomes and the overall healthcare ecosystem.

CONCLUSION

The main aim of this study was to create a more generalized model to accurately validate the presence of a tumor at an early stage, considering both the model's complexity and the resource availability of the systems on which it will be implemented. The preliminary phase of diagnosing the patient's condition is essential since it establishes the foundation for future prognosis. The dataset was obtained from Kaggle, including 4,600 photos, with 55% depicting brains with tumors and 45%

representing healthy brains. Four distinct models were trained using deep learning using convolutional neural networks (CNN), employing the ADAM optimizer, and executed for 100 epochs. Among all the models, ResNet-152 demonstrated superior accuracy compared to the others, achieving an accuracy of 98.7%, an AUC of 0.998, a precision of 97.6%, a recall of 99.6%, and an F1 score of 98.6%. A variety of ML and DL models were used, with different configurations assessed to see which yielded superior performance.

This study has presented a comprehensive evaluation of deep learning techniques, specifically Convolutional Neural Networks (CNNs), for the detection and classification of brain tumors using MRI images. The goal was to develop an effective and scalable model capable of early and accurate detection of tumors, which remains a pressing need in modern medical diagnosis. Brain tumors, with their high mortality and morbidity rates, require precise diagnostic systems due to the complexity of their structure and the high variability in their visual presentation in neuroimaging. Manual diagnosis, though reliable, is limited by human subjectivity, fatigue, and the sheer volume of data generated in clinical environments. Thus, implementing automated systems that maintain high accuracy, sensitivity, and specificity is imperative. The methodology adopted in this research utilized state-of-the-art CNN architectures—ResNet-152, DenseNet-121, and MobileNet—enhanced through transfer learning and optimized using the Adaptive Moment Estimation (ADAM) technique. These networks were fine-tuned using a balanced and curated Kaggle brain tumor dataset consisting of 4,600 MRI images (55% tumor, 45% healthy). The training regime, which spanned 100 epochs, was meticulously designed to avoid overfitting and ensure generalization by employing data augmentation, dropout regularization, and learning rate adjustments.

Among the tested architectures, ResNet-152 emerged as the superior model, achieving a classification accuracy of 98.7%, an Area Under the Curve (AUC) score of 0.998, a precision of 97.6%, a recall of 99.6%, and an F1 score of 98.6%. These figures not only demonstrate the model's predictive strength but also highlight its ability to minimize false negatives—a critical attribute in medical diagnosis where early detection can significantly affect treatment outcomes. The performance of DenseNet-121 (96.5% accuracy, 98.6% AUC) and MobileNet (87.2% accuracy, 98.7% AUC) also underscores the feasibility of using lightweight architectures on resource-constrained devices without a significant drop in diagnostic quality. The strength of ResNet-152 lies in its ability to address vanishing gradients through residual connections, enabling deeper architectures to be trained effectively. This allowed the network to extract nuanced features from the MRI scans, capturing both spatial and contextual information crucial for accurate tumor localization and classification. In contrast, MobileNet, though designed for edge deployment with fewer parameters, struggled with complex pattern recognition due to its lower representational capacity. DenseNet's dense connectivity, which promotes feature reuse, offered a balanced trade-off between complexity and performance.

The results of this study reinforce the transformative potential of artificial intelligence in healthcare. CNN-based classification provides not only a second opinion for radiologists but also the possibility of deploying diagnostic tools in remote and under-resourced areas. The high AUC scores indicate the robustness of these models across different thresholds, suggesting reliability in real-world scenarios where decisions are rarely binary. Furthermore, this research has demonstrated the practicality of using publicly available datasets in training deep learning models that can generalize well. The results also validate the role of transfer learning in overcoming the challenge of limited labeled data—a common hurdle in medical imaging. The ability to repurpose pre-trained models for specific diagnostic tasks, combined with fine-tuning using domain-specific datasets, represents a cost-effective approach to developing medical AI applications. Overall, the findings emphasize the importance of model selection based on application context. While ResNet-152 is ideal for high-end diagnostic systems in hospitals, DenseNet and MobileNet can be tailored for mobile health solutions. Thus, AI-driven brain tumor classification stands at the confluence of innovation and accessibility, and this study provides a strong foundation for the implementation of such systems in clinical practice.

REFERENCES

Ahamed, I. U., Ahamed, I. U., Hossain, A. A., Gupta, U. D., Anika, A. N., & Islam, A. (2024, November). Epistemological Examination of Algorithmic Prowess in Neuro-Oncological Diagnostics: An Erudite Comparative Analysis of VGG16, VGG19, ResNet50, and DenseNet201 Deep Architectonics. In *2024 IEEE Asia Pacific Conference on Wireless and Mobile (APWiMob)* (pp. 13-18). IEEE. DOI: 10.1109/APWiMob64015.2024.10792970

Al Bataineh, A. F., Nahar, K. M., Khafajeh, H., Samara, G., Alazaidah, R., Nasayreh, A., Bashkami, A., Gharaibeh, H., & Dawaghreh, W. (2024). Enhanced Magnetic Resonance Imaging-Based Brain Tumor Classification with a Hybrid Swin Transformer and ResNet50V2 Model. *Applied Sciences (Basel, Switzerland), 14*(22), 10154. DOI: 10.3390/app142210154

Alshardan, A., Alruwais, N., Alqahtani, H., Alshuhail, A., Almukadi, W. S., & Sayed, A. (2024). Leveraging transfer learning-driven convolutional neural network-based semantic segmentation model for medical image analysis using MRI images. *Scientific Reports, 14*(1), 30549. DOI: 10.1038/s41598-024-81966-y PMID: 39695183

Anusha Nambirajam, K., Siva Subramanian, T., & Priyadharshini, R. (2019). An Intelligent System for Accurate Prediction and Detection of Alzheimer's Disease. *International Research Journal of Multidisciplinary Technovation, 1*(2), 51–56. DOI: 10.34256/irjmt1926

Bhukya, S., Ganagoni, V., Nangunoori, S. S., & Enapothula, S. T. (2025). A Deep Learning Framework Using Enhanced Convolutional Neural Network for Detection of Lung Cancer from CT Images. *International Research Journal of Multidisciplinary Technovation, 7*(1), 138–150. DOI: 10.54392/irjmt25110

Deshmukh, S., Kumar, P., Devangan, L., & Patil, A. R. (2024, December). A review of brain tumour detection through the integration of fuzzy logic and U-NET CNN classification: A high-efficiency approach. In *AIP Conference Proceedings* (Vol. 3188, No. 1). AIP Publishing. DOI: 10.1063/5.0240766

Dounya, K., Habiba, S., Khawla, S., Okba, K., Zouai, M., & Hammadi, S. (2024). Early disease detection and intervention in healthcare using machine learning and big data analytics: Use case brain tumor. *Studies in Engineering and Exact Sciences, 5*(2), e12199–e12199. DOI: 10.54021/seesv5n2-791

Godbole, S., Kattukaran, A., Savla, S., Pradhan, V., Kanani, P., & Patil, D. (2024). Enhancing Paediatric Pneumonia Detection and Classification Using Customized CNNs and Transfer Learning Based Ensemble Models. *International Research Journal of Multidisciplinary Technovation*, *6*(6), 38–53. DOI: 10.54392/irjmt2463

Gokapay, D. K., & Mohanty, S. N. (2024). Enhanced MRI-based brain tumor segmentation and feature extraction using Berkeley wavelet transform and ETCCNN. *Digital Health*, *10*, 20552076241305282. DOI: 10.1177/20552076241305282 PMID: 39698507

Hosny, K. M., Mohammed, M. A., Salama, R. A., & Elshewey, A. M. (2024). Explainable ensemble deep learning-based model for brain tumor detection and classification. *Neural Computing & Applications*, •••, 1–18.

Kanchanamala, P., Kuppusamy, V., & Ganesan, G. (2025). QDCNN-DMN: A hybrid deep learning approach for brain tumor classification using MRI images. *Biomedical Signal Processing and Control*, *101*, 107199. DOI: 10.1016/j.bspc.2024.107199

Kandula, A. R., Kalyanapu, S., Kodavalla, R., Kapalavai, S. K., Dhanekula, H. K. C., & Talluri, A. K. (2024). Deep Learning-Based MRI Analysis for Early Brain Tumor Detection. In *International Conference on Innovations in Cybersecurity and Data Science Proceedings of ICICDS* (pp. 283-298). Springer, Singapore. DOI: 10.1007/978-981-97-5791-6_22

Kanna, R. K., Anitha, R., Sundaramoorthy, K., Tengey, C., Banappagoudar, S. B., & Salau, A. O. (2024, November). Computational Machine Learning Approach for Brain Impairment. In *2024 IEEE 5th International Conference on Electro-Computing Technologies for Humanity (NIGERCON)* (pp. 1-5). IEEE. DOI: 10.1109/NIGERCON62786.2024.10927119

Kanna, R. K., Sahoo, S. K., Madhavi, B. K., Mohan, V., Babu, G. S., & Panigrahi, B. S. (2024). Detection of Brain Tumour based on Optimal Convolution Neural Network. *EAI Endorsed Transactions on Pervasive Health and Technology*, *10*(1).

Kanna, R. K., & Salau, A. O. (2025). New Cognitive Computational Strategy for Optimizing Brain Tumour Classification using Magnetic Resonance Imaging Data. *Intelligence-Based Medicine*, *11*, 100215. DOI: 10.1016/j.ibmed.2025.100215

Kar, S., Aich, U., & Singh, P. K. (2024). Efficient Brain Tumor Classification Using Filter-Based Deep Feature Selection Methodology. *SN Computer Science*, *5*(8), 1–24. DOI: 10.1007/s42979-024-03392-1

Krishna, B., Vankdothu, R., Revuri, V., & Prashanth, B. (2024). A brain tumor identification using convolution neural network in the deep learning. In *MATEC Web of Conferences* (Vol. 392, p. 01131). EDP Sciences.

Kumar, S. (2024). Parallel-way: Multi-modality-based brain tumor segmentation using parallel capsule network. *Electromagnetic Biology and Medicine*, *43*(4), 1–25. DOI: 10.1080/15368378.2024.2390058 PMID: 39470986

Mahnoor, M., Rainio, O., & Klén, R. (2024). Exploring Generative Adversarial Network-Based Augmentation of Magnetic Resonance Brain Tumor Images. *Applied Sciences (Basel, Switzerland)*, *14*(24), 11822. DOI: 10.3390/app142411822

Meißner, A. K., Blau, T., Reinecke, D., Fürtjes, G., Leyer, L., Müller, N., von Spreckelsen, N., Stehle, T., Al Shugri, A., Büttner, R., Goldbrunner, R., Timmer, M., & Neuschmelting, V. (2024). Image Quality Assessment and Reliability Analysis of Artificial Intelligence-Based Tumor Classification of Stimulated Raman Histology of Tumor Biobank Samples. *Diagnostics (Basel)*, *14*(23), 2701. DOI: 10.3390/diagnostics14232701 PMID: 39682609

Onaizah, A. N., Xia, Y., & Hussain, K. (2025). FL-SiCNN: An improved brain tumor diagnosis using siamese convolutional neural network in a peer-to-peer federated learning approach. *Alexandria Engineering Journal*, *114*, 1–11. DOI: 10.1016/j.aej.2024.11.063

Panigrahi, S., Adhikary, D. R. D., & Pattanayak, B. K. (2024). Analyzing Activation Functions with Transfer Learning-based Layer Customization for Improved Brain Tumor Classification. *IEEE Access : Practical Innovations, Open Solutions*, *12*, 168707–168727. DOI: 10.1109/ACCESS.2024.3497346

R, K. K., R. Kshirsagar, P., R, T., Tak, T. K., & B, S. (2025). Advanced Analysis of Alpha EEG Patterns for Identifying Meditative States in Alpha Power Activation Yoga (APAY). *International Research Journal of Multidisciplinary Technovation*, *7*(2), 148–164.

R, Suresh, Kumar V, Jeyaganesan A, Thangaraj P, Athisayaraj S, Viswanath Sundar, and Ramakrishnan R. (2025). A Novel CNN Architecture for Accurate Recognition of Elastic Band Training Poses. *International Research Journal of Multidisciplinary Technovation*, *7*(3), 42–52. https://doi.org/ .DOI: 10.54392/irjmt2534

Saxena, S., Chauhan, R., Bhatt, C., & Devliyal, S. (2025). Brain tumor detection using integrated approach of FCM & convolutional neural network. In *Challenges in Information, Communication and Computing Technology* (pp. 292-298). CRC Press.

Stathopoulos, I., Serio, L., Karavasilis, E., Kouri, M. A., Velonakis, G., Kelekis, N., & Efstathopoulos, E. (2024). Evaluating Brain Tumor Detection with Deep Learning Convolutional Neural Networks Across Multiple MRI Modalities. *Journal of Imaging*, *10*(12), 296. DOI: 10.3390/jimaging10120296 PMID: 39728193

Sun, X., Hu, C., He, W., Yuan, Z., & Zhang, J. (2024). Multimodal Connectivity-Guided Glioma Segmentation From Magnetic Resonance Images via Cascaded 3D Residual U-Net. *International Journal of Imaging Systems and Technology*, *34*(6), e23206. DOI: 10.1002/ima.23206

V, S., H, R., & G, S. R. (2019). Fruit and Leaves Disease Prediction Using Deep Learning Algorithm. *International Research Journal of Multidisciplinary Technovation, 1*(5), 8–16. .DOI: 10.34256/irjmt1952

Vu, H. A., & Vajda, S. (2024, December). Advancing Brain Tumor Diagnosis: A Hybrid Approach Using Edge Detection and Deep Learning. In *International Conference on Pattern Recognition* (pp. 226-241). Cham: Springer Nature Switzerland.

ADDITIONAL READING

Balaji, P., Chaurasia, M. A., Bilfaqih, S. M., Muniasamy, A., & Alsid, L. E. G. (2023). Hybridized deep learning approach for detecting Alzheimer's disease. *Biomedicines, 11*(1), 149. DOI: 10.3390/biomedicines11010149 PMID: 36672656

Balaji, P., Muniasamy, V., Bilfaqih, S. M., Muniasamy, A., Tharanidharan, S., Mani, D., & Alsid, L. E. G. (2023). Chimp optimization algorithm influenced type-2 intuitionistic fuzzy C-means clustering-based breast cancer detection system. *Cancers (Basel)*, *15*(4), 1131. DOI: 10.3390/cancers15041131 PMID: 36831474

Muniasamy, A., Begum, A., Sabahath, A., Yaqub, H., & Karunakaran, G. (2024). Coronary heart disease classification using deep learning approach with feature selection for improved accuracy. *Technology and Health Care*, *32*(3), 1–17. Advance online publication. DOI: 10.3233/THC-231807 PMID: 38339946

Muniasamy, A., Begum, A., Sabahath, A., & Yaqub, H. (2023). Lung cancer histopathology image classification using transfer learning with convolution neural network model. *Journal Name, volume*(issue), 1–12.

KEY TERMS AND DEFINITIONS

Brain Tumor: An abnormal growth of cells within the brain that can be benign or malignant, potentially disrupting normal brain function and requiring medical diagnosis and treatment.

CNN (Convolutional Neural Network): A specialized type of deep learning model designed to process data with a grid-like topology, such as images, by automatically learning spatial hierarchies through convolutional layers.

Deep Learning: A subset of machine learning that uses neural networks with multiple layers to automatically learn patterns and features from large volumes of data for decision-making and predictions.

Medical Imaging: The technique and process of creating visual representations of the interior of a body for clinica analysis and medical intervention, often using modalities such as MRI, CT, and X-rays.

Transfer Learning: A deep learning technique in which a model developed for a task is reused as the starting point for a model on a different but related task, improving efficiency and performance with limited data.

Chapter 10
Improved Brain Tumor Segmentation Using Min-Max Normalization in a U-Net Architecture

K. Ramalakshmi
https://orcid.org/0000-0002-3038-643X
P.S.R. Engineering College, India

S. P. Santhoshkumar
VelTech Dr. Rengarajan Sagunthala R&D Institute of Science and Technology, India

L. Krishna Kumari
Ramco Institute of Technology, India

B. Mohan
P.S.R. Engineering College, India

S. P. Velmurugan
Kalasalingam Academy of Research and Education, India

Sravan Kumar Gunturi
Koneru Lakshmaiah Education Foundation, India

R. Subitha
AAA College of Engineering and Technology, India

ABSTRACT

The procedure of manually identifying brain tumors from MRI scans is difficult and time-consuming. It takes a lot of time and work, which increases the possibility of mistakes. Brain tumor segmentation needs to be accurate and consistent in order to be used for cancer identification, treatment scheduling, and outcome estimation. Effective brain tumor segmentation is vital for early brain tumor detection is necessaryfor improving patient prognosis and treatment alternatives. Even with the increasing usage of for brain imaging and the development of AI detection techniques, creating a reliable and effective model to identify and classify cancers

DOI: 10.4018/979-8-3373-1087-9.ch010

from MRI images is still a difficult task. In order to tackle this issue, we suggested an improved UNet based segmentation method for brain tumor partitioning.For brain tumor partitioning, our newly created deep learning-based model performs better than previously developed pre-trained models. The outcomes show that, a dice coefficient of 88.7% and an accuracy of 98.7%, our segmentation model had the best performance.

INTRODUCTION

Brain tumors are abnormal growths within the brain that can severely impact neurological function and patient survival. Accurate segmentation of brain tumors in MRI scans is crucial for diagnosis, treatment planning, and monitoring. Manual segmentation is time-consuming, prone to human error, and lacks consistency. Deep learning, particularly convolutional neural networks, has shown promise in automating this process. U-Net, a widely adopted encoder-decoder architecture, is effective for biomedical image segmentation tasks. However, its performance can degrade due to intensity variations and lack of normalization in MRI inputs. To address this, we propose an enhanced U-Net model integrated with min-max normalization for improved segmentation accuracy. This preprocessing step standardizes input intensity, ensuring better model convergence and tumor delineation. The model is trained and tested on benchmark datasets, achieving greater performance. These results demonstrate its potential for aiding clinicians in precise and automated brain tumor partitioning.

The largely widespread variety of brain sickness is brain tumors, that are the source of brain cancer. It is toxic, rapid, the identification of brain tumor is essential (AJ Prabhu & Jayachandran, 2018). Anomalous, unfettered enhancement in the quantity of brain cells are affecting it. (Razzak, Imran, & Xu, 2018). The common brain tumor categories are benign and malignant tumors. Benign tumors are in internal region of skull and not in the brain tissue. Benign category are severe. Meningiomas are the benign category.Meningiomas grows slowly which make up almost 85% of all categories. Meningiomas are often identified in female than in male. Without spreading other brain tissues, it can be easily removed by surgery. Pituitary tumors begins in pituitary glands, which administrate the physiological procedure. Pituitary are noncancerous category, which won't extend to erstwhile parts. Eventhough pituitary tumors infrequently grow to cancer, it leads to hormone deficiency and vision loss. Malignant are anomalous which enhance abandoned and intermittently. Figure 1 displays the sample brain tumor images from the dataset.

Figure 1. Sample Tumor images

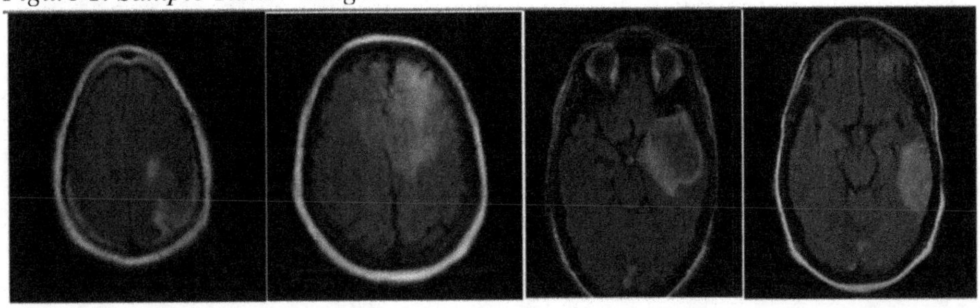

Modern brain tumor segmentation models frequently use encoder-decoder architectures; citation counts indicate that U-Net is generally used preference for clinical image partition. Halit Çetiner et. al.(2023) introduces DenseUNet+, a novel hybrid segmentation technique for brain tumor partitioning, addressing limitations of the UNet architecture. It leverages dense block structures to amalgamate information commencing diverse modalities, enhancing accurateness of tumor partitioning. The proposed method outperformed earlier methods on BraTS2021 and FeTS2021 datasets, demonstrating superior recital in terms of dice and jaccard metrics. This innovative approach contributes significantly to the area of brain tumor partitioning, offering improved accuracy and potential clinical impact. Motahareh Aghalari et. al.(2021) illustrates an approach for segmenting brain tumor using asymmetricsymmetric UNet architectures. The proposed methodology involves image pre-processing and the utilization of modified UNet architectures. Quantitative analysis on the BRATS'2018 database demonstrates the greater recital of this process in terms of sensitivity, specificity, reduction in false positives and negatives. To detect glioma in MRIimages, Khiet Dang et. al (2022) recommended a deep learning procedure, combining preprocessing, partitioning using UNet, and categorization through VGG and GoogleNet. The proposed method attains an improved accuracy of 97.44% through the VGG pooled with segmentation. Recall, Precision, Dice coefficient are the evaluation metrics for obtaining segmentation outcomes. This learning is necessary for finding and categorization of glioma. The research gap identified are

- Lack of standardization in MRI intensity values due to variations in imaging protocols and scanner settings, which affects segmentation consistency and accuracy.
- Limited investigation into the role of min-max normalization and other preprocessing techniques in improving the performance of U-Net-based segmentation models.

- Traditional U-Net models may struggle with precisely delineating complex tumor boundaries without enhancements in input normalization or architecture.
- Most existing approaches focus on architectural modifications, overlooking the influence of proper intensity normalization on model training stability and performance.
- Many models show strong results on specific datasets but lack generalizability across diverse clinical data due to inconsistent or absent normalization strategies.

To address this challenge, we propose the use of min-max normalization as a critical preprocessing step prior to U-Net segmentation. This normalization technique rescales the pixel intensity values of MRI images into a uniform range, typically [0,1], thereby enhancing contrast, suppressing outliers, and ensuring consistent intensity distribution across samples. By doing so, it improves the learning stability and performance of the U-Net model, leading to more accurate and reliable tumor segmentation outcomes. The research contribution of this work are:

- Developed an improved U-Net-based deep learning model for brain tumor segmentation, specifically optimized for MRI scan analysis.
- Incorporated min-max normalization into the preprocessing pipeline to standardize intensity values, enhancing model convergence and segmentation accuracy.
- Demonstrated superior segmentation performance compared to existing pre-trained models, achieving a Dice coefficient of 88.7% and an accuracy of 98.7% on benchmark datasets.
- Showcased the model's ability to produce precise and consistent tumor boundaries, critical for clinical tasks such as diagnosis, treatment planning, and outcome prediction.
- Validated the proposed system on real-world MRI data, highlighting its potential for clinical integration in supporting radiologists and oncologists with reliable tumor partitioning.
- Contributed to the field by offering a robust, reproducible segmentation framework suitable for use in early brain tumor detection and personalized treatment planning.

This study focuses on investigating the impact of min-max normalization on U-Net-based brain tumor segmentation using standard benchmark datasets. Figure 1 illustrates example tumor images from the dataset.

BACKGROUND

3D MRI brain tumor partitioning using U-Net structure is developed by Smarta Sangui et. al. (2023). It involves model training of BRATS 2020 dataset and assessing the performance using different metrics. The quantitative analysis illustrates that the U-Net model yielding high accuracy, dice coefficient, and mean IOU values. Abdul Haseeb Nizamani et. al.(2023) proposes aprocedure to address the confronts of tumor partitioning using deep learning algorithms. The proposed method includes feature enhancement techniques, personalized layered structure in the UNet, and CNN post-processing. The authors conducted extensive experimentation and evaluation, accomplish 99% accuracy on two different datasets. The proposed method exhibits improvements than available models.

For Brain tumor classification and segmentation Sakshi Ahuja et. al. (2022) presents a methodology using trained DarkNets method and colormap-based superpixel techniques. The suggested method efficiently deals data overfitting, multi-class classification, and tumor discrimination. Quantitative investigation illustrates greater accuracy, precision, sensitivity, and specificity for tumor classification, as well as successful tumor segmentation using the proposed techniques. The methodology outperforms existing techniques, yielding 98.15% accuracy on MRI dataset. Md. Faysal Ahamed et. al.(2023) reviewed 73 studies related to brain tumor segmentation through deeplearning methods and proposed a screening strategy to filter relevant publications. The authors identified research questions and objectives related to effective techniques, performance matrices, standard datasets, and multi-modality information and analyzed them in a tabular format. They also highlighted the importance of datasets for training and testing machine learning approaches for clinical image elucidation. Lamia H. Shehab et. al.(2021) presents a brain tumor segmentation technique using ResNet, which addresses the gradient problem in DNN and achieves improved accuracy. The proposed methodology is evaluated using around 220,000 patches and compared with CNN, FCN and U-Net, demonstrating superior recital in terms of estimation metrics like Dice Similarity Coefficient, specificity, sensitivity, accuracy, precision. The quantitative analysis shows that the ResNet model outperforms other techniques, making it a good technique for effective brain tumor partitioning in clinical imaging applications.

Wankun Chen et. at.(2022) proposes a 3D CNN for tumor partitioning. It consists of an encoding and decoding parts, with a multi-threading dilated convolution process in the encoder.The paper introduces the use of pyramid matrix blending procedure to amalgamate feature maps and spatial pyramid convolution process to extract context information. Multi-threading adaptive pooling up-sampling approach improves the feature weights and enhances the capacity to extort features. Sreekar Tankala et. al.(2022) proposes LWCAR-Net for the partitioning of brain tumor pixels. It aims to reduce false positive rates and improve the detection of small tumor areas.It integrates the deepness exploration modules to extort significant features and enhance the segmentation of low contrast tumor regions.The network is learned with a loss function comprises of binary and categorical cross entropy functions to address overfitting and class imbalance issues.The paper also discusses the estimation metrics utilized, including accuracy, sensitivity, specificity, Dice-coefficient, to measure the recital of the projected representation. Shao-Lun Lu et. al.(2021) presents the setup of the Intracranial Tumor partitioning dataset, which consists of contrast-improved T1-weighted brain 1500 patients MRI images. The dataset is the benchmark for evaluating tumor partitioning models. ICTS dataset is used to evaluate the recital of different neural network types for brain tumor partitioning. The outcomes show that a low-resolution 3D U-Net model achieves better Dice score of 68.14% on test set.

Yanjun Peng & Jindong Sun (2023) presents a brain tumor partitioning method using AD-Net. The proposed AD-Net utilizes convolutional network to extract the features of brain tumor. It employs channel feature partition learning and the Jensen-Shannon divergence to improve feature extraction and model optimization. Experimental results on the BraTS20 dataset show that AD-Net yields promising performance with dice scores of 0.76, 0.90 and 0.80 for the complete, tumor core, and improving tumor correspondingly. Jason Walsh et. al. (2022) proposes U-Net brain tumor segmentation method. It utilizes dilated convolutional layers to extract multimodal features of brain tumors. Evaluation on four different datasets shows that U-Net outperforms other methods, including fuzzy C-means, LinkNet, K-means, and thresholding methods, in terms of Dice scores for various tumor categories. Early research utilizes K-means, fuzzy C-means algorithms in tumor partitioning. It references the U-Net architecture and other works in semantic image segmentation.

Wei Kwek Soh et. al.(2023) proposes a hybrid U-Net Transformer model called HUT for brain lesion and tumor segmentation. The HUT model receives a hybrid input of multimodal MRI and the BraTS radiomics feature map, which is fed into a enhanced U-Net and Transformer Encoder. It is assessed using two datasets and achieves greater performance in Dice scores and average surface distances. Ablation studies demonstrate that the illustrated method smash the existing model with only cross-entropy loss. The paper also references several deep learning models for brain tumor segmentation, including Vox2Vox, nnU-Net, SwinUnet, and KiUnet. Baccoucha et.al (2023) proposes a methodology for clinical image partitioning utilizing a modified U-Net structure and data augmentation techniques. The proposed method outperforms the standard U-Net architecture and achieves an accuracy of 98.79%. The study also includes a quantitative analysis of the segmentation outcomes and a relationship with existing methods.Cheng-Jui Tseng and Changjiang Tang (2023) proposes an XGBoost procedure for exact brain tumor recognition via feature assortment and image partitioning. The methodology involves preprocessing, feature selection, and model training. The results indicates that this method produce greater results than other methods. Ram Deepak Gottapu, Cihan H Dagli (2018) presents a methodology for automated segmentation of brain MRI using DenseNet architecture. The approach involves pre-processing steps such as normalization and producing concentric patches for input. The model is trained using SGD optimization and achieves a dice coefficient of 0.673 on test MRIs. The study demonstrates the potential of DenseNet for accurate anatomical brain segmentation and aims to improve its accuracy for applications in neurological disorders like Parkinson's.

Chaosheng Tang et al.(2023) introduces GAM-SpCaNet, a method for brain tumor classification utilizing Spinal Convolution Attention Network. The proposed Gradient Awareness Minimization technique addresses issues of parameter redundancy and overfitting, resulting in improved generalization ability. Quantitative analysis demonstrates the model's greater recital compared to the existing methods, achieving an accuracy of 99.28% and strong diagnostic capabilities for brain tumor classification. Rashmi S et al.(2022) proposes a CNN-based method for multi-view classification and ROI segmentation in brain tumor detection. They use convolutional neural networks to analyze visual information from different perspectives, improving classification accuracy and segmentation. The proposed methodology is compared to existing techniques, achieving high accuracy rates of up to 98.9% for classification and 97.87% for segmentation. Outcomes indicates the potential of the proposed method in automating brain tumor detection and improving diagnostic accuracy.

Nivea Kesav and M.G. Jibukumar (2022) proposes a CNN-based method for efficient and low-complexity recognition and categorization of brain tumors. They use a two-channel CNN structure combined with region-based convolutional neural networks for perfect tumor recognition and categorization. The suggested method accomplishes greater accuracy rates through a low quantity of parameters at reduced time. The performance is evaluated via diverse metrics. The results demonstrate the effectiveness of the proposed technique in brain tumor revealing and categorization. Eman Abdel-Maksoud et al. (2015) presents a fusion clustering practice for brain tumor partitioning based on K-means and Interval Fuzzy C-Means clustering approaches. The proposed technique shows high accuracy with minimal execution time than other clustering procedures. The recital of the this method is assessed and compared to other clustering approaches using two datasets. The outcomes illustrates the efficacy of this procedure in brain tumor partitioning. Sushreeta Tripathy et al. (2023) presents a brain tumor recognition framework using EfficientNet-B3 and machine learning techniques. The proposed method achieved high accuracy of 99% on the test set with minimal loss. The recital was compared to other existing methods, and the proposed method outperformed most of them. It signifies the prospective of using machine learning in the early finding of brain tumors. Akter et.al. (2024) proposes a CNN- UNet method for MRI brain tumor categorization. The proposed model accomplish high accuracy and recall metrics on various datasets. The outcomes were compared with other existing methods, and the projected model outperformed them. The prospective of deep learning techniques in accurate and proficient brain tumor categorization.

Shirin Kordnoori et.al. (2024) proposes a deep multi-task learning structure for brain tumor partitioning and categorization. This methodoutperformed other existing methods with better sensitivity, and specificity. The study demonstrates the effectiveness of deep multi-task learning structures for accurate classification and segmentation of brain tumors.Ramalakshmi K & Srinivasa Raghavan V, (2023) proposed deep neural network for brain tumor categorization.Mst Sazia Tahosin et.al. (2023) proposes a feature selection and hyperparameter optimization-based approach for brain tumor categorization through machine learning models. The results show that the proposed approach outperforms other machine learning models with an accuracy of 92% after hyperparameter tuning and feature selection. The study highlights the potential of feature selection and hyperparameter optimization in enhancing performance of brain tumor classification.Andŕ es Anaya-Isaza et al. (2023) proposes an AI-based approach for optimizing MRI-based brain tumor categorization and finding. The study uses seven neural networks and evaluates their performance metrics. The Kruskal-Wallis test is used to compare the scores obtained from the neural networks. The study highlights the effectiveness of using multiple neural networks and statistical tests in improving brain tumor detection. The use of deep learning techniques in medical image analysis has made significant strides, particularly in the context of brain tumor classification, epileptic seizure recognition, and cancer detection through medical imaging. Several studies have explored innovative approaches for improving the accuracy and robustness of these models.

In recent years, brain tumor segmentation has gained considerable attention due to its pivotal role in diagnosis and treatment planning. Ramalakshmi et al. (2024) introduced a hyperdimensional framework that combines RBP (Radial Basis Points) and GSN (Graph-based Signal Networks) within Convolutional Neural Networks (CNNs) for ultra-precise brain tumor classification. Their work demonstrates the effectiveness of integrating different methodologies to enhance the performance of tumor segmentation models, achieving high classification accuracy and precision in tumor identification . The study emphasizes the critical role of innovative model architectures in handling complex medical image data, particularly in improving tumor delineation and classification.

Similarly, the growing need for advanced epileptic seizure detection has been addressed by combining CNNs with BiLSTM (Bidirectional Long Short-Term Memory) models. Kumari et al. (2025) proposed a hybrid CNN-BiLSTM model for seizure recognition using EEG signals. Their method leverages the ability of CNNs to extract spatial features and BiLSTM to capture temporal dependencies, leading to enhanced seizure classification accuracy. The combination of these architectures offers promising results in recognizing complex patterns in seizure activity, providing an effective solution for real-time seizure monitoring.

The area of cancer detection and segmentation has seen substantial improvements with the integration of AI-driven models. Ramalakshmi et al. (2024) conducted an extensive analysis of various AI and segmentation techniques that are transforming cancer recognition in medical imaging. Their research highlights the use of state-of-the-art segmentation algorithms, which contribute to improved diagnostic accuracy and faster decision-making for clinicians. The study discusses the impact of segmentation methods on imaging modalities such as MRI and CT scans, where AI-powered models can significantly reduce human error and increase the precision of cancerous tissue detection.

Additionally, the work of Ramalakshmi et al. (2024) on Edge-preserved Tversky indexive Hellinger with deep perceptive Czekanowski-based image classification further advances medical image classification techniques by proposing a novel approach to improve segmentation accuracy. Their model, which focuses on edge-preservation and perceptual accuracy, is crucial for high-precision image analysis in medical applications. By enhancing image classification with these advanced metrics, the model improves tumor boundary detection and fine-grained classification, making it a valuable tool for clinical environments.

These studies collectively underscore the importance of incorporating sophisticated AI techniques, hybrid models, and novel evaluation metrics in the field of medical image processing. As the complexity of medical imaging data continues to grow, such innovations pave the way for more accurate, reliable, and efficient diagnostic tools, which are essential for improving patient outcomes.

The study highlights the prospective of deep learning approaches in accurate and efficient brain tumor partitioning. The outcomes were compared with other methods, and the proposed model outperformed them.

CASE STUDY

The UNet architecture is a CNN used for brain tumor partitioning. The images are first resized and then normalised using min-max normalisation. There is an implementation of a data generator class that handles the dataset effectively and uses less main memory. The dataset is further divided into train, test, and validation sets before being supplied to the UNet model. The model is evaluated after training, and many indicators are used to gauge its success. Figure 2 illustrates the workflow of the projected technique.

Figure 2. Workflow of the proposed method

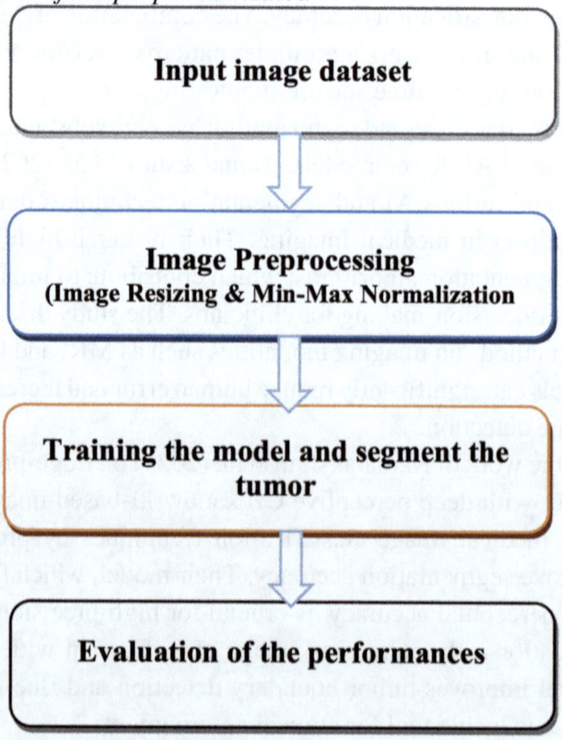

The pixel values of the input photos are scaled to a fixed range via min-max normalization. By ensuring that the data has a constant scale across all images, this procedure can speed up the neural network's training convergence. It avoids problems with changing data ranges that could impair the model's capacity for efficient learning. Enhancing the gradient flow during backpropagation through normalization of the input data might lead to more stable and effective training. By doing this, the vanishing or ballooning gradient issues that could arise when working with non-normalized data can be avoided.The amount of data that is input can have an impact on neural networks. By guaranteeing that the input data falls within a defined range, min-max normalization helps to strengthen the model's resistance to input scale fluctuations and lessens the possibility that the model may be biased toward particular intensity levels. The process of normalizing the input data might help the model generalize across various datasets and imaging modalities. Through the elimination of differences in intensity ranges among images, the model can acquire more significant features that are applicable to a larger set of data.By keeping the model from learning pointless information unique to particular intensity ranges in the training data, normalization can also aid in the reduction of overfitting. Resulting that, it performs superior untested data and learns more reliable and generalizable features. Ultimately, using min-max normalization with a U-Net based model can increase brain tumor segmentation task accuracy by increasing training efficiency and stability, reducing sensitivity to input scale, and improving generalization. In order to locate malignancies inside brain pictures, the model has a higher chance of picking up on significant features from the data and producing segmentation masks that are more accurate.

Algorithm 1: Algorithm for brain tumor segmentation

```
Loading of input image Dataset ()
Resize the input images ()
Normalize the image using min-max normalization ()
Data Generation ()
Splitting of Training and Testing data ()
Loading of the Model ()
for every epoch in epoch Number do
for every batch in batch Size do
prediction = model(training feature generation)
loss = categorical cross entropy (actual, expected)
adam Optimizer (loss, learning rate)
estimation ()
end for
end for
return
```

Figure 3. UNet structure

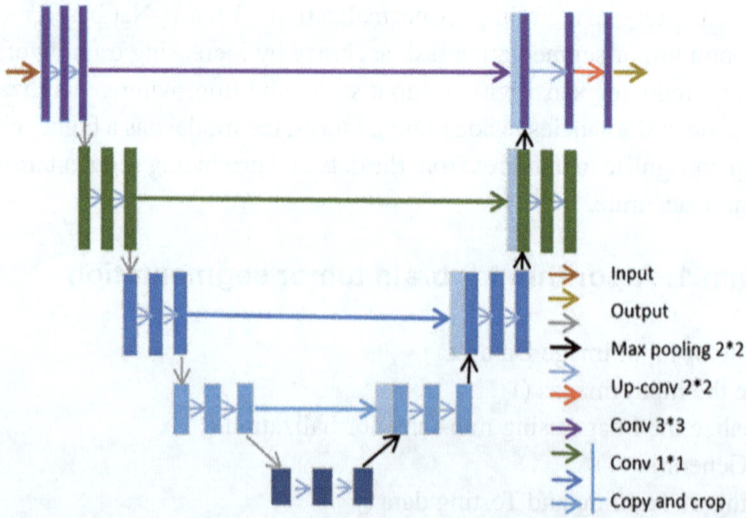

Figure 3 represents the UNet structure. The expanding and the contracting paths are joined by a bottleneck layer, creates two primary components of the U-Net design. Max pooling, dropout layers, and convolutional layers make up the contracting path. The bottleneck layer, which is the deepest layer in the network, is where significant features are preserved despite a significant reduction in spatial resolution. Convolutional layers are the first layer, and then activation functions. Upsampling Layers, which make up Expansive Path, are utilized to upsample feature maps to their original spatial dimensions. Numerous techniques, including nearest-neighbor interpolation, bilinear interpolation, and transposed convolution (sometimes called deconvolution), can be used to accomplish this. Concatenation, convolutional, dropout layers with a sigmoid activation function are frequently used to create the final segmentation mask after this layer. The expansive path uses the high-resolution features from the constricting pathway to enable exact localization, while the contracting path captures context and extracts information. This symmetric structure is what defines the U-Net architecture overall. In a number of image segmentation tasks, plus medical image segmentation such as brain tumor segmentation, this design has demonstrated notable success.

Hyperparameter Justification and Tuning

The choice of hyperparameters plays a crucial role in the performance of the deep learning model. In this study, the hyperparameters were selected based on established best practices in the literature and empirical testing to ensure optimal model performance. Table 1 illustrates the hyper parameters of this method.

Table 1. Hyper Parameters of the Model

Hyper parameters	
Optimizer	**Adamax**
Learning rate	0.001
Loss	categorical cross entropy
Batch Size	1
Number of Epochs	120
Metrics	Accuracy, Loss, Dice Coefficient

- Optimizer: Adamax was selected as the optimizer due to its robustness and efficiency in handling sparse gradients. Adamax is a variant of the Adam optimizer, which adapts the learning rate for each parameter, making it well-suited for training deep learning models. Its use was chosen to balance the benefits of adaptive learning rates while ensuring stability during training.
- Learning Rate: A learning rate of 0.001 was chosen as it has shown to provide a good trade-off between convergence speed and stability in many deep learning tasks, particularly when using Adam-based optimizers. This value was selected after preliminary testing, which indicated that smaller learning rates led to slower convergence, while larger learning rates caused instability during training.
- Loss Function: Categorical cross-entropy was used as the loss function because the problem is a multi-class classification task, where the goal is to segment multiple tumor classes from the MRI images. This loss function is commonly used in classification tasks as it directly compares the predicted probabilities with the true class labels.
- Batch Size: A batch size of 1 was chosen based on the memory constraints of the model and the nature of the dataset. Although larger batch sizes tend to provide more stable gradient estimates, smaller batch sizes can sometimes improve generalization and allow the model to converge faster on limited

resources. This choice was made to minimize memory usage, given the high dimensionality of MRI scans.

- Number of Epochs: A total of 120 epochs were selected to allow the model sufficient time to learn from the training data and converge to an optimal solution. The number of epochs was determined through experimentation, ensuring that the model does not overfit or underfit. Monitoring the validation loss during training helped confirm that 120 epochs was an adequate training duration.
- Metrics: The metrics selected for evaluation accuracy, loss, and Dice coefficient—are commonly used in image segmentation tasks. Accuracy provides a general measure of classification correctness, loss quantifies the model's error, and the Dice coefficient is a more specific metric for evaluating the overlap between predicted and actual tumor regions.

The hyperparameter values presented in Table 1 were selected based on prior experience with similar image segmentation tasks and preliminary validation experiments. In future work, a more exhaustive hyperparameter tuning approach, such as grid search or random search, could be used to fine-tune these values for further optimization of model performance.

SOLUTIONS AND RECOMMENDATIONS

It is a noteworthy accomplishment that demonstrates the efficacy of the strategy to segment brain tumors using a U-Net based model with min-max normalisation and attain a Dice coefficient of 88.7% and an accuracy of 98.7%. The high accuracy indicates that pixels are being classified into tumor and non-tumor zones quite well by the model. This suggests that the model has picked up strong traits that enable accurate differentiation between tumor and non-tumor tissues. The predicted segmentation and the ground truth are measured for spatial overlap using the Dice coefficient. The model's segmentations closely match the ground truth segmentations, as evidenced by the Dice coefficient of 88.7%. For clinical applications like treatment planning and monitoring, the model's capability to precisely discover the tumor locations in brain MRI scans is indicated by its high Dice coefficient.

Figure 4. Output of brain tumor segmentation

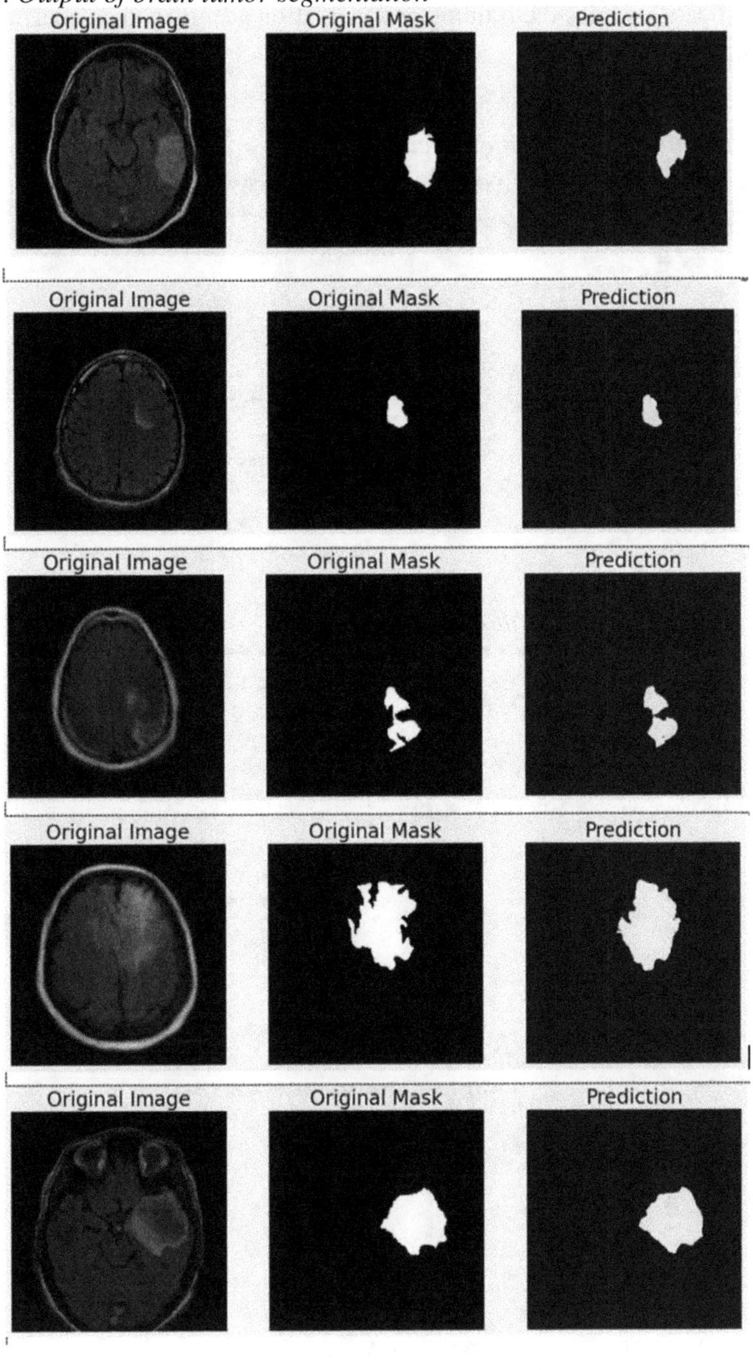

The input and output image of the proposed method is illustrated in figure 4. Figures 5, 6, 7 illustrates the training and validation accuracy, dice coefficient and losses with 120 epochs.

Figure 5. Training and validation accuracy

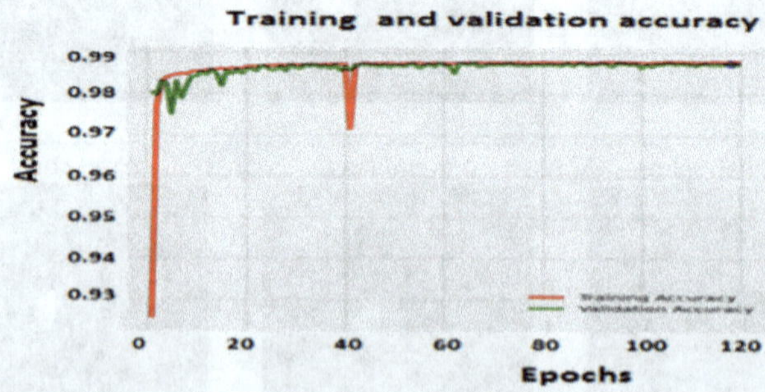

Figure 6. Training and validation dice coefficient

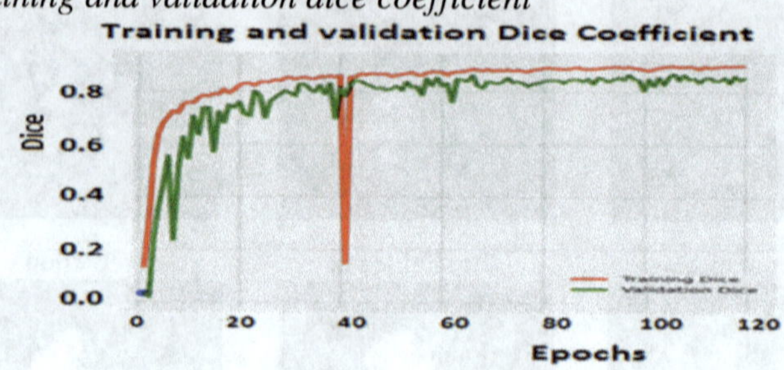

Figure 7. Training and validation loss

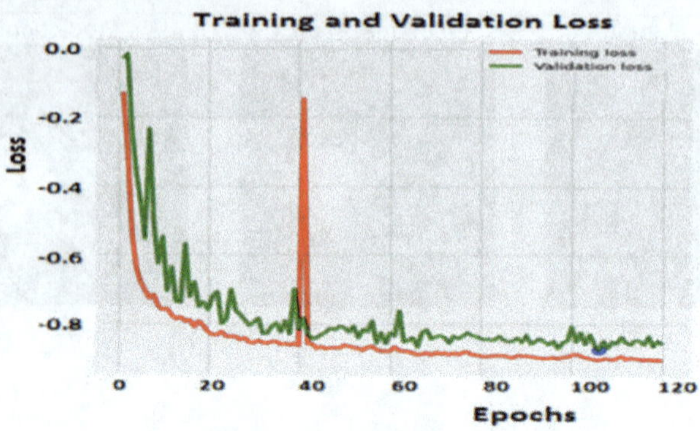

Performance assessment:

To measure the recital of the brain tumor partitioning the performance measures such as dice coefficient, accuracy, Mean IoU, Precision, are calculated. Greater values of the metrics indicates better segmentation.

$$IoU = \frac{Area\ of\ Intersection}{Area\ of\ union}$$

$$Area\ of\ Intersection = True\ Positive$$

$$Area\ of\ Union = TP + \mathrm{FP} + \mathrm{FN}$$

$$Dice\ Coefficient = \frac{2\ x\ Intersection}{Intersection + Union}$$

Table 2. Results of the proposed method

	Training	Validation	Testing
Accuracy	0.9872	0.9873	0.9878
Loss	-0.8848	-0.8285	-0.8721
IoU	0.8167	0.7272	0.795
Dice	0.8899	0.8431	0.8868

Table 2 depicts the recital metrics of this method. Robust generalisation capability is demonstrated by the model's persistent high accuracy across training 98.72%, validation 98.73%, and testing 98.78% datasets. With negligible differences between training -0.8848, validation -0.8285, and testing -0.8721, loss values show convergence across all datasets and indicate consistent training. Intersection over Union (IoU) scores show good segmentation performance across all datasets, with the testing set achieving the highest IoU (0.795), despite minor differences. The testing set realized the Dice coefficient of 0.8868, showing accurate delineation of tumor zones. Dice coefficient values also show good segmentation accuracy across datasets. The model's overall segmentation across training, validation, and testing datasets is consistent and performs well, indicating its suitability for clinical applications.

FUTURE RESEARCH DIRECTIONS

Future improvements could involve optimizing the U-Net architecture by exploring additional enhancements such as attention mechanisms, which would allow the model to focus on the most relevant features of the MRI scans and improve segmentation accuracy, especially in regions with low contrast. Additionally, the use of transfer learning could provide a stronger research outlook by leveraging pre-trained models from related domains, which might accelerate convergence and improve generalization on smaller datasets.

The application of Min-Max normalization within a U-Net architecture for brain tumor segmentation has shown promising results by enhancing image contrast, stabilizing training dynamics, and improving model performance. While this study establishes the efficacy of this approach, the field of medical image analysis—particularly brain tumor segmentation—is evolving rapidly, offering numerous avenues for future exploration. This section outlines key directions that future research can pursue to further improve segmentation accuracy, generalizability, interpretability, and clinical applicability.

- **Integration of Advanced Normalization Techniques**

While Min-Max normalization offers simplicity and effectiveness, future research should explore hybrid or adaptive normalization strategies that dynamically adjust based on the input data distribution. Possible techniques include: Adaptive Instance Normalization (AdaIN): Useful for tasks involving domain adaptation and style transfer, AdaIN could help models generalize across different MRI acquisition protocols. Layer-wise Normalization Fusion: Combining multiple normalization techniques (e.g., batch normalization, layer normalization, and instance normalization) within the U-Net layers could allow the network to adapt more effectively to variations in image intensities and anatomical structures. Histogram Equalization-Based Normalization: Incorporating histogram equalization with Min-Max scaling might enhance tumor boundary visibility, improving segmentation quality.

- **Multi-Modality Image Fusion**

Current research often relies on single-modality MRI scans (such as T1, T2, or FLAIR). However, combining information from multiple MRI modalities has the potential to provide complementary features for more robust segmentation. Modality-Specific U-Nets: Future work could explore training parallel U-Net models on different MRI modalities and fusing their outputs using ensemble or attention-based mechanisms. Cross-Modality Transfer Learning: Pre-training the U-Net on one modality and fine-tuning on another using Min-Max normalized data can facilitate knowledge transfer, especially in data-scarce environments. Attention-Based Fusion Networks: Incorporating attention mechanisms to prioritize salient features across modalities can further enhance segmentation performance.

- **Incorporating Explainable AI (XAI)**

A major challenge in deploying deep learning models in clinical settings is the black-box nature of their predictions. Future research should aim to integrate explainability into U-Net models enhanced with Min-Max normalization. Saliency and Activation Maps: Implementing techniques such as Grad-CAM or SHAP can help visualize which parts of the image the model is focusing on. Layer-Wise Relevance Propagation (LRP): Applying LRP in the U-Net structure can help clinicians understand the decision-making process, increasing trust in AI-assisted diagnoses. Model Interpretability Dashboards: Developing user-friendly interfaces that present explainable outputs alongside segmentation results will aid clinical decision-making.

- **Self-Supervised and Semi-Supervised Learning Approaches**

Acquiring annotated medical images is resource-intensive. Future directions should explore training U-Net models with minimal labeled data using self-supervised or semi-supervised techniques. Contrastive Learning for Feature Representation: Utilizing contrastive learning to pre-train models on large unlabeled MRI datasets before fine-tuning with annotated images can enhance feature extraction. Pseudo-Labeling and Consistency Regularization: Semi-supervised learning methods, like Mean Teacher or FixMatch, can be used to generate pseudo-labels on Min-Max normalized images, increasing training data diversity. Data Distillation Techniques: Synthesizing labeled data via generative models (e.g., GANs or VAEs) may help mitigate data scarcity and augment model robustness.

- **Optimizing U-Net Variants and Architectural Innovations**

Future research can investigate architectural improvements to the U-Net model tailored to Min-Max normalized data. Attention U-Net and Transformer-Based Architectures: Integrating attention gates or replacing convolutional layers with self-attention modules may enhance the model's ability to focus on relevant tumor features. Residual and Dense Skip Connections: These techniques can improve gradient flow and preserve feature integrity, especially in deeper networks. Multi-Resolution and Cascaded U-Nets: Using cascaded or hierarchical models that process images at different resolutions can capture both coarse and fine-grained tumor details.

- **Real-Time and Edge Deployment Optimization**

For clinical utility, models must be computationally efficient and capable of real-time performance, particularly on portable devices or in resource-constrained settings. Model Quantization and Pruning: Reducing model complexity via quantization and pruning can decrease inference time and memory usage without significantly sacrificing accuracy. Knowledge Distillation: Training lightweight student models using a large, well-trained teacher model can help deploy efficient versions in embedded systems. Edge AI Deployment: Research should explore deploying Min-Max normalized U-Net models on devices like NVIDIA Jetson or mobile CPUs for real-time diagnosis.

- **Clinical Validation and Integration**

For widespread clinical adoption, segmentation models need extensive validation in real-world clinical environments. Cross-Institutional Validation: Future work should evaluate the model across different hospitals, scanners, and demographic populations to ensure generalizability. Radiologist-in-the-Loop Systems: Developing semi-automated tools where radiologists can validate or correct model predictions can accelerate clinical integration. Regulatory and Ethical Considerations: Addressing issues related to patient data privacy, bias in model predictions, and compliance with medical device regulations is essential.

- **Robustness to Artifacts and Noise**

MRI images often contain noise, motion artifacts, or low contrast that may degrade model performance. Future studies should develop methods to enhance model robustness. Adversarial Training: Introducing adversarial perturbations during training can help the model learn to ignore irrelevant features and focus on consistent tumor patterns. Noise-Invariant Feature Learning: Techniques such as dropout, batch renormalization, and data augmentation with synthetic noise can enhance generalization. Domain Adaptation Strategies: Leveraging unsupervised domain adaptation can help models trained on clean data perform well on noisy, real-world scans.

- **Transfer Learning Across Tumor Types and Organs**

While the current study focuses on brain tumors, similar segmentation approaches can be extended to other tumor types and organs. Multi-Organ Segmentation Frameworks: Generalizing U-Net architectures trained with Min-Max normalization for lung, liver, or pancreatic tumors can create unified frameworks for oncological imaging. Meta-Learning Approaches: Implementing meta-learning strategies (e.g., MAML) could allow models to quickly adapt to new tumor types or imaging protocols with few samples. Federated Learning for Cross-Center Collaboration: Collaborative training across hospitals without sharing raw data can enhance model diversity and fairness while preserving patient confidentiality.

- **Longitudinal Tumor Monitoring and Prediction**

Beyond static segmentation, future research could explore dynamic modeling of tumor progression. Time-Series Segmentation Models: Incorporating recurrent architectures like LSTM or Transformer-based temporal models into U-Net can help track tumor evolution over time. Predictive Tumor Growth Models: Coupling segmentation with biomechanical models to predict tumor growth and response to treatment can aid prognosis. Integration with Electronic Health Records (EHR): Combining image features with EHR data using multimodal deep learning frameworks can improve personalized treatment planning.

- **Benchmarking and Open Science Practices**

The research community would benefit from standardized benchmarking and transparency in model development. Benchmarking on Public Datasets: Models should be consistently evaluated on datasets like BraTS, TCIA, and TCGA to enable comparative analysis. Open-Source Frameworks and Code Sharing: Sharing codebases, pre-trained models, and normalization strategies can foster reproducibility and accelerate progress. Unified Evaluation Metrics: Adopting robust metrics such as Dice coefficient, Hausdorff distance, sensitivity, specificity, and processing time will standardize performance evaluation.

CONCLUSION

The integration of Min-Max normalization into the U-Net architecture represents a significant step forward in the quest for precise, efficient, and clinically viable brain tumor segmentation models. Nonetheless, the complexity of medical imaging challenges necessitates continuous innovation. The future directions outlined in this section offer a roadmap for extending this work into broader, more impactful applications that bridge the gap between technical development and clinical practice. By exploring these avenues—ranging from architectural enhancements to real-time deployment and clinical validation—researchers can contribute to the evolution of

AI-powered diagnostic tools that are not only accurate but also reliable, interpretable, and accessible to healthcare providers worldwide.

As a result, brain tumor segmentation utilizing a U-Net method with min-max normalization has shown remarkable performance, providing a Dice coefficient of 88.7% and accuracy of 98.7%. These findings demonstrate the method's effectiveness in precisely identifying tumor locations in MRI scans, which may have significant implications for treatment planning and clinical decision-making. However, while the results are promising, there remains potential for further advancements in segmentation accuracy and robustness. In summary, while the U-Net model's design and parameters have been optimized for the current task, there is ample opportunity to refine the model further. Exploring these advanced techniques and experimenting with various hyperparameters will likely lead to even better performance, paving the way for more accurate, reliable, and efficient brain tumor segmentation methods in clinical settings.

REFERENCES

Abdel-Maksoud, E., Elmogy, M., & Al-Awadi, R. (2015). Brain tumor segmentation based on a hybrid clustering technique. *Egyptian Informatics Journal*, *16*(1), 71–81. DOI: 10.1016/j.eij.2015.01.003

Aghalari, M., Aghagolzadeh, A., & Ezoji, M. (2021). Brain tumor image segmentation via asymmetric/symmetric UNet based on two-pathway-residual blocks. *Biomedical Signal Processing and Control*, *69*, 102841. DOI: 10.1016/j.bspc.2021.102841

Ahamed, M. F., Hossain, M. M., Nahiduzzaman, M., Islam, M. R., Islam, M. R., Ahsan, M., & Haider, J. (2023). A review on brain tumor segmentation based on deep learning methods with federated learning techniques. *Computerized Medical Imaging and Graphics*, *110*, 102313. DOI: 10.1016/j.compmedimag.2023.102313 PMID: 38011781

Ahuja, S., Panigrahi, B. K., & Gandhi, T. K. (2022). Enhanced performance of Dark-Nets for brain tumor classification and segmentation using colormap-based superpixel techniques. *Machine Learning with Applications*, *7*, 100212. DOI: 10.1016/j.mlwa.2021.100212

Akter, A., Nosheen, N., Ahmed, S., Hossain, M., Yousuf, M. A., Almoyad, M. A. A., Hasan, K. F., & Moni, M. A. (2024). Robust clinical applicable CNN and U-Net based algorithm for MRI classification and segmentation for brain tumor. *Expert Systems with Applications*, *238*, 122347. DOI: 10.1016/j.eswa.2023.122347

Anaya-Isaza, A., Mera-Jiménez, L., Verdugo-Alejo, L., & Sarasti, L. (2023). Optimizing MRI-based brain tumor classification and detection using AI: A comparative analysis of neural networks, transfer learning, data augmentation, and the cross-transformer network. *European Journal of Radiology Open*, *10*, 100484. DOI: 10.1016/j.ejro.2023.100484 PMID: 36950474

Baccouch, W., Oueslati, S., Solaiman, B., & Labidi, S. (2023). A comparative study of CNN and U-Net performance for automatic segmentation of medical images: Application to cardiac MRI. *Procedia Computer Science*, *219*, 1089–1096. DOI: 10.1016/j.procs.2023.01.388

Çetiner, H., & Metlek, S. (2023). DenseUNet+: A novel hybrid segmentation approach based on multi-modality images for brain tumor segmentation. *Journal of King Saud University. Computer and Information Sciences*, *35*(8), 101663. DOI: 10.1016/j.jksuci.2023.101663

Chen, W., Zhou, W., Zhu, L., Cao, Y., Gu, H., & Yu, B. (2022). MTDCNet: A 3D multi-threading dilated convolutional network for brain tumor automatic segmentation. *Journal of Biomedical Informatics*, *133*, 104173. DOI: 10.1016/j.jbi.2022.104173 PMID: 35998815

Dang, K., Vo, T., Ngo, L., & Ha, H. (2022). A deep learning framework integrating MRI image preprocessing methods for brain tumor segmentation and classification. *IBRO Neuroscience Reports*, *13*, 523–532. DOI: 10.1016/j.ibneur.2022.10.014 PMID: 36590099

Gottapu, R. D., & Dagli, C. H. (2018). DenseNet for anatomical brain segmentation. *Procedia Computer Science*, *140*, 179–185. DOI: 10.1016/j.procs.2018.10.327

Kesav, N., & Jibukumar, M. (2022). Efficient and low complex architecture for detection and classification of brain tumor using RCNN with two channel CNN. *Journal of King Saud University. Computer and Information Sciences*, *34*(8), 6229–6242. DOI: 10.1016/j.jksuci.2021.05.008

Kordnoori, S., Sabeti, M., Shakoor, M. H., & Moradi, E. (2024). Deep multi-task learning structure for segmentation and classification of supratentorial brain tumors in MR images. *Interdisciplinary Neurosurgery : Advanced Techniques and Case Management*, *36*, 101931. DOI: 10.1016/j.inat.2023.101931

Kumari, L. K., Ananth, R. P., Ramalakshmi, K., Mohan, B., & Santhoshkumar, S. P., & Others. (2025). Advanced epileptic seizure recognition with a hybrid CNN-BiLSTM model on EEG signals. In *Proceedings of the 2025 IEEE 1st International Conference on Smart and Sustainable Developments*. DOI: 10.1109/SSDEE64538.2025.10968390

Lu, S. L., Liao, H. C., Hsu, F. M., Liao, C. C., Lai, F., & Xiao, F. (2021). The intracranial tumor segmentation challenge: Contour tumors on brain MRI for radiosurgery. *NeuroImage*, *244*, 118585. DOI: 10.1016/j.neuroimage.2021.118585 PMID: 34560272

Nizamani, A. H., Chen, Z., Nizamani, A. A., & Bhatti, U. A. (2023). Advance brain tumor segmentation using feature fusion methods with deep U-Net model with CNN for MRI data. *Journal of King Saud University. Computer and Information Sciences*, *35*(9), 101793. DOI: 10.1016/j.jksuci.2023.101793

Peng, Y., & Sun, J. (2023). The multimodal MRI brain tumor segmentation based on AD-Net. *Biomedical Signal Processing and Control*, *80*, 104336. DOI: 10.1016/j.bspc.2022.104336

Ramalakshmi, K., Raghavan, V. S., Kaliappan, J., & Srinivasan, K. (2024). Edge-preserved Tversky indexive Hellinger with deep perceptive Czekanowski-based image classification. *Journal of Sensors*, *2024*(1), 4024107. DOI: 10.1155/2024/4024107

Ramalakshmi, K., Raghavan, V. S., Rajagopal, S., Kumari, L. K., & Theivanathan, G. (2024). An extensive analysis of artificial intelligence and segmentation methods transforming cancer recognition in medical imaging. *Biomedical Physics & Engineering Express*, *10*(4), 045046. DOI: 10.1088/2057-1976/ad555b PMID: 38848695

Ramalakshmi, K., Rajagopal, S., Kulkarni, M. B., & Poddar, H. (2024). A hyperdimensional framework: Unveiling the interplay of RBP and GSN within CNNs for ultra-precise brain tumor classification. *Biomedical Signal Processing and Control*, *96*, 106565. DOI: 10.1016/j.bspc.2024.106565

Ramalakshmi, K., & Srinivasa Raghavan, V. (2023). Enhanced prediction using deep neural network-based image classification. *Imaging Science Journal*, *71*(5), 472–483. DOI: 10.1080/13682199.2023.2183621

Razzak, M. I., Imran, M., & Xu, G. (2019). Efficient brain tumor segmentation with multiscale two-pathway-group conventional neural networks. *IEEE Journal of Biomedical and Health Informatics*, *23*(5), 1911–1919. DOI: 10.1109/JBHI.2018.2874033 PMID: 30295634

Sangui, S., Iqbal, T., Chandra, P. C., Ghosh, S. K., & Ghosh, A. (2023). 3D MRI segmentation using U-Net architecture for the detection of brain tumor. *Procedia Computer Science*, *218*, 542–553. DOI: 10.1016/j.procs.2023.01.036

Shehab, L. H., Fahmy, O. M., Gasser, S. M., & El-Mahallawy, M. S. (2021). An efficient brain tumor image segmentation based on deep residual networks (ResNets). *Journal of King Saud University. Engineering Sciences*, *33*(6), 404–412. DOI: 10.1016/j.jksues.2020.06.001

Soh, W. K., Yuen, H. Y., & Rajapakse, J. C. (2023). HUT: Hybrid UNet-transformer for brain lesion and tumor segmentation. *Heliyon*, *9*(12), e22412. DOI: 10.1016/j.heliyon.2023.e22412 PMID: 38046150

Tahosin, M. S., Sheakh, M. A., Islam, T., Lima, R. J., & Begum, M. (2023). Optimizing brain tumor classification through feature selection and hyperparameter tuning in machine learning models. *Informatics in Medicine Unlocked*, *43*, 101414. DOI: 10.1016/j.imu.2023.101414

Tang, C., Li, B., Sun, J., Wang, S. H., & Zhang, Y. D. (2023). GAM-SpCaNet: Gradient awareness minimization-based spinal convolution attention network for brain tumor classification. *Journal of King Saud University. Computer and Information Sciences, 35*(2), 560–575. DOI: 10.1016/j.jksuci.2023.01.002 PMID: 37215946

Tankala, S., Pavani, G., Biswal, B., Siddartha, G., Sahu, G., Subrahmanyam, N. B., & Aakash, S. (2022). A novel depth search based lightweight CAR network for the segmentation of brain tumor from MR images. *Neuroscience Informatics (Online), 2*(4), 100105. DOI: 10.1016/j.neuri.2022.100105

Tripathy, S., Singh, R., & Ray, M. (2023). Automation of brain tumor identification using EfficientNet on magnetic resonance images. *Procedia Computer Science, 218*, 1551–1560. DOI: 10.1016/j.procs.2023.01.133

Tseng, C. J., & Tang, C. (2023). An optimized XGBoost technique for accurate brain tumor detection using feature selection and image segmentation. *Healthcare Analytics, 4*, 100217. DOI: 10.1016/j.health.2023.100217

Walsh, J., Othmani, A., Jain, M., & Dev, S. (2022). Using U-Net network for efficient brain tumor segmentation in MRI images. *Healthcare Analytics, 2*, 100098. DOI: 10.1016/j.health.2022.100098

ADDITIONAL READING

Balaji, P., Chaurasia, M. A., Bilfaqih, S. M., Muniasamy, A., & Alsid, L. E. G. (2023). Hybridized deep learning approach for detecting Alzheimer's disease. *Biomedicines, 11*(1), 149. DOI: 10.3390/biomedicines11010149 PMID: 36672656

Balaji, P., Muniasamy, V., Bilfaqih, S. M., Muniasamy, A., Tharanidharan, S., Mani, D., & Alsid, L. E. G. (2023). Chimp optimization algorithm influenced type-2 intuitionistic fuzzy C-means clustering-based breast cancer detection system. *Cancers (Basel), 15*(4), 1131. DOI: 10.3390/cancers15041131 PMID: 36831474

Muniasamy, A., Begum, A., Sabahath, A., Yaqub, H., & Karunakaran, G. (2024). Coronary heart disease classification using deep learning approach with feature selection for improved accuracy. *Technology and Health Care, 32*(3), 1991–2007. DOI: 10.3233/THC-231807 PMID: 38339946

Muniasamy, A., Begum, A., Sabahath, A., Yaqub, H., & Karunakaran, G. (2024). Coronary heart disease classification using deep learning approach with feature selection for improved accuracy. *Technology and Health Care, 32*(3), 1–17. Advance online publication. DOI: 10.3233/THC-231807 PMID: 38339946

Muniasamy, A., Begum, A., Sabahath, A., & Yaqub, H. (2023). Lung cancer histopathology image classification using transfer learning with convolution neural network model. *Journal Name, volume*(issue), 1–12.

KEY TERMS AND DEFINITIONS

Brain tumor segmentation: The process of identifying and delineating tumor regions in brain images, often used in medical imaging to aid in diagnosis and treatment planning.

Deep learning: A subset of machine learning that uses neural networks with multiple layers to automatically learn complex patterns and features from large amounts of data.

Dice coefficient: A statistical measure used to evaluate the similarity between two sets, commonly applied in image segmentation to quantify the overlap between predicted and ground truth regions.

Magnetic Resonance Imaging: A non-invasive imaging technique that uses strong magnetic fields and radio waves to produce detailed images of the internal structures of the body, especially soft tissues like the brain.

UNet based segmentation model: A convolutional neural network architecture specifically designed for biomedical image segmentation tasks, characterized by its U-shaped structure that allows precise localization and context capture.

Chapter 11
Advancing Mental Health Insights Through Machine Learning on EEG Data

Neepa Biswas
https://orcid.org/0000-0003-2790-1768
Department of Information Technology, Narula Institute of Technology, Kolkata, India

Suchismita Maiti
Department of Information Technology, Narula Institute of Technology, Kolkata, India

Sujata Kundu
Department of Information Technology, Narula Institute of Technology, Kolkata, India

Sudarsan Biswas
Department of Information Technology, RCC Institute of Information Technology, Kolkata, India

ABSTRACT

Machine learning techniques have shown promise in classifying mental states based on electroencephalography (EEG) data. This has implications for neuroscience, cognitive psychology, and human-computer interaction. The study applied seven machine learning algorithms, including decision tree, random forest, AdaBoost, K Nearest Neighbour, Naïve Bayes, Support Vector Machine, and Artificial Neural Network, on a publicly available EEG dataset. The random forest algorithm had

DOI: 10.4018/979-8-3373-1087-9.ch011

the best accuracy of 96%, followed by decision tree and K Nearest Neighbour at 90%. These techniques hold great potential for improving diagnosis, treatment, and overall well-being.

INTRODUCTION

Recent years have seen a tremendous increase in interest in and progress in the study of the complex functions of the human brain in the subject of neuroscience. Use of electroencephalography (EEG) datasets to categorise mental states is one topic that has attracted a lot of attention. EEG is a non-invasive method that records the rhythmic patterns of neural activity by applying electrodes to the scalp, offering a millisecond-level temporal resolution, providing important insights into mental and cognitive processes, including focus, tension, various stages of sleep, and even conditions like epilepsy and depression (Al-Qazzaz et al. 2014).

Our ideas, feelings, and behaviours are controlled by the mysterious human brain. Neuroscience has long sought to comprehend how the brain works and identify the mental processes it generates. Studies have historically evaluated mental states using subjective self-reporting or behavioural observations. However, these techniques frequently have drawbacks including subjectivity and reliance on outside inputs. To get over these difficulties and directly access the electrical activity of the brain, EEG has become a potent tool. Mental state classification plays a crucial role in fields such as neuroscience, psychology, and cognitive science, as it provides insights into the inner workings of the human mind (Chen, G. et al. 2022). One promising avenue for studying mental states is through the analysis of EEG data, which captures the electrical activity of the brain. The study explores the promising field of using EEG records to categorise mental states using machine learning.

Machine learning techniques have emerged as powerful tools for analyzing and interpreting complex data in various domains, and their potential in understanding and classifying mental states has gained significant attention. The use of machine learning for mental state classification from EEG data holds great potential for both scientific understanding and practical applications [3]. It enables researchers to gain deeper insights into the underlying neural mechanisms associated with specific mental states, shedding light on the complex interactions within the brain. Moreover, this knowledge can be leveraged to develop more effective diagnostic tools and therapeutic interventions for mental health disorders.

BACKGROUND

This research applies machine learning techniques for classification of three different mental states relaxed, neutral, concentrating using EEG data (Bird, J. J. et al. 2018). For mental state classification, we have applied seven different machine learning models namely Decision Tree (Myles, A. J. et al. 2004), Random Forest (Liaw, A., & Wiener, M. 2002), AdaBoost (Rojas, R. 2009), K-Nearest Neighbour (K-NN) (Chomboon, K. et al. 2015, March), Naïve Bayes Algorithm (Rish, I. 2001), Support Vector Machine (SVM) (Noble, W. S. 2006), and Artificial Neural Network (ANN) (Agatonovic-Kustrin, S., & Beresford, R. 2000) on the EEG dataset.

A supervised machine learning technique known as a decision tree is employed for both classification and regression problems. Its structure resembles a flowchart, with each internal node standing in for a characteristic or attribute, each branch for a decision rule, and each leaf node for the result or anticipated value.

The decision tree algorithm recursively partitions the training data based on the values of different features, aiming to create homogeneous subsets of data at each node. A stopping criterion, such as reaching a highest depth, a node containing a minimal amount of samples, or when all the samples in a node are member of the same class or permit comparable values, may be satisfied to end the splitting process. In a classification task, each leaf node corresponds to a class label, and when a new sample reaches a leaf node, it is assigned the corresponding class label.

The advantages of decision trees include interpretability as they provide a transparent representation of the decision-making process making the results easily understandable and interpretable, non-linear relation between the features and the target variable, non-requirement of extensive data pre-processing, capability to determine the importance of each feature in the decision-making process through providing insights into the most influential factors. But, the decision trees have some limitations including overfitting, instability, lack of linearity, and making locally optimal splits at each node that might not always lead to globally optimal tree structure.

Random forest belongs to an ensemble learning method which combines multiple decision trees to attain predictions. It is a popular machine learning algorithm used for both classification and regression tasks. Random forest builds a collection of decision trees and aggregates their predictions to obtain a final prediction.

The key idea behind random forest is to introduce randomness into the tree-building process. The steps for working of random forest include random sampling in which subsets of training data are randomly divided into multiple bootstrap samples with replacement, and the bootstrap samples are used to train individual decision trees; feature randomness in which at each split in a decision tree, random forest considers only a random subset of features instead of all the features, thereby incorporating randomness and preventing any single feature from dominating the tree building process; tree building in which each decision tree is grown like a regular decision tree, and until a stopping requirement is satisfied, the tree construction algorithm recursively splits the data depending on the chosen features.; aggregation in which the predictions from each decision tree is combined to obtain the final prediction, or the most common predictions from the individual trees are chosen as the overall prediction.

Random forest has several advantages like robustness, high accuracy, versatility, and based on how much each characteristic contributes to the total forecast, it is providing a measure of feature relevance. The limitations of random forest include difficulty in interpretation of specific decision making process of each decision tree within the ensemble, and higher computational complexity as it deals with large number of trees and high-dimensional data, thereby requiring more time and resources in training and evaluating a random forest model compared to a single decision tree.

An ensemble learning approach called AdaBoost (Adaptive Boosting) combines a number of weak classifiers to produce a powerful classifier. Although it can be expanded to multi-class classification jobs, its primary use is for binary classification tasks. AdaBoost assigns weights to each training example and iteratively trains weak classifiers on the weighted data to emphasize the misclassified samples in subsequent iterations.

The steps for AdaBoost are as follows: Initializing weights where equal weights are assigned to all the training examples initially; training of weak classifiers in which a weak classifier that is a simple model performing slightly better than random guessing (e.g., a one-level decision tree) is weighted by the example weights and trained on the weighted training data; updating of weights where the weights of the misclassified samples are increased in order to make them more influential in the next iteration, thereby allowing subsequent weak classifiers to focus on the previously misclassified samples; combining of weak classifiers in which every weak classifier is weighted based on its performance, and the final prediction is determined by combining the predictions of all weak classifiers using their respective weights; repetition where the three steps namely training of weak classifiers, updating of weights, and combining the weak classifiers are repeated for a predefined number of iterations or until the desired level of performance is achieved.

The advantages for AdaBoost classifier include improved accuracy, versatility, robustness to overfitting, and providing a measure of feature importance. The limitations include sensitivity to noisy data and outliers, computational expensiveness, and lack of interpretability. Despite the limitations, the AdaBoost classifier remains a popular and effective algorithm for boosting weak classifiers and achieving high predictive accuracy.

K-NN is a supervised machine learning algorithm treated for both classification and regression tasks. An algorithm for supervised machine learning that is used for classification and regression applications is K-NN. Based on the similarity of occurrences in the training data, this non-parametric approach provides predictions. In K-NN, the "K" refers to the number of nearest neighbours that are considered for making predictions. The K-NN algorithm functions in two phases: training phase and prediction phase. In the training phase, the algorithm simply stores the labelled examples from the training data. In the prediction phase, the algorithm measures the distance (e.g., Euclidean distance) between a given new, unlabelled instance and all the instances in the training data; then, it selects the K-instances with the smallest distances (nearest neighbours) to the new instance; finally, for the classification tasks, the algorithm assigns the class label that is most frequent among the K nearest neighbours as the predicted class for the new instance. The choice of the value for K is crucial in the K-NN algorithm. A small K value may lead to overfitting and increased sensitivity to noise, while a large K value may cause underfitting and loss of local patterns. The optimal value for K depends on the dataset and should be chosen through experimentation or cross-validation.

K-NN is intuitive, easy to understand, and often serves as a baseline algorithm for classification tasks. However, it has limitations, including curse of dimensionality in which the distance between the instances becomes less meaningful in high dimensional spaces attributed due to increased features; memory intensiveness as K-NN requires storing of entire training datasets which may be large in size; higher computational time complexity during prediction as growing of the size of the training dataset increases the prediction time complexity with each prediction requiring calculating distances from all training instances.

Based on the Bayes theorem and the presumption of feature independence, the Naive Bayes algorithm is a supervised machine learning technique. It is commonly used for classification tasks and is particularly effective with high-dimensional data. The algorithm works in five phases: the training phase during which the algorithm learns the statistical properties of the features and their relationship to the class labels from the labelled training data; the probability estimation phase in which using Bayes' Theorem, the Naive Bayes method determines the likelihood of each class label given the observed feature values, with the goal being to find the class label that has the highest probability given the inputs; the independence assumption phase in which the method presumes that the features are conditionally independent of one another with the given class label; the feature probability estimation phase when the algorithm determines the likelihood of each feature value for each class label independently through estimation of the probability distributions of the features that can be modelled using different techniques depending on whether the features are categorical or continuous; the class prediction phase in which the algorithm combines the probabilities of the characteristics and the prior probabilities of the class labels to determine the posterior probability of every class label for the input instance and to choose the class label having the highest probability as the predicted class,

SVM is a supervised machine learning algorithm applied for classification and regression tasks. It is helpful in treating both linearly separable and nonlinearly separable data. SVM constructs a hyperplane or a set of hyperplanes in a high-dimensional space that optimally separates the instances of different classes. SVM algorithm works in two stages: training phase and prediction phase. In the training phase, SVM maps the input instances to a high-dimensional feature space using a kernel function, given a labelled training dataset. This transformation allows SVM to find a hyper-plane that can separate the instances of different classes effectively. SVM aims to discover the hyper-plane that expands the margin, which is the distance between the nearest instances of each class and the hyper-plane. These instances are termed as support vectors. Maximizing the margin helps in achieving better generalization performance. In cases where a linear separation is not possible, SVM uses a technique called the kernel trick. It applies a nonlinear transformation to the input data implicitly, allowing SVM to find nonlinear decision boundaries in the original feature space. During the prediction phase, SVM maps new instances to the same high-dimensional feature space using the same kernel function for making predictions about new instances. The predicted class label is determined by which side of the hyper-plane the instance falls on. A class label is given to instances on one side of the hyper-plane, and a different class label is given to instances on the opposite side.

Advantages of SVM include effectiveness in high dimensional space, flexibility with kernel functions, and good generalization performance. Limitations of SVM include sensitivity to noisy data and higher computational complexity when the dataset is large or when complex kernel functions are used.

ANNs are a variety of machine learning model which takes its clues from the design and operation of biological neural networks in the human brain. ANNs are highly flexible and capable of learning complex patterns and relationships from data. They have been used effectively for a variety of activities, including classification, regression, image recognition, natural language processing, and more. The key components of ANN include neurons, weights, activation function, forward propagation, loss function, backward propagation, hyper-parameters etc.

ANNs offer several advantages, including their ability to learn from complex and high-dimensional data, adaptability to various problem domains, and potential for parallel and distributed computing. However, training ANNs can be computationally expensive and requires substantial amounts of labeled training data. Additionally, ANNs can be challenging to interpret compared to simpler models like linear regression or decision trees. Table 1 depicts a comparative study on the seven machine learning models for classification tasks.

Table 1. Pros and Cons of the six supervised machine learning models considered for the study

Machine Learning Algorithm	Pros	Cons
Decision Tree	- Interpretable and easy to understand - Can handle both categorical and numerical data - Does not require much data preprocessing - Can handle missing values	- Prone to overfitting - Sensitive to small variations in data - Unstable with small changes in data
Random Forest	- Handles overfitting through ensemble of trees - Robust to noise and outliers - Effective feature selection - Handles both categorical and numerical data	- Complexity increases with the number of trees - Black box model - Requires more computational resources
AdaBoost	- Improves weak learners through iterations - Reduces overfitting - Handles both categorical and numerical data - Can work with different base models	- Sensitive to outliers and noisy data - Can be computationally expensive
K-NN	- Simple and easy to implement - No training phase required - Works well with small datasets - Non-parametric and versatile	- Sensitive to irrelevant and noisy features - Computationally expensive for large datasets - Requires proper scaling of features
Naïve Bayes	- Efficient and fast - Handles high-dimensional data well - Performs well with small training sets	- Assumption of independence may not hold - Sensitive to irrelevant features
SVM	- Effective in high-dimensional spaces - Memory efficient - Handles both linear and non-linear relationships - Robust to overfitting	- Choice of kernel function can be challenging - Computationally expensive for large datasets - Requires proper feature scaling
ANN	- Powerful in capturing complex relationships in data - Can learn non-linear relationships	- Requires large amount of training data and computational resources - Prone to overfitting

RELATED WORK

A substantial corpus of study has been conducted in recent years that uses EEG datasets to categorise different mental states. Researchers have made tremendous progress in creating reliable models that can distinguish between distinct emotional and cognitive states using EEG data. An overview of several significant research and approaches used in the discipline is provided in this section.

The study in (Guo, K. et al. 2019) used SVM and fuzzy cognitive graph (FCM) to recognise emotions. The technique identifies emotions by combining facial expressions and EEG waves. The DEAP dataset was used for the experiment. The experiment's guiding idea is that after denoising the data, the researchers divides it into short-time data, which they subsequently compressed for dimensionality reduction. In order to identify the process, the wavelet transform approach was employed to extract features.

In another study (Kumar, D. K., & Nataraj, J. L. 2019), the authors compared the SEED-IV dataset with DEAP dataset experimentally using SVM. The DEAP dataset was produced by the 32-channel Twente and Geneva devices with signal frequency 500HZ. The SEED-IV dataset consisted of EEG signals recorded while 15 individuals watched 2-minute film clips at 1000 Hz. The signals were initially reduced in frequency using filters and MATLAB, after which features were retrieved using discrete wavelet transform, and finally emotions were identified using SVM. The findings indicate that the SVM approach performs well in terms of accuracy on both datasets.

A common deep learning algorithm is the convolutional neural network (CNN). It is ideal for situations involving enormous amounts of data due to its distinctive structure. In a one-dimensional convolutional neural network, the researchers in a study (Yang, H. et al. 2019) suggested a multi-column CNN emotion identification model made up of numerous recognition modules depending on pooling layers and CNN model. The DEAP data set was pre-processed with lower frequency, and the EEG signals were analysed and sampled using a bandpass filter many times before being used as the input of the recognition module. To guarantee the correctness of the outcomes, the recognition findings have been weighted with averaged by each module's outcomes. According to the findings, the model successfully reached to high valence rates of 90.01% and arousal rates of 90.65%.

Several traditional emotion detection models, including DNN, CNN, LSTM, and CNN-LSTM, were analysed in a study (Zhang, Y et al. 2020). Through the use of several samples and a band-pass filter, the researchers decreased the data frequency to 4-45 Hz. Adam was employed to modify the neural network's topology and optimise its parameters as researchers categorised emotions based on intensity and arousal. According to the experimental findings, the classification accuracies of CNN in addition with combined CNN-LSTM model were 82.24% and 88.87% respectively on standard dataset and 90.12% and 94.17% respectively on the original dataset. The findings indicate that CNN and combined CNN-LSTM work quite well in classifying emotions.

Wavelet Transform and RNN were combined in an emotional model put forth in the study (Djamal, E. C., & Putra, R. D. 2020) that can recognise emotions including melancholy, relaxation, and enjoyment. The EEG signals were dissected into brain waves associated with mood using a wavelet transform, and an RNN model for recognition was created. The information was gathered from the EEG waves produced by emotional audio-visual stimuli in 10 healthy persons. The findings of the trial indicated that, respectively, 92%, 53%, and 97% of people could recognise happy, relaxation, and melancholy.

A cyclic convolution network model (ACRNN) with an attention mechanism was put up combining CNN and RNN (Tao, W. et al. (2020).). In the ACRNN model, CNN was largely used to extract emotional characteristics from EEG data that are spatial in nature, while RNN was mostly used to extract emotional features from EEG data that are temporal in nature. Experimental data included DREAMER and DEAP. Adam was used to modify the model's structure and optimise the neural network parameters. The model was created using Python and the TensorFlow framework. The RNN's Softmax function concluded the classification of emotions. The outcomes demonstrate the superior performance of CNN and CNN-LSTM in classifying emotions.

A Bi-LSTM-based model for categorising emotions. Bi-LSTM, which is based on LSTM, combining the forward and backward information of the input sequence was proposed in (Yu, C., & Wang, M. 2022). A DEAP dataset was used for the experiment. The researchers chose 15 channels of emotion-related EEG data, decreased the frequency to 128HZ, and then filtered the data with a filter before feeding it into the Bi-LSTM's Softmax layer for detection and classification. Another Bi-LSTM based model was proposed in (Algarni, M. et al. 2022). In this study, emotions were divided into three primary categories: arousal, valence, and liking. Valence, arousal, and like had average accuracy rates of 99.45%, 96.87%, and 99.68% respectively.

The growing prevalence of mental health issues has driven significant research into machine learning (ML) and deep learning (DL) techniques for mental disorder diagnosis and prediction. Karimian (2025) presents a concise review highlighting the potential of ML algorithms in identifying and predicting various mental health conditions, emphasizing the importance of data-driven approaches in psychological diagnostics. The paper outlines several ML models and their comparative effectiveness across diverse datasets.

Focusing on physiological signals, Singh et al. (2024) explore the use of EEG sensors coupled with ML models for mental health assessment. Their work demonstrates that EEG signals offer a non-invasive, real-time insight into brain activity, which, when processed using ML algorithms, can accurately detect signs of mental stress and emotional imbalance.

Abir et al. (2025) extend this investigation by employing both machine learning and deep learning techniques for EEG-based prediction of psychiatric disorders. Their study showcases the superiority of deep neural networks, particularly convolutional neural networks (CNNs) and recurrent neural networks (RNNs), in extracting complex patterns from EEG signals, leading to enhanced prediction accuracy.

Rahul et al. (2024) provide a systematic review centered on schizophrenia classification using EEG data and ML/DL methods. They analyze various algorithms applied in the domain, noting that deep learning approaches, especially hybrid and ensemble models, offer promising results for automated diagnosis. Their review also stresses the necessity of large, balanced datasets for model robustness and generalizability.

Complementing these findings, Badr et al. (2024) discuss the application of deep learning for mental stress evaluation through EEG signals. Their comprehensive review emphasizes advancements in neural computing and explores architectures like CNNs, LSTMs, and hybrid models. They highlight challenges such as signal noise, subject variability, and the requirement for domain-specific feature engineering.

Even though a lot of progress has been made, further study and technology development are still required to increase the reliability, consistency, and usefulness of EEG-based mental state classification. Researchers can get important insights into the intricate processes of the human brain by fusing the capabilities of EEG with powerful machine learning algorithms, thereby improving our understanding of these processes. The effects of classifying mental states based on EEG datasets are extensive. The early detection and diagnosis of neurological and mental diseases in clinical settings could be facilitated by EEG-based classification, allowing for prompt interventions and individualised care.

METHODOLOGY

The EEG dataset that has been used in this study is a publicly available dataset. The data were collected using the sensor named Muse Headband. The commercial sensing device records activity of brain through five dry application sensors such as NZ (reference point), TP9, AF7, AF8, and TP10. Interference of electromyography signals was eliminated though assignment of non-verbal tasks requiring little or no movement. The subjects were instructed to keep their eyes open during the experimental data collection. Three different kinds of stimuli were formulated for consideration of three different states: relaxed, neutral, and concentrating. Data acquisition for the relaxed task was performed while the subjects were hearing low-tempo music. In this case, the sound effects were designed in such a way that the subjects might meditate relaxing their muscles and were in resting mode. Similar test was performed for data acquisition for neutral mental state, except that no kind of stimulus was given. The experiment was done before performing any other tests for preventing the lasting effects of relaxing or concentrating states. Data acquisition for the concentrating state was done with the subjects being instructed to follow the "shell game" in which under one of three cups, a ball was hidden and then switched. The task for this experiment was to try and follow under which cup, the ball has been hidden.

Dataset description

The EEG data is labelled by means of three different mental states and is presumptively the time series associated with one or more electrodes over the course of an experiment. The dataset is free from noise and artefacts such as muscle and movement artefacts, blinking, and electrical interference. The following steps have been followed for application of machine learning algorithms on the EEG dataset that is being used here.

Feature extraction

This step is for extraction of relevant features from the EEG data. The purpose of feature extraction is to obtain important information from the EEG signal that can distinguish among relaxed, neutral, and concentrating mental states. The EEG signal is segmented into a series of windows with one-second length, with the succeeding windows overlapping by 0.5 second. The EEG signal data that is used here contain a number of statistical features, and result in generation of a high-dimensional attribute space. The statistical features that have been generated for every time window are described as follows.

The sample standard deviation and sample mean have been derived for every EEG signal, contributing to eight features. Another eight features have been extracted from sample kurtosis and sample skewness of each signal. Eight features were extracted from the minimum and maximum value of each signal. Ten features were extracted from the sample variance of every signal along with co-variances of all pairs of EEG signals. Four features were extracted from the eigenvalues of the co-variance matrix. Ten features were extracted from the upper triangular elements of the matrix logarithm obtained from the covariance matrix. Three hundred features were extracted through applying Fast Fourier Transform on every signal to obtain the count of the frequency components of individual signal. Forty features were obtained from the frequency values of the ten most energetic components of the Fast Fourier Transform. All these features were extracted considering the full-time window.

Sixteen features were extracted considering two half-windows – eight features for all the signals corresponding to the change in the sample standard deviations and sample means between the first and second half windows, and another eight features for all the signals signifying the change in minimum and maximum values between the first and second half windows. While considering the quarter-windows, 56 features were extracted from all the signals based on the sample mean of every quarter-window, along with all paired differences of sample means between two quarter windows. One hundred and twelve features were extracted from all the signals based on the minimum (maximum) values of every quarter window, in addition to the paired differences of minimum (maximum) values between the quarter windows.

After all the features were extracted from the EEG signals, the final dataset contains 2479 data objects, with each data object being characterized by 989 features and a single class label of either relaxed, or neutral, or concentrating. All these features have been used in this study for classification of mental states.

Model Selection

Model selection is the process of deciding which machine learning model is best for a specific task or issue. It entails assessing and contrasting several models according to their effectiveness, complexity, understanding, and other pertinent characteristics. In this study, six different supervised machine learning models namely Decision Tree, Random Forest, AdaBoost, K-NN, Naïve Bayes Algorithm, and SVM have been applied on the collected EEG dataset.

Training the Model

In this phase, training data is fed into the selected machine learning model. The labelled dataset is divided into a training set and a testing set. Usually, the training dataset contains 70%-80% of the labelled dataset. The model learns from the input features and their corresponding target labels to adjust its internal parameters or weights. During the training phase, a loss function is defined for quantifying the discrepancy between the model's predictions and the true labels. The goal is to minimize the loss during training. Moreover, an optimization algorithm is chosen for adjusting the model's parameters to minimize the loss function. Also, tuning of the models' hyper-parameters like learning rate, regularization strength, tree depth, etc. is further done to achieve better performance from the trained model.

Testing the Model

Testing of the model involves evaluating the model's performance and assessing how well it generalizes to unseen data. The model is tested with the testing dataset that accounts for 20%-30% of the labelled dataset. The trained model is used to make predictions on the testing dataset.

Prediction

Given an unseen data, a trained model's prediction is evaluated using some metrics like accuracy, precision, recall, and F1-score. The predicted labels or outcomes are compared with the ground truth labels or the outcomes from the testing dataset. The results of the evaluation metrics for the trained model determines the performance of the model on the testing dataset. Based on the predictions on the testing datasets, it may be needed to train the model again or hyper-tuning of the model parameters.

Figure 1 depicts the proposed methodology.

Figure 1. Schematic diagram of the proposed methodology

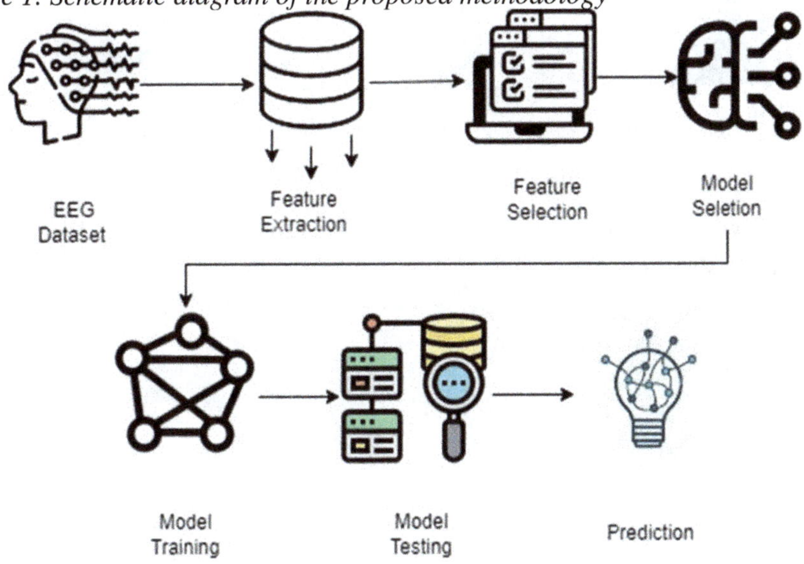

RESULT AND DISCUSSION

The experiment has been done on applying seven different supervised machine learning models namely decision tree, random forest, AdaBoost, K-NN, Naïve Bayes, SVM, and ANN on the EEG dataset to classify three mental states: *relaxed*, *neutral*, and *concentrating*. In the considered dataset, the *relaxed* mental state is denoted with numeric value '0', the *neutral* mental state is denoted as numeric value '1', and the *concentrating* mental state is denoted with numeric value '2'. So, the mental state classification problem in this study is to distinguish different kinds of EEG signals into three different classes denoted by three different numeric values. As stated previously, the dataset contains 989 features along with the target label, and the number of objects is 2479. Three different such features are 'lag1_mean_0', 'lag1_covM_0_2', and 'lag1_freq_010_0' whose histogram plots are shown in Figure 2(a), 2(b), and 2(c) respectively.

Figure 2. Histogram plot for the features

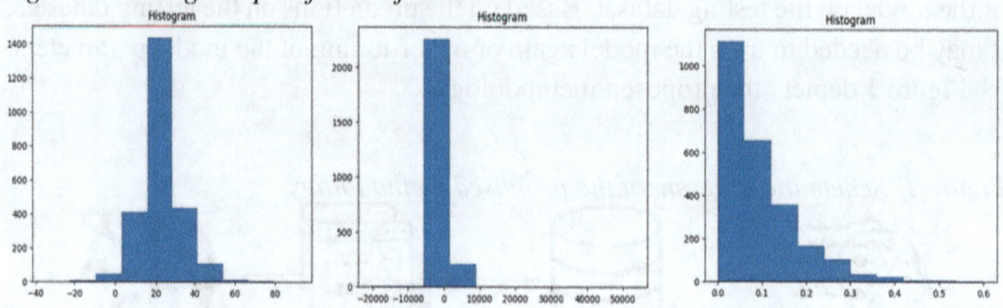

(a) feature 'lag1_mean_0'; (b) feature 'lag1_covM_0_2'; (c) feature 'lag1_freq_010_0

The categorical distribution of the target labels in the considered EEG dataset is graphically shown in Figure 3.

Figure 3. Label-wise distribution of the EEG dataset

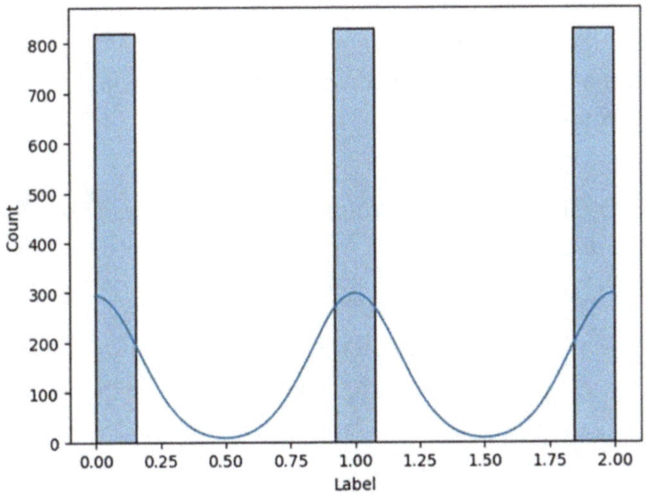

The performance of the machine learning models have been evaluated based on four performance metrics: recall, precision, accuracy, and F1-score. Table 2 shows the performance of six machine learning models except ANN on the EEG dataset.

Table 2. Performance of six machine learning models

Machine Learning Model	Recall	Precision	Accuracy	F1-Score
Decision Tree	90%	89%	89.31%	90%
Random Forest	96%	99%	96.37%	98%
AdaBoost	72%	73%	77.02%	73%
K-NN	90%	92%	91.53%	91%
Naïve Bayes	92%	60%	71.57%	73%
SVM	98%	49%	60.28%	65%

From Table 2, it can be easily conceived that Random forest is the best performing model among all the models, followed by K-NN and Decision Tree. For Random forest model, the overall accuracy level is 96.37%, whereas for the K-NN algorithm, it is 91.53%, and for Decision tree model, the overall accuracy level is 89.13%.

In case of applying ANN on the EEG dataset, a sequential model has been built with three dense layers, first one with 32 neurons, second one with 64 neurons, and the third one with 3 neurons. For the first two layers, *relu* activation function has been used, and for the third layer, *softmax* activation function has been used. The 'sparse_categorical_crossentropy' loss function has been used. The batch size is 32, and the number of epochs is 15. The accuracy has been obtained as 91.13%. Figure 4 shows the graphical plot for the training vs validation accuracy. Comparing the accuracy levels of all the seven implemented machine learning models, the Random forest model is found to be the best model for mental state classification from the EEG dataset.

Figure 4. The graphical plot for the training vs validation accuracy for ANN model applied on EEG dataset

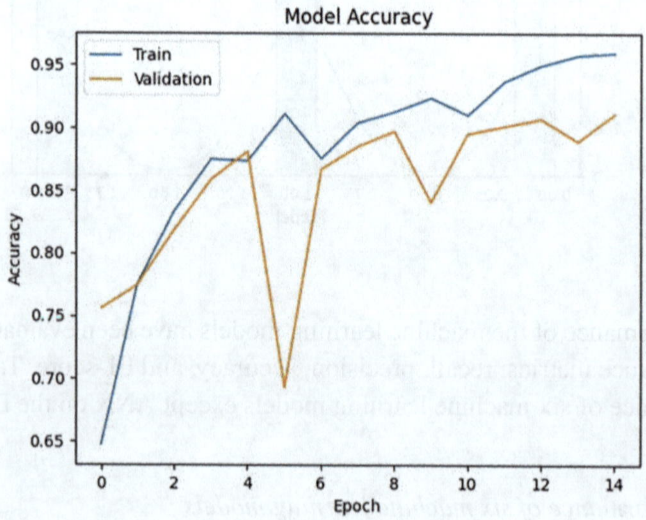

From Table 2, it can be said that Random forest, K-NN, Decision tree algorithms can be applied for mental state classification from EEG dataset, as the accuracy levels of the algorithms lie within 89% to 97%. The accuracy level of AdaBoost is nearly 80%, with the accuracy of the Naïve Bayes algorithm being around 70%. The performance of SVM is not convincing, as its overall accuracy level is around 60%.

FUTURE RESEARCH DIRECTIONS

There are a number of directions for further study in the area of mental state classification using EEG datasets, notwithstanding the tremendous progress that has been made: Accounting for the disparities in mental states between individuals is a significant difficulty. The accuracy and reliability of mental state classification would be increased by creating personalised models that can adjust to unique neurophysiological properties and consider changes in brain activity across individuals.

Classification on a finer scale: A more thorough comprehension of the complicated nature of cognitive processes would be possible by extending the classification system to encompass more precise mental states. Applications in clinical settings, mental wellness programmes, and human-computer interactions might benefit from the ability to distinguish between distinct subcategories of emotions or different levels of attention and focus. Long-term monitoring of mental states may help in the early identification of mental diseases and offer patients individualised interventions. For real-world applications, it is essential to make sure that EEG-based mental state classification models are reliable and generalizable. To verify a model's usefulness and reliability in various contexts, it should be tested among a variety of groups, considering variables like age, gender, and cultural differences. Understanding the complexity of the human brain and enhancing numerous applications in healthcare, neuropsychology, and human-computer interfaces are made possible by the classification of mental states using EEG datasets. The creation of precise, individualised, and real-time mental state classification systems will be facilitated by ongoing research and advancements in machine learning algorithms, feature extraction methods, and interdisciplinary collaborations, ultimately benefiting both individuals and society as a whole.

Additionally, the advancement of brain-computer interfaces (BCIs) holds promise for enabling direct brain-to-external device connection, allowing people with motor limitations to reclaim their freedom. Additionally, real-time stress monitoring and the facilitation of mindfulness and meditation practises are just a couple of the potential uses for EEG-based mental state classification in terms of mental wellness.

In the realm of cognitive psychology, machine learning-facilitated EEG analysis enables empirical validation of theories related to human thought processes, mental workload, and behavioral responses. It allows researchers to create predictive models that can link specific EEG signal features (e.g., frequency bands, power spectral densities) to psychological states. For instance, distinguishing between states of high cognitive engagement versus mental fatigue could support real-time mental workload assessment in educational or occupational environments.

More prominently, the application of EEG classification models in human-computer interaction (HCI) represents a significant technological advancement. The ability to read mental commands and translate them into actionable outputs—such as controlling external devices or virtual environments—paves the way for the development of Brain-Computer Interfaces (BCIs). These interfaces serve as critical tools for enabling communication and control for individuals with motor impairments, allowing them to interact with assistive technologies using only their thoughts. Beyond assistive applications, BCIs powered by EEG classification are finding use in gaming, virtual reality, smart home control, and adaptive user interfaces that respond dynamically to a user's mental and emotional states.

Another area of future exploration is real-time classification and deployment in wearable EEG devices. Integrating high-performing machine learning algorithms into portable EEG systems can revolutionize mental health monitoring and neuro-feedback therapies. For example, real-time emotion recognition could be used to alert individuals experiencing acute stress or anxiety, prompting timely interventions. Similarly, detecting early signs of cognitive decline or neurological disorders such as Alzheimer's or epilepsy through continuous EEG monitoring could lead to earlier diagnosis and improved treatment outcomes.

The future of EEG-based mental state classification lies in continued interdisciplinary collaboration—combining insights from neuroscience, data science, psychology, and engineering to refine algorithms, enhance interpretability, and ensure ethical deployment. Addressing challenges such as data privacy, model generalizability, and hardware limitations will be essential in transitioning these techniques from experimental to everyday use. As machine learning continues to evolve and EEG technology becomes more accessible, the potential for transformative impact on healthcare, education, and human experience becomes ever more promising.

CONCLUSION

Brain-computer interfaces and neuro-feedback systems, which use real-time applications of mental state classification based on EEG data, have created new opportunities for strengthening human-computer interactions. An important development in bridging the gap between the human brain and technology is the capacity to read mental commands and operate external equipment based on EEG signals. Using EEG datasets to categorise mental states is a fascinating and quickly developing area in neuroscience. On the basis of EEG data, the study builds reliable models that can distinguish between various cognitive and emotional states. Accurate classifications have been made possible by applying random forest or K-NN models on the EEG dataset.

The classification of mental states using electroencephalography (EEG) data has emerged as a transformative approach at the intersection of neuroscience, machine learning, and human-computer interaction (HCI). This study explored the application of seven distinct machine learning algorithms—Decision Tree, Random Forest, AdaBoost, K-Nearest Neighbour (K-NN), Naïve Bayes, Support Vector Machine (SVM), and Artificial Neural Network (ANN)—on a publicly available EEG dataset, with the primary objective of assessing their effectiveness in classifying human cognitive and emotional states.

Among the classifiers evaluated, the Random Forest algorithm demonstrated the highest accuracy of 96%, substantially outperforming other models and showcasing its robust performance in handling high-dimensional, noisy EEG data. Decision Tree and K-NN also achieved commendable accuracies of 90%, suggesting their suitability for scenarios that demand simplicity, interpretability, and fast computation. These results underscore the capacity of machine learning models, particularly ensemble-based techniques like Random Forest, to extract meaningful patterns from EEG signals, which are inherently complex, non-linear, and variable across individuals.

This study contributes to a growing body of research focused on decoding mental states from neural data, and its implications are far-reaching. First, from a neuroscience perspective, the ability to identify distinct cognitive and affective states through EEG signals aids in understanding how different mental conditions manifest in brain activity. This supports efforts to map neural signatures of emotions, attention, memory, and cognitive load—critical elements in both clinical and experimental settings.

The machine learning techniques employed in this study not only demonstrate strong classification capabilities but also emphasize the importance of feature selection and model tuning in achieving high accuracy. EEG data is notoriously noisy and susceptible to artifacts from eye movements, muscle activity, and external electrical sources. Preprocessing steps such as filtering, artifact removal, and feature extraction are therefore critical in ensuring model reliability. Moreover, the study highlights the comparative strengths and limitations of each algorithm. For example, while Random Forest excels in accuracy and handles overfitting through ensemble learning, models like Naïve Bayes may underperform in complex, non-linear data scenarios due to their strong independence assumptions.

An important takeaway from this research is the need for model interpretability, especially in healthcare and neuroscience domains. Clinicians and researchers require models that not only provide accurate predictions but also offer insights into the decision-making process. Tree-based models like Decision Trees and Random Forests inherently offer a degree of transparency, allowing for feature importance analysis, which can reveal which aspects of EEG signals are most predictive of certain mental states. This can guide future research into the neurophysiological basis of emotions and cognition.

Furthermore, this study opens avenues for personalized mental state classification models. EEG signals are highly individualistic, affected by factors such as age, gender, neurophysiology, and mental health history. While generalized models are useful for establishing baseline performance, future research should focus on adaptive or transfer learning approaches that allow models to personalize predictions based on individual EEG profiles. Federated learning, for instance, could enable the development of decentralized, privacy-preserving models that learn across multiple subjects while maintaining data security—a crucial consideration in medical and psychological applications.

In conclusion, the application of machine learning algorithms to EEG data has created new opportunities for decoding the human mind and enhancing human-computer symbiosis. The results of this study demonstrate that algorithms such as Random Forest and K-Nearest Neighbour can effectively classify mental states with high accuracy, enabling practical applications in diverse domains from assistive technology to cognitive training. These advances represent an important step toward bridging the gap between brain activity and digital systems, making thought-driven technology an attainable reality.

REFERENCES

Abir, S. I., Shoha, S., Hossain, M. M., Sultana, N., Saha, T. R., Sarwer, M. H., & Hasan, M. (2025). Machine Learning and Deep Learning Techniques for EEG-Based Prediction of Psychiatric Disorders. *Journal of Computer Science and Technology Studies*, *7*(1), 46–63. DOI: 10.32996/jcsts.2025.7.1.4

Agatonovic-Kustrin, S., & Beresford, R. (2000). Basic concepts of artificial neural network (ANN) modeling and its application in pharmaceutical research. *Journal of Pharmaceutical and Biomedical Analysis*, *22*(5), 717–727. DOI: 10.1016/S0731-7085(99)00272-1 PMID: 10815714

Al-Qazzaz, N. K., Ali, S. H. B. M., Ahmad, S. A., Chellappan, K., Islam, M. S., & Escudero, J. (2014). Role of EEG as biomarker in the early detection and classification of dementia. *TheScientificWorldJournal*, *2014*(1), 906038. DOI: 10.1155/2014/906038 PMID: 25093211

Algarni, M., Saeed, F., Al-Hadhrami, T., Ghabban, F., & Al-Sarem, M. (2022). Deep learning-based approach for emotion recognition using electroencephalography (EEG) signals using Bi-directional long short-term memory (Bi-LSTM). *Sensors (Basel)*, *22*(8), 2976. DOI: 10.3390/s22082976 PMID: 35458962

Badr, Y., Tariq, U., Al-Shargie, F., Babiloni, F., Al Mughairbi, F., & Al-Nashash, H. (2024). A review on evaluating mental stress by deep learning using EEG signals. *Neural Computing & Applications*, *36*(21), 12629–12654. DOI: 10.1007/s00521-024-09809-5

Bird, J. J., Manso, L. J., Ribeiro, E. P., Ekart, A., & Faria, D. R. (2018, September). *A study on mental state classification using eeg-based brain-machine interface. In 2018 international conference on intelligent systems (IS)*. IEEE.

Chen, G., Helm, H. S., Lytvynets, K., Yang, W., & Priebe, C. E. (2022). Mental state classification using multi-graph features. *Frontiers in Human Neuroscience*, *16*, 930291. DOI: 10.3389/fnhum.2022.930291 PMID: 35880106

Chomboon, K., Chujai, P., Teerarassamee, P., Kerdprasop, K., & Kerdprasop, N. (2015, March). An empirical study of distance metrics for k-nearest neighbor algorithm. In *Proceedings of the 3rd international conference on industrial application engineering* (Vol. 2, p. 4). DOI: 10.12792/iciae2015.051

Djamal, E. C., & Putra, R. D. (2020). Brain-computer interface of focus and motor imagery using wavelet and recurrent neural networks. *Telkomnika*, *18*(5), 2748–2756. DOI: 10.12928/telkomnika.v18i5.14899

Guo, K., Yu, H., Chai, R., Nguyen, H., & Su, S. W. (2019, July). A hybrid physiological approach of emotional reaction detection using combined FCM and SVM classifier. In *2019 41st Annual International Conference of the IEEE Engineering in Medicine and Biology Society (EMBC)* (pp. 7088-7091). IEEE. DOI: 10.1109/EMBC.2019.8857698

Karimian, M. (2025). A Short Review on Diagnosing and Predicting Mental Disorders with Machine Learning. *International Journal of Applied Data Science in Engineering and Health, 1*(1), 20–27.

Kumar, D. K., & Nataraj, J. L. (2019). Analysis of EEG based emotion detection of DEAP and SEED-IV databases using SVM.

Liaw, A., & Wiener, M. (2002). Classification and regression by randomForest. *R News, 2*(3), 18–22.

Myles, A. J., Feudale, R. N., Liu, Y., Woody, N. A., & Brown, S. D. (2004). An introduction to decision tree modeling. *Journal of Chemometrics: A Journal of the Chemometrics Society, 18*(6), 275-285.

Noble, W. S. (2006). What is a support vector machine? *Nature Biotechnology, 24*(12), 1565–1567. DOI: 10.1038/nbt1206-1565 PMID: 17160063

Rahul, J., Sharma, D., Sharma, L. D., Nanda, U., & Sarkar, A. K. (2024). A systematic review of EEG based automated schizophrenia classification through machine learning and deep learning. *Frontiers in Human Neuroscience, 18*, 1347082. DOI: 10.3389/fnhum.2024.1347082 PMID: 38419961

Rish, I. (2001, August). An empirical study of the naive Bayes classifier. In *IJCAI 2001 workshop on empirical methods in artificial intelligence* (Vol. 3, No. 22, pp. 41-46).

Rojas, R. (2009). AdaBoost and the super bowl of classifiers a tutorial introduction to adaptive boosting. *Freie University, Berlin. Tech. Rep, 1*(1), 1–6.

Singh, M., Vyas, C., & Mazumdaar, B. D. (2024, February). Mental Health Assessment Using EEG Sensor and Machine Learning. In *International Conference On Innovative Computing And Communication* (pp. 199-216). Singapore: Springer Nature Singapore. DOI: 10.1007/978-981-97-3817-5_13

Tao, W., Li, C., Song, R., Cheng, J., Liu, Y., Wan, F., & Chen, X. (2020). EEG-based emotion recognition via channel-wise attention and self-attention. *IEEE Transactions on Affective Computing, 14*(1), 382–393. DOI: 10.1109/TAFFC.2020.3025777

Wang, X. W., Nie, D., & Lu, B. L. (2014). Emotional state classification from EEG data using machine learning approach. *Neurocomputing*, *129*, 94–106. DOI: 10.1016/j.neucom.2013.06.046

Yang, H., Han, J., & Min, K. (2019). A multi-column CNN model for emotion recognition from EEG signals. *Sensors (Basel)*, *19*(21), 4736. DOI: 10.3390/s19214736 PMID: 31683608

Yu, C., & Wang, M. (2022). Survey of emotion recognition methods using EEG information. *Cognitive Robotics*, *2*, 132–146. DOI: 10.1016/j.cogr.2022.06.001

Zhang, Y., Chen, J., Tan, J. H., Chen, Y., Chen, Y., Li, D., Yang, L., Su, J., Huang, X., & Che, W. (2020). An investigation of deep learning models for EEG-based emotion recognition. *Frontiers in Neuroscience*, *14*, 622759. DOI: 10.3389/fnins.2020.622759 PMID: 33424547

ADDITIONAL READING

Balaji, P., Chaurasia, M. A., Bilfaqih, S. M., Muniasamy, A., & Alsid, L. E. G. (2023). Hybridized deep learning approach for detecting Alzheimer's disease. *Biomedicines*, *11*(1), 149. DOI: 10.3390/biomedicines11010149 PMID: 36672656

Balaji, P., Muniasamy, V., Bilfaqih, S. M., Muniasamy, A., Tharanidharan, S., Mani, D., & Alsid, L. E. G. (2023). Chimp optimization algorithm influenced type-2 intuitionistic fuzzy C-means clustering-based breast cancer detection system. *Cancers (Basel)*, *15*(4), 1131. DOI: 10.3390/cancers15041131 PMID: 36831474

Muniasamy, A., Begum, A., Sabahath, A., Yaqub, H., & Karunakaran, G. (2024). Coronary heart disease classification using deep learning approach with feature selection for improved accuracy. *Technology and Health Care*, *32*(3), 1–17. Advance online publication. DOI: 10.3233/THC-231807 PMID: 38339946

Muniasamy, A., Begum, A., Sabahath, A., & Yaqub, H. (2023). Lung cancer histopathology image classification using transfer learning with convolution neural network model. *Journal Name, volume*(issue), 1–12.

KEY TERMS AND DEFINITIONS

EEG Data: The spontaneous biological potential of the brain on the scalp is amplified and recorded to produce the signal pattern known as an EEG. This potential, which is usually obtained by applying non-invasive electrodes to the scalp, has been demonstrated to represent the macroscopic activity of the brain surface.

Emotion Detection: The practice of determining someone's emotional state via their body language, tone of voice, facial expressions, or text is known as emotion detection. Software that analyzes data using machine learning techniques and artificial intelligence (AI) is frequently used to implement it.

Machine Learning: A branch of artificial intelligence (AI) called machine learning (ML) enables machines to learn from their experiences and get better over time without explicit programming. To evaluate vast volumes of data, identify patterns, and reach conclusions, it employs algorithms.

Mental State Classification: Predicting or categorizing an individual's mental state based on their brain activity is the focus of the machine learning field of mental state categorization. It can be used to identify and alter negative thought patterns that influence emotions and behavior.

Model Performance Evaluation: Model performance evaluation is the process of assessing how well a machine learning model performs at the task it was designed for. It's an important part of model development, testing, and deployment.

Chapter 12
Challenges and Future Directions: Emerging Trends and Limitations in ML and Optimization for Healthcare

Anandhavalli Muniasamy
https://orcid.org/0000-0001-8940-3954
College of Computer Science, King Khalid University, Saudi Arabia

Gauthaman Karunakaran
https://orcid.org/0000-0002-0213-7735
Government Pharmacy College, Sajong, India

ABSTRACT

Machine learning (ML) and optimization have the potential to transform healthcare, but several challenges hinder their widespread adoption. This chapter explores the limitations in ML and optimization, including data quality issues, model generalization, and computational constraints. Key challenges include the integration of diverse datasets from electronic health records (EHRs), wearable devices, and imaging, and the need for models that generalize across populations. The chapter focuses the importance of interpretable models for clinicians and addresses ethical concerns. Emerging trends offer solutions, such as multimodal data integration, explainable AI, federated learning, hybrid models, and real-time edge computing. The chapter also highlights the focus on personalized healthcare and predictive modeling while emphasizing ethical, social, equity consideration. Chapter concludes with future directions include innovations in model architecture, quantum computing, and interdisciplinary collaboration to ensure the responsible development of ML and optimization in healthcare.

DOI: 10.4018/979-8-3373-1087-9.ch012

INTRODUCTION

Machine learning (ML) and optimization techniques have significantly transformed the healthcare industry, enabling improved disease diagnosis, treatment planning, drug discovery, and hospital resource management. These advancements have been driven by the rapid growth of computational power, the availability of large-scale healthcare datasets, and the integration of artificial intelligence (AI) with traditional medical practices. However, despite these promising developments, several challenges continue to hinder the widespread adoption and effectiveness of ML and optimization in healthcare. Issues such as data privacy concerns, algorithmic bias, model interpretability, and the integration of AI-driven systems with existing healthcare workflows remain critical obstacles that require further research and technological innovations (Yu et al., 2018).

One of the fundamental limitations in ML-based healthcare applications is the need for high-quality, diverse, and well-annotated medical datasets. Many healthcare institutions face difficulties in sharing patient data due to strict regulatory policies such as the Health Insurance Portability and Accountability Act (HIPAA) in the United States and the General Data Protection Regulation (GDPR) in Europe (Rieke et al., 2020). These restrictions hinder the development of robust and generalizable ML models that can work effectively across different populations and medical conditions. Additionally, biases in training data can lead to disparities in model performance, disproportionately affecting underrepresented patient groups and exacerbating existing healthcare inequalities (Obermeyer et al., 2019).

Another key challenge is the interpretability and explainability of ML models in clinical decision-making. Many state-of-the-art ML models, such as deep neural networks, operate as "black boxes," making it difficult for clinicians to understand the reasoning behind their predictions. This lack of transparency can lead to trust issues and reluctance among healthcare professionals to adopt AI-based tools in critical decision-making processes. Consequently, there is a growing need for explainable AI (XAI) techniques that can enhance the interpretability of ML models while maintaining high predictive performance.

Looking ahead, emerging trends in ML and optimization for healthcare aim to address these limitations by leveraging federated learning, transfer learning, and hybrid AI-human decision systems. Federated learning offers a privacy-preserving approach to training ML models on decentralized data sources, reducing the risks associated with data sharing and regulatory compliance (Bengani et al., 2024). Transfer learning enables the adaptation of pre-trained models to new medical domains with limited labeled data, thereby enhancing model generalizability (Raghu et al., 2019). Additionally, hybrid AI-human systems integrate ML predictions with clinician expertise, ensuring that AI-driven insights complement, rather than replace, human judgment in medical decision-making (Topol, 2019).

The integration of Machine Learning (ML) and optimization techniques into healthcare has revolutionized the way medical data is analyzed, diagnoses are made, and treatments are personalized. From predictive analytics to robotic surgery, ML and optimization have enabled significant advancements in patient care, operational efficiency, and medical research. However, despite these remarkable achievements, the field faces numerous challenges that hinder its full potential. These challenges range from data quality and interpretability issues to ethical concerns and computational limitations. At the same time, emerging trends such as federated learning, explainable AI (XAI), and quantum computing are paving the way for transformative solutions.

Machine Learning and optimization have already demonstrated their potential to transform healthcare. For instance, ML algorithms have been used to predict patient outcomes, optimize treatment plans, and even discover new drugs (Topol, 2019). Optimization techniques, on the other hand, have been applied to resource allocation, scheduling, and logistics in healthcare systems, leading to improved efficiency and reduced costs (Brailsford et al., 2019). Figure 1 illustrates the diverse applications of ML and optimization in healthcare, ranging from clinical decision support to operational management.

Despite these successes, several limitations persist. One of the most significant challenges is the quality and availability of data. Healthcare data is often fragmented, incomplete, or biased, which can lead to inaccurate models and suboptimal decisions (Johnson et al., 2016). Additionally, the "black-box" nature of many ML algorithms raises concerns about interpretability and trust, particularly in high-stakes medical decisions (Caruana et al., 2015). Ethical issues, such as data privacy and algorithmic bias, further complicate the adoption of these technologies (Obermeyer et al., 2019). Figure 2 summarizes the key limitations of ML and optimization in healthcare. Obermeyer et al. (2019) highlight algorithmic bias in healthcare, the discussion must go further by critically evaluating mitigation strategies like adversarial debiasing and reweighting. Adversarial debiasing offers robust bias reduction but is complex and resource-intensive, whereas reweighting is simpler and scalable but may miss nuanced biases. The effectiveness of each method depends on the dataset and clinical context, emphasizing the need for context-specific fairness strategies in healthcare AI.

To address these limitations, several emerging trends are gaining traction. Federated learning, for example, allows ML models to be trained across multiple decentralized datasets without sharing raw data, thereby addressing privacy concerns (Bengani et al., 2024). Explainable AI (XAI) techniques are being developed to make ML models more transparent and interpretable, fostering trust among healthcare providers and patients (Arrieta et al., 2020). Quantum computing, though still in its infancy, holds the potential to solve complex optimization problems that are currently intractable with classical computers.

This chapter explores the current limitations of ML and optimization in healthcare, highlighting the barriers that prevent widespread adoption and scalability. Additionally, it delves into the emerging trends that promise to address these challenges, offering a glimpse into the future of healthcare innovation. By understanding these limitations and trends, stakeholders can better navigate the complexities of implementing ML and optimization in healthcare, ensuring that these technologies are both effective and equitable.

This chapter is structured as follows: Section 2 provides the background details of evolution of ML and optimization in healthcare. Section 3 explores an in-depth analysis of the current limitations of ML and optimization in healthcare, including data quality, interpretability, ethical concerns, and computational challenges. Section 3 explores the emerging trends that are poised to address these limitations, with a focus on federated learning, explainable AI, and quantum computing. Finally, Section 4 discusses the future directions and opportunities for research and implementation in this rapidly evolving field and the chapter ends with conclusion section.

BACKGROUND

Historical Evolution of ML and Optimization in Healthcare

The historical evolution of machine learning (ML) and optimization in healthcare has been marked by a gradual yet transformative integration of computational methods into medical practice and decision-making. Initially, rule-based expert systems such as MYCIN in the 1970s demonstrated the potential of artificial intelligence in clinical diagnostics, albeit with limited scalability and adaptability. The 1990s saw the rise of statistical learning and data-driven models, enabling early predictive analytics in areas such as disease prognosis and treatment planning. As electronic health records (EHRs) and large-scale biomedical datasets became more prevalent in the 2000s, optimization techniques were increasingly applied to resource allocation, scheduling, and operational efficiency within hospitals. In recent years, the convergence of deep learning, reinforcement learning, and evolutionary algorithms has fueled rapid advancements in medical imaging, personalized medicine, and drug discovery. Despite this progress, challenges remain in ensuring model interpretability, data privacy, and ethical deployment—highlighting the need for continuous refinement and responsible innovation. Table 1 provides the historical evolution of machine learning (ML) adoption in healthcare, highlighting the shift from rule-based systems to deep learning and the emergence of transformer models in genomics.

Table 1. Historical evolution of machine learning (ML) adoption in healthcare

Era	Key Developments
1950s–1970s	**Rule-Based Systems:** Early AI in healthcare relied on expert systems like MYCIN, which used predefined rules for diagnosis and treatment recommendations.
1980s–1990s	**Introduction of Machine Learning:** Statistical methods and algorithms began to be explored, allowing systems to learn from data, though still limited by data quality and computational resources.
2000s	**Rise of Deep Learning:** Advancements in neural networks, particularly deep learning models, led to significant improvements in tasks like medical imaging, speech recognition, and natural language processing.
2010s	**Dominance of Deep Learning:** Deep learning models, such as convolutional neural networks (CNNs), achieved human-level performance in various applications, including radiology and genomics.
2017	**Transformer Architecture Introduced:** The paper "Attention Is All You Need" introduced the transformer model, revolutionizing natural language processing and setting the stage for its application in genomics.
2018–2020	**Transformer Models in Genomics:** Models like AlphaFold utilized transformer architectures to predict protein structures, marking a significant advancement in computational biology.
2022–Present	**Transformer Models in Bioinformatics:** Transformer models are increasingly applied in bioinformatics for tasks such as sequence analysis and functional genomics, enhancing predictive accuracy and personalized medicine approaches.

Key developments in ML and optimization in healthcare

Key developments in machine learning (ML) and optimization in healthcare have significantly reshaped clinical practice, diagnostics, and operational efficiency. Advanced ML algorithms such as deep neural networks, convolutional neural networks (CNNs), and transformers have revolutionized medical image analysis, enabling accurate detection of conditions like cancer, diabetic retinopathy, and COVID-19 from imaging data. Natural language processing (NLP) has facilitated the extraction of meaningful insights from unstructured clinical notes and EHRs, enhancing clinical decision support systems. In parallel, optimization techniques have played a pivotal role in streamlining healthcare operations, including patient scheduling, supply chain management, and treatment planning. Reinforcement learning and metaheuristic algorithms have further contributed to adaptive treatment strategies and resource allocation. The integration of ML with optimization frameworks has led to the emergence of intelligent systems capable of delivering personalized care while improving cost-effectiveness and patient outcomes.

ML has enabled a diverse range of intelligent and compassionate features in healthcare, showcasing its broad applications and services. By integrating advanced technologies such as artificial intelligence (AI) and cloud-based data systems, ML enhances healthcare delivery. Notably, it has facilitated the creation of electronic medical records (EMRs) at a reasonable cost, significantly benefiting the healthcare sector. Additionally, ML contributes to other critical areas, including the generation of smart reports, digital documentation, and efficient record-keeping, all of which underscore its transformative impact on healthcare services. Figure 1 highlights these advancements, illustrating the integration and impact of ML in healthcare.

Figure 1. Smart features of machine learning for healthcare domain.

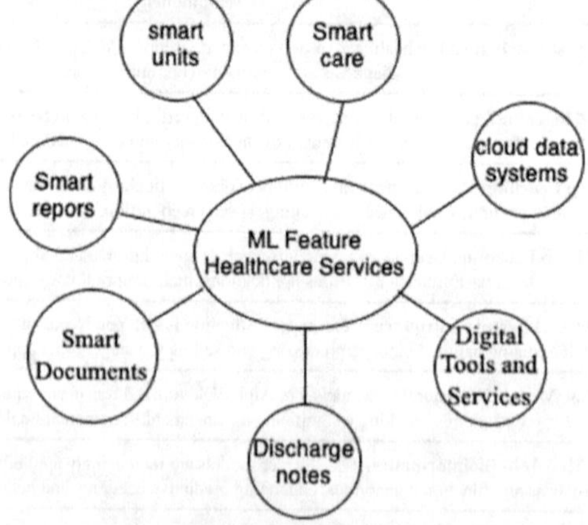

ML-supported applications in the healthcare sector are categorized into several key areas. Smart Units, including Fit Bits and Smart Watches, enable real-time monitoring of patient vitals such as heart rate, blood pressure, and physical activity (Muniasamy, A, 2025). Smart Care integrates Electronic Medical Records (EMRs) and cost-reduction strategies, leveraging ML-driven automation and predictive analytics to enhance hospital workflows and efficiency. Support through Smart Documents refers to AI-powered tools that facilitate documentation, clinical decision-making, and automated report generation, reducing administrative workload (Esteva et al., 2019). Smart Reportsimprove diagnostics and reporting by analyzing medical imaging, pathology reports, and lab results, enhancing accuracy and speeding up diagnoses (Litjens et al., 2017). Discharge Notes are streamlined using ML to ensure consistency and accuracy while reducing manual documentation efforts (Luo et al., 2021). Digital Tools and Services encompass AI tools that aid in disease prediction, drug discovery, and personalized treatment planning (Topol, 2019). Lastly, Cloud Data Systems leverage ML-driven cloud computing to provide secure, scalable, and interoperable health data storage and analysis, facilitating improved collaboration among healthcare professionals (Rieke et al., 2020). Table 2 provides a structured overview of how ML features are optimized in healthcare, along with supporting references for further exploration.

Table 2. Overview of Smart ML features with optimization healthcare

ML Feature	Description	Optimization Techniques	References
Smart Units	Real-time monitoring of patient vitals (e.g., heart rate, blood pressure).	- Reinforcement Learning (RL): Optimizes real-time data collection and analysis. - Edge Computing:Reduces latency and improves efficiency in wearable devices.	Rancea et al., 2024; Alabbasy et al., 2022; Haripriya et al., 2025; Tripathy et al., 2024
Smart Care	Integration of EMRs and cost-reduction strategies using predictive analytics.	- Gradient Boosting Machines (GBM):Optimizes predictive models for hospital workflows. - Linear Programming (LP): Optimizes resource allocation and cost reduction.	Shilo et al., 2020; Bhatt et al., 2021
Smart Documents	AI-powered tools for documentation, clinical decision-making, and report generation.	- Natural Language Processing (NLP):Optimizes text extraction and summarization. - Convolutional Neural Networks (CNNs):Enhances document classification.	Esteva et al., 2019; Nguyen et al., 2019;
Smart Reports	Improves diagnostics and reporting through medical imaging and lab result analysis.	- Deep Learning (DL):Optimizes image recognition and anomaly detection. - Transfer Learning:Reduces training time and improves accuracy in diagnostics.	Litjens et al., 2017; Kim et al., 2020
Discharge Notes	Streamlines discharge documentation for consistency and accuracy.	- Recurrent Neural Networks (RNNs):Optimizes sequential data processing for notes. - Text Generation Models (e.g., GPT): Automates note generation.	Luo et al., 2021; Ganzinger et al., 2025
Digital Tools and Services	AI tools for disease prediction, drug discovery, and personalized treatment.	- Genetic Algorithms (GA): Optimizes drug discovery and treatment planning. - Bayesian Optimization:Enhances hyperparameter tuning in predictive models.	Acosta et al., 2022; Liu et al., 2022; Nguyen et al., 2019; Bhatt et al., 2021
Cloud Data Systems	ML-driven cloud computing for secure, scalable, and interoperable health data.	- Distributed Computing:Optimizes data storage and processing across cloud systems. - Federated Learning:Ensures data privacy while improving collaborative analysis.	Rieke et al., 2020; Haripriya et al., 2025

Figure 2. Pillars of machine learning for healthcare services

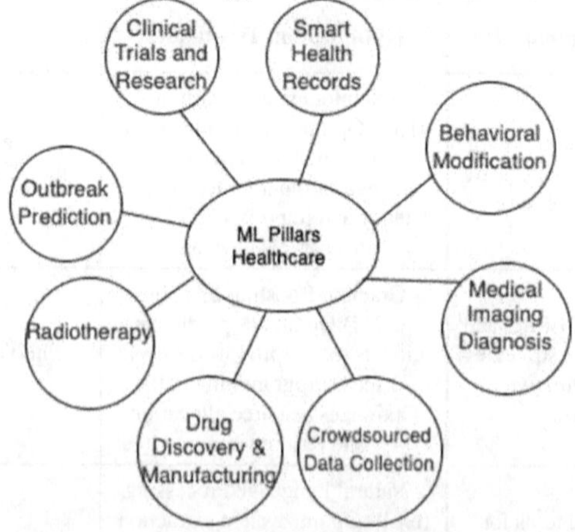

Figure 2 highlights various ML-driven applications that enhance healthcare advancements. Drug Discovery and Manufacturing benefits from ML by predicting molecular interactions, optimizing chemical synthesis, and identifying potential drug candidates, significantly reducing development time and costs (Vamathevan et al., 2019). Medical Imaging Diagnosis leverages deep learning models to assist radiologists in detecting diseases like cancer, pneumonia, and neurological disorders through automated analysis of medical images (Litjens et al., 2017). Behavioral Modification utilizes AI-driven mobile applications and wearables to monitor patient behavior, offering personalized recommendations for managing chronic conditions such as diabetes and mental health disorders (Triantafyllidis & Tsanas, 2019). Smart Health Records automate the organization, retrieval, and predictive analysis of electronic health records (EHRs), improving data accuracy and reducing administrative burden (Rajkomar et al., 2018). Clinical Trials and Research are optimized by ML, which streamlines patient recruitment, trial design, and data analysis, enhancing the efficiency of medical studies (Topol, 2019). Crowdsourced Data Collection incorporates patient-generated data from wearable sensors and online health forums, advancing public health research and personalized treatment (Rieke et al., 2020). Better Radiotherapy benefits from ML's ability to predict optimal radiation doses, increasing treatment accuracy and minimizing side effects for cancer patients (Hosny et al., 2018). Lastly, Outbreak Prediction relies on AI models to analyze epidemiological data, social media trends, and genomic sequences, enabling early detection and containment of disease outbreaks such as COVID-19 (Chimmula & Zhang, 2020). Table 3 highlights various ML-driven applications that enhance healthcare advancements

Table 3. Overview of how ML Pillars with Optmization in healthcare

ML Feature	Description	Optimization Techniques	References
Drug Discovery and Manufacturing	Predicts molecular interactions, optimizes chemical synthesis, and identifies drug candidates.	- **Graph Neural Networks (GNNs):**Optimizes molecular property prediction.	Vamathevan et al., 2019; Saebi et al., 2021; Haripriya et al., 2025
		- **Reinforcement Learning (RL):** Enhances chemical synthesis optimization.	
Medical Imaging Diagnosis	Assists radiologists in detecting diseases through automated image analysis.	- Convolutional Neural Networks (CNNs):Optimizes image recognition and classification. - **Transfer Learning:**Improves accuracy with limited labeled data.	Litjens et al., 2017; Wu et al., 2024; Tripathy et al., 2024
Behavioral Modification	AI-driven tools for monitoring patient behavior and offering personalized recommendations.	- Reinforcement Learning (RL): Optimizes personalized feedback systems. - **Federated Learning:**Ensures privacy in behavioral data analysis.	Triantafyllidis et al., 2019; Bhatt et al., 2021
Smart Health Records	Automates EHR organization, retrieval, and predictive analysis.	- Natural Language Processing (NLP):Optimizes data extraction and summarization. - Gradient Boosting Machines (GBM):Enhances predictive analytics.	Rajkomar et al., 2018; Nguyen et al., 2019
Clinical Trials and Research	Streamlines patient recruitment, trial design, and data analysis.	- Bayesian Optimization: Optimizes trial design and patient recruitment. - **Meta-Learning:**Improves efficiency in multi-task learning for trial data.	Acosta et al., 2022; Liu et al., 2022; Nguyen et al., 2019
Crowdsourced Data Collection	Incorporates patient-generated data for public health research and personalized treatment.	- Federated Learning:Ensures privacy in distributed data analysis. - **Active Learning:**Reduces labeling effort for large datasets.	Rieke et al., 2020; Haripriya et al., 2025

continued on following page

Table 3. Continued

ML Feature	Description	Optimization Techniques	References
Better Radiotherapy	Predicts optimal radiation doses for cancer treatment.	- Deep Reinforcement Learning (DRL):Optimizes dose prediction and treatment planning. - **Convolutional Neural Networks (CNNs):**Enhances tumor segmentation and dose mapping.	Hosny et al., 2018; Kim et al., 2020
Outbreak Prediction	Analyzes epidemiological data, social media trends, and genomic sequences for early detection.	- Recurrent Neural Networks (RNNs):Optimizes time-series data analysis. - **Graph Neural Networks (GNNs):**Enhances genomic sequence analysis.	Chimmula et al., 2020; Rancea et al., 2024; Alabbasy et al., 2023; Gupta et al., 2024

Debates in Federated Learning: Privacy vs. Model Performance

Federated learning (FL) enables institutions to collaboratively train machine learning models without sharing raw data, thereby enhancing privacy. However, this approach can lead to challenges such as non-independent and identically distributed (non-IID) data across institutions, which may degrade model performance . Privacy-preserving techniques like differential privacy (DP) and secure aggregation are employed to protect data during training. While these methods bolster privacy, they can introduce noise or computational overhead, potentially compromising model accuracy . Furthermore, FL models may still be vulnerable to inference attacks, where adversaries deduce sensitive information from model updates . Thus, achieving an acceptable balance between privacy and performance necessitates careful consideration of privacy budgets, noise levels, and the specific requirements of healthcare applications.

Lessons from Failed Implementations

IBM Watson Health's ambitious foray into healthcare AI, particularly through its Watson for Oncology system, offers critical lessons in the complexities of AI deployment in clinical settings. One significant shortcoming was its reliance on hypothetical patient scenarios rather than real-world data, leading to recommendations that were not only impractical but, in some cases, unsafe. For instance, Watson suggested chemotherapy for a patient with severe bleeding, a treatment contraindicated for such a condition . Additionally, the system was trained predominantly on data from Memorial Sloan Kettering Cancer Center, resulting in a bias toward practices and treatment protocols specific to that institution. This narrow training base limited Watson's applicability and effectiveness across diverse healthcare environments with varying resources and standards . Moreover, the AI's decision-making process was often opaque, earning it the label of a 'black-box' system, which eroded trust among clinicians . These issues underscore the necessity for diverse, real-world data, transparency in AI processes, and rigorous clinical validation to ensure the safe and effective integration of AI in healthcare.

Challenges of ML and Optimization for Healthcare

While ML and optimization hold immense promise, several limitations hinder their widespread and effective application in healthcare.

- **Data Challenges**
  - o Issues with data availability, quality, and heterogeneity: Healthcare data is often siloed within different institutions or departments, making it difficult to access and aggregate large datasets necessary for training robust ML models.Data quality can be a major concern, with issues such as missing values, errors, inconsistencies, and variability in data formats.Heterogeneity refers to the diverse nature of healthcare data, which can include structured data (e.g., EHRs), unstructured data (e.g., clinical notes), and multimodal data (e.g., images, genomic data). Integrating and processing these diverse data types is a significant challenge. (Rieke, 2020)
  - o Incomplete or biased datasets: Healthcare datasets may not be representative of the entire population, leading to biased models that perform poorly on certain subgroups. For instance, datasets may overrepresent certain demographics or disease severities. Incomplete datasets, with missing data points, can also affect model accuracy and reliability. (Rajkomar, 2018)
  - o Integration of data from disparate sources such as electronic health records (EHRs), wearable devices, and imaging: Combining data from various sources is technically challenging due to differences in data formats, coding systems, and data governance policies. Ensuring interoperability between different systems is crucial for seamless data integration.(Shilo, S, 2020)
- **Model Generalization**
  - o Challenges in developing models that generalize across populations with diverse demographics and medical conditions: ML models trained on a specific dataset may not perform well on data from different populations

or healthcare settings. This is due to variations in patient characteristics, disease prevalence, treatment protocols, and healthcare systems.Generalization is a key challenge in ensuring that ML models are robust and can be deployed effectively in real-world clinical practice. (Topol et al., (2019).

- **Interpretability and Explainability**
  - o Need for transparent models that clinicians can trust and use confidently in critical decision-making: Many ML models, particularly deep learning models, are "black boxes," meaning that it is difficult to understand how they arrive at their predictions. Clinicians need to understand the reasoning behind a model's output to trust it and use it appropriately. Explainable AI (XAI) is an emerging field that aims to develop more transparent and interpretable ML models. (Litjens et al., 2017)
- **Computational Constraints**
  - o Resource-intensive nature of ML models and optimization algorithms, particularly in real-time settings: Training and deploying complex ML models, especially deep learning models, requires significant computational resources, including powerful hardware and software. Optimization algorithms can also be computationally intensive, especially for large-scale problems.In real-time settings, such as during surgery or in intensive care units, there may be limitations on the computational resources available, which can hinder the use of certain ML and optimization techniques.(Hosny, A.,2018)
- **Ethical and Regulatory Issues**
  - o Bias in algorithms, patient privacy concerns, and compliance with evolving regulatory frameworks like HIPAA and GDPR: ML algorithms can perpetuate or amplify existing biases in the data they are trained on, leading to unfair or discriminatory outcomes. Patient privacy is a major concern when using healthcare data for ML, and it is essential to comply with regulations such as HIPAA (in the US) and GDPR (in Europe) to protect patient information. There is a need for clear regulatory frameworks to govern the development, deployment, and use of ML and optimization in healthcare. (Vamathevan, J., 2019) [REMOVED INCLUDEPICTURE FIELD]

CASE STUDY: USE CASES OF MACHINE LEARNING IN HEALTHCARE

1. Disease Diagnosis and Prediction

ML models can analyze medical imaging, lab results, and patient history to detect diseases at an early stage. Some key applications include:

- Cancer Detection: ML algorithms, such as convolutional neural networks (CNNs), can analyze radiology scans (X-rays, MRIs, CT scans) to detect cancerous cells with high accuracy.
- Heart Disease Prediction: ML models analyze patient data, including blood pressure, cholesterol levels, and lifestyle factors, to assess the risk of cardiovascular diseases.
- Diabetes Management: Predictive models help monitor glucose levels and recommend personalized treatment plans.

2. Personalized Treatment and Precision Medicine

ML enables personalized treatment plans by analyzing patient genetics, medical history, and response to previous treatments. Applications include:

- Drug Response Prediction: ML models assess how a patient will respond to a particular drug based on genetic markers.
- Genomics and Proteomics: ML helps in sequencing DNA and identifying genetic disorders for targeted therapies.
- Clinical Decision Support Systems (CDSS): AI-driven systems assist doctors in choosing the best treatment options.

3. Medical Imaging and Radiology

ML enhances medical imaging interpretation, reducing diagnostic errors. Examples include:

- Automated Image Analysis: AI-powered software detects abnormalities in medical scans, assisting radiologists.
- Early Disease Detection: ML models identify patterns in images that indicate diseases before symptoms appear.

4. Predictive Analytics for Patient Care

ML helps hospitals and healthcare providers predict patient deterioration and optimize care plans:

- Sepsis Prediction: Early detection of sepsis through ML analysis of patient vitals and lab results.
- Hospital Readmission Prediction: ML identifies patients at high risk of readmission, allowing proactive intervention.
- ICU Monitoring: Continuous patient monitoring with ML algorithms helps detect critical conditions in real time.

5. Drug Discovery and Development

ML accelerates the drug discovery process by analyzing chemical compounds, predicting their effectiveness, and identifying potential side effects. Applications include:

- Molecular Modeling: AI-driven simulations predict how molecules interact with biological targets.
- Clinical Trial Optimization: ML identifies the best candidates for clinical trials, reducing costs and time.

6. Healthcare Operations and Resource Management

ML optimizes hospital workflows, reducing costs and improving efficiency:

- Appointment Scheduling: Predictive analytics help optimize patient appointments and reduce wait times.
- Medical Supply Chain Optimization: AI-driven demand forecasting ensures hospitals have the necessary medical supplies.
- Insurance Fraud Detection: ML detects fraudulent claims and billing anomalies.
- MIMIC-III: Demonstrates the challenges of data integration and the importance of fairness in healthcare AI.
- Federated Learning: Highlights privacy-preserving techniques and collaborative frameworks for responsible AI development.
- RSNA Pneumonia Detection: Showcases the role of explainable AI and hybrid models in medical imaging.

- AI for Healthcare Projects: Focuses on personalized healthcare and ethical AI development.
- CORD-19: Illustrates the use of NLP for outbreak prediction and collaborative research.

Table 4 shows the dataset resources along with key themes, use cases and its respective limitations.

Table 4. Detailed Breakdown of Key Themes, Use Cases, and References

Resource	Key Themes	Example Use Case	References	Limitations
MIMIC-III Dataset	- Data integration and representation - Explainable AI - Fairness and equity - Predictive healthcare	Develop a sepsis prediction model using structured (lab results) and unstructured (clinical notes) data.	Johnson et al.. 2016; Rancea et al., 2024	Data is limited to a single geographic region and time period; potential biases in documentation and population demographics may affect generalizability.
Federated Learning for Healthcare	- Federated learning - Privacy-preserving techniques - Collaborative frameworks	Train a hospital readmission prediction model using federated learning across multiple institutions.	Rieke et al. (2020).	Communication overhead, system heterogeneity, and limited interpretability of models; potential trade-offs between privacy and model performance.
RSNA Pneumonia Detection Challenge	- Medical imaging diagnosis - Explainable AI - Hybrid models	Build a deep learning model to detect pneumonia from chest X-rays, ensuring interpretability for radiologists.	Litjens, G., et al. (2017). Wu et al., 2024	Imaging data may not reflect diverse populations or acquisition settings; limited generalizability across hospitals and imaging protocols.
AI for Healthcare Projects	- Personalized and predictive healthcare - Ethical AI - Hybrid models	Predict patient survival using clinical data while addressing biases and ensuring fairness.	Acosta et al. (2022). Liu et al., 2022	Data sparsity and heterogeneity can affect model accuracy; ethical challenges in aligning AI recommendations with patient autonomy and clinical practice.
CORD-19 Dataset	- Outbreak prediction - Explainable AI - Collaborative frameworks	Extract insights from COVID-19 research papers using NLP to understand transmission patterns and treatment options.	Wang et al., (2020). Chimmula, V. K. R., et al. (2020).	Dataset quality depends on the timeliness and accuracy of published papers; evolving terminology and scientific uncertainty can hinder NLP model reliability.

MIMIC-III: Demonstrates the challenges of data integration and the importance of fairness in healthcare AI. Federated Learning: Highlights privacy-preserving techniques and collaborative frameworks for responsible AI development. RSNA Pneumonia Detection: Showcases the role of explainable AI and hybrid models in medical imaging. AI for Healthcare Projects: Focuses on personalized healthcare and ethical AI development. CORD-19: Illustrates the use of NLP for outbreak prediction and collaborative research.

SOLUTIONS AND RECOMMENDATIONS

This section highlights the emerging trends in ML and optimization techniques for healthcare.

1. Advances in Data Integration and Representation

The integration of structured and unstructured data through multimodal learning is revolutionizing healthcare analytics. By combining diverse data sources such as electronic health records (EHRs), medical imaging, wearable device data, and genomic information, ML models can generate comprehensive insights for improved decision-making. Optimization techniques like transfer learning **and** graph neural networks (GNNs) enable the fusion of heterogeneous data, enhancing predictive accuracy and enabling personalized treatment plans. For example, multimodal learning has been used to predict patient outcomes by integrating clinical notes, lab results, and imaging data, leading to more accurate diagnoses and treatment recommendations. Recent advancements in data representation, such as embeddings and knowledge graphs, further improve the interpretability and usability of integrated datasets.

2. Explainable and Trustworthy AI

The development of interpretable ML models is critical for building trust and ensuring ethical AI deployment in healthcare. Techniques such as SHAP and LIME provide transparency by explaining model predictions, which is essential for gaining clinician and patient trust. Optimization methods like rule-based systems and decision trees are being integrated with deep learning to create hybrid models that balance accuracy and interpretability. Explainable AI (XAI) is particularly important in high-stakes applications such as cancer diagnosis and treatment planning, where understanding the rationale behind predictions is crucial. Recent trends also focus on ethical AI frameworks to address biases and ensure fairness in healthcare applications. (Band et al., 2023, Abujaber & Nashwan, 2024, Bhatt et al., 2021)

While the review references key studies on explainable AI (XAI) methods such as SHAP and LIME, it lacks a critical comparison of their practical strengths and weaknesses, particularly in clinical settings. SHAP, based on Shapley values, provides consistent, globally interpretable outputs and is well-suited for high-stakes environments like diagnostics or treatment planning, where reliability and theoretical soundness are critical. However, it is computationally intensive and may be less practical for real-time applications. LIME, on the other hand, offers faster, local approximations and is easier to implement, making it attractive for interactive use by clinicians, but its explanations can vary across runs and may not always capture global model behavior. By contrasting these methods, it becomes evident that the choice of XAI tool should be guided by the specific clinical use case, balancing interpretability, computational feasibility, and the need for either local or global explanation fidelity.

3. Federated Learning and Privacy-Preserving Techniques

Federated learning (FL) is emerging as a decentralized approach to train ML models without compromising patient data privacy. By enabling model training across distributed devices (e.g., hospitals, wearables) while keeping data localized, FL addresses privacy concerns and regulatory requirements like HIPAA and GDPR. Optimization techniques such as differential privacy and secure multi-party computation (SMPC) further enhance data security during model aggregation. FL has been successfully applied in healthcare for tasks like disease prediction, medical imaging analysis, and personalized treatment planning. Recent advancements focus on improving FL efficiency and scalability, making it a promising solution for collaborative healthcare research. (Rieke, N., et al., 2020, Wang, L., et al., 2020)

4. Hybrid Models

The integration of ML with domain knowledge and optimization techniques is enhancing the performance and reliability of healthcare models. Hybrid models combine the strengths of data-driven ML approaches (e.g., deep learning) with rule-based systems and expert knowledge to improve accuracy and generalizability. For example, in radiology, hybrid models integrate deep learning with radiologists' expertise to enhance diagnostic accuracy. Optimization techniques like Bayesian optimization and genetic algorithms are used to fine-tune these models, ensuring they are both robust and interpretable. Recent trends also focus on incorporating physics-informed neural networks (PINNs) to embed domain-specific constraints into ML models. (Sirocchi et al. (2024), Nguyen et al., 2019)

5. Edge Computing and Real-Time Analytics

The deployment of ML models and optimization algorithms on edge devices is enabling faster, localized decision-making in healthcare. Edge computing reduces latency by processing data closer to the source (e.g., wearables, IoT devices), making it ideal for real-time applications like patient monitoring and emergency response. Optimization techniques such as model compression and quantization are used to deploy lightweight ML models on resource-constrained devices. Recent advancements focus on federated edge learning, which combines the benefits of edge computing and federated learning for privacy-preserving, real-time analytics. (Rancea et al., 2024; Alabbasy et al. 2023, Gupta, R., et al., 2024).

6. Personalized and Predictive Healthcare

The shift toward precision medicine and predictive modeling is transforming healthcare by enabling customized patient care. ML models analyze patient-specific data, including genetic, lifestyle, and clinical information, to predict disease risks and recommend personalized treatments. Optimization techniques like Bayesian networks and reinforcement learning are used to refine predictive models and adapt them to individual patient needs. Recent trends focus on integrating multi-omics data(genomics, proteomics, etc.) and leveraging deep learning for more accurate predictions. These advancements are paving the way for proactive healthcare interventions and improved patient outcomes. (Acosta et al. (2022), Liu et al., 2022, Bhatt et al., 2021)

Table 5 outlines the Emerging trends in ML and optimization techniques.

Table 5. Emerging trends in ML and optimization techniques

Topic	References
Advances in Data Integration	Haripriya et al., 2025; Tripathy et al., 2024
Explainable and Trustworthy AI	Band et al., 2023; Bhatt et al., 2021
Federated Learning	Rieke et al., 2020; Haripriya, et al., 2025
Hybrid Models	Sirocchi et al., 2022; Kim et al., 2022; Nguyen et al., 2019

continued on following page

Table 5. Continued

Topic	References
Edge Computing	Rancea et al., 2024; Alabbasy et al., 2023
Personalized and Predictive Care	Acosta et al., 2022; Liu et al., 2022; Bhatt et al., 2021

The table 6 summarizes the key challenges in implementing ML and optimization techniques in healthcare while providing actionable solutions to overcome them.

Table 6. Challenges and solutions in ML and optimization

Challenge Aspect	Challenges	Solutions
Ethical, Social, and Equity Challenges	Algorithmic bias leading to disparities in healthcare outcomes.	Develop bias-mitigation techniques, use diverse datasets, and promote fairness-aware ML algorithms.
Fairness and Equity in ML Models	Lack of transparency in ML models, making clinical decisions less interpretable.	Implement explainable AI (XAI) methods and encourage model validation by multidisciplinary teams.
Access to Advanced Healthcare Tech	Disparities in access to AI-powered medical technologies, especially in underprivileged regions.	Promote affordable AI solutions, expand digital healthcare infrastructure, and support government policies.
Regulatory Compliance and Ethics	Privacy concerns and compliance with regulations such as HIPAA and GDPR.	Strengthen data governance policies, adopt federated learning for secure data sharing, and enforce AI ethics guidelines.
Collaborative AI Development	Lack of interdisciplinary collaboration leading to biased or incomplete AI models.	Foster partnerships between healthcare professionals, technologists, and policymakers to co-develop AI solutions.
Economic and Cost Barriers	High implementation costs of AI-driven healthcare solutions.	Encourage public-private partnerships, increase funding for AI research, and develop cost-effective AI models.

Overview of how ML and optimization techniques are addressing ethical, social, and equity challenges in healthcare.

This section emphasizes the importance of fairness, equity, and collaboration in the development and deployment of AI technologies. Fairness and Equity: Techniques like adversarial debiasing and fairness metrics are essential for creating equitable ML models. Access to Technologies: Federated learning and edge computing are bridging the gap in access to advanced healthcare technologies. Collaborative Frameworks: Participatory design and ethical AI frameworks ensure responsible and inclusive AI development.

1. Ensuring Fairness and Equity in ML and Optimization Models:

Ensuring fairness and equity in ML and optimization models is critical to avoid perpetuating biases and disparities in healthcare. Techniques such as fairness-aware algorithms, bias mitigation strategies, and equity-focused optimization are being developed to address biases in datasets and model predictions. For example, adversarial debiasing and reweighting methods are used to ensure that ML models do not disproportionately favor or disadvantage specific demographic groups. Recent advancements also focus on algorithmic auditing and fairness metrics to evaluate and improve model performance across diverse populations. By incorporating fairness constraints into optimization frameworks, researchers aim to create models that deliver equitable outcomes for all patients, regardless of race, gender, or socioeconomic status. (Rancea et al., 2024, Tripathy et al., 2024, Hardt, M., et al., 2021, Rajkomar, A., et al., 2018)

2. Addressing Disparities in Access to Advanced Healthcare Technologies:

Disparities in access to advanced healthcare technologies, such as AI-driven diagnostic tools and personalized treatment systems, remain a significant challenge. ML and optimization techniques are being used to develop low-cost, scalable solutions that can be deployed in underserved regions. For instance, federated learning enables the use of distributed datasets from diverse populations, improving model generalizability and accessibility. Additionally, edge computing and lightweight ML models are being optimized for resource-constrained settings, ensuring that advanced technologies can reach remote and low-income areas. Recent efforts also focus on policy frameworks and public-private partnerships to bridge the digital divide and promote equitable access to healthcare innovations. (Rieke, N., et al., 2020, Gupta et al., 2022, Bhatt et al., 2021)

3. Promoting Collaborative Frameworks for Responsible AI Development:

Promoting collaborative frameworks for responsible AI development involves engaging stakeholders from diverse backgrounds, including clinicians, policymakers, ethicists, and patients. Multi-stakeholder collaboration ensures that AI systems are designed with ethical considerations, transparency, and accountability in mind. Techniques such as participatory design and co-creationare being used to incorporate diverse perspectives into the development process. Optimization methods like constraint-based modeling and ethical AI frameworks are applied to align AI systems with societal values and regulatory requirements. Recent initiatives also emphasize the importance of open-source tools and standardized guidelines to foster transparency and reproducibility in AI research. By fostering collaboration, the healthcare community can build AI systems that are not only technically robust but also socially responsible. (Abujaber & Nashwan, 2024, Nguyen et al., 2019, Liu et al., 2022).

To emphasize the socio-technical factors influencing AI adoption in healthcare, Greenhalgh et al. (2017) highlight that successful integration of AI in hospitals necessitates a comprehensive understanding of organizational culture, workflow dynamics, and stakeholder engagement, beyond mere technical readiness. From a clinical psychology perspective, trust in AI systems is pivotal; studies indicate that clinicians' acceptance of AI recommendations is significantly influenced by the system's transparency and the perceived reliability of its outputs. Moreover, health economics literature underscores the importance of rigorous cost-benefit analyses to evaluate AI interventions' value propositions, ensuring that resource allocation aligns with improved patient outcomes and system efficiency.

FUTURE RESEARCH DIRECTIONS

The future directions highlight the immense potential of ML and optimization techniques in revolutionizing healthcare, paving the way for more efficient, accurate, and ethical medical solutions.

- **Innovations in Model Architecture and Optimization Methods to Address Scalability and Robustness**

Advancements in machine learning architectures and optimization techniques are driving improvements in the scalability, efficiency, and robustness of healthcare applications. The integration of transformer models, federated learning, and reinforcement learning is enhancing the ability of ML systems to process large-scale and heterogeneous medical data while ensuring privacy and security. Optimization methods, such as metaheuristic algorithms and adaptive learning rates, are refining model performance by minimizing computational costs and improving convergence speeds. Additionally, hybrid AI approaches combining deep learning with traditional statistical models are proving effective in enhancing prediction accuracy and reducing bias in medical decision-making. These innovations will enable healthcare systems to leverage ML for real-time applications, ensuring reliability and trustworthiness in critical scenarios such as diagnostics, personalized treatment, and resource allocation.

- **Potential of Quantum Computing to Revolutionize Optimization in Healthcare**

Quantum computing holds transformative potential in optimizing complex healthcare challenges by exponentially increasing computational power. Traditional optimization problems, such as drug discovery, genomics, and treatment planning, often require extensive processing time due to the vast search space of possible solutions. Quantum algorithms, such as quantum annealing and variational quantum eigensolvers, can drastically accelerate computations by efficiently handling multidimensional optimization problems. In medical imaging, quantum-enhanced ML models can optimize feature selection, improving diagnostic accuracy and reducing false positives. Additionally, quantum-driven simulations can facilitate personalized medicine by modeling intricate biological interactions at an unprecedented scale. While quantum computing in healthcare is still in its early stages, ongoing research and advancements in quantum hardware and hybrid quantum-classical models present immense opportunities for tackling previously intractable medical challenges.

- **Growing Importance of Interdisciplinary Collaboration Among Clinicians, Data Scientists, and Policymakers**

The successful implementation of ML and optimization techniques in healthcare depends on seamless collaboration among clinicians, data scientists, and policymakers. Interdisciplinary teamwork ensures that AI models are developed with domain expertise, addressing real-world clinical needs while maintaining ethical and regulatory compliance. Clinicians contribute medical knowledge to guide ML model design, while data scientists refine algorithms to enhance interpretability and efficiency. Policymakers play a crucial role in setting guidelines for data privacy, bias mitigation, and equitable access to AI-driven healthcare solutions. The adoption of AI governance frameworks and regulatory sandboxes fosters responsible AI development, ensuring transparency and accountability. Moreover, international collaborations and open-source initiatives can accelerate innovation by sharing standardized datasets and best practices, ultimately leading to more inclusive and effective healthcare AI solutions.

- **Importance of educating users about ML technologies**

An often overlooked yet critical aspect of integrating machine learning (ML) into healthcare is the need to adequately train and educate healthcare professionals on how to effectively use these tools. While advanced ML models can offer powerful insights and decision support, their true potential can only be realized when clinicians and administrators understand their capabilities, limitations, and interpretability. Training programs that focus on the fundamentals of ML, model interpretation, data literacy, and ethical considerations are essential to bridge the gap between technical innovation and practical application. Empowering healthcare professionals with this knowledge not only enhances trust in AI-driven systems but also promotes more informed and collaborative decision-making, ultimately leading to better patient outcomes and safer deployment of technology in clinical environments.

CONCLUSION

Machine learning (ML) and optimization techniques are transforming healthcare by enhancing diagnostics, treatment planning, and operational efficiency, but face challenges including data quality, model generalization, interpretability, computational constraints, and ethical/regulatory hurdles, necessitating robust data governance, explainable AI, and adherence to privacy frameworks. This chapter explores these current limitations, highlighting barriers to widespread adoption and scalability, while also delving into emerging trends that promise to address them, offering a glimpse into the future of healthcare innovation. Future opportunities lie in advancing model architectures, leveraging technologies like quantum computing, and fostering interdisciplinary collaboration to ensure responsible AI deployment. Addressing data privacy, algorithmic biases, ethical dilemmas, and access disparities through federated learning, explainable AI, hybrid models, and edge computing is crucial for developing fair, transparent, and accountable AI systems. Ultimately, collaborative frameworks among clinicians, researchers, policymakers, and patients are essential to create ethical, equitable, and patient-centered AI solutions that improve global healthcare efficiency. By understanding these limitations and trends, stakeholders can better navigate the complexities of implementing ML and optimization in healthcare, ensuring that these technologies are both effective and equitable.

REFERENCES

Abujaber, A. A., & Nashwan, A. J. (2024). Ethical framework for artificial intelligence in healthcare research: A path to integrity. *World Journal of Methodology*, *14*(3), 94071. DOI: 10.5662/wjm.v14.i3.94071 PMID: 39310239

Acosta, J. N., Falcone, G. J., Rajpurkar, P., & Topol, E. J. (2022). Multimodal biomedical AI. *Nature Medicine*, *28*(9), 1773–1784. DOI: 10.1038/s41591-022-01981-2 PMID: 36109635

Alabbasy, F. M., Abohamama, A. S., & Alrahmawy, M. F. (2023). Compressing medical deep neural network models for edge devices using knowledge distillation. *Journal of King Saud University. Computer and Information Sciences*, *35*(7), 101616. DOI: 10.1016/j.jksuci.2023.101616

Arrieta, A. B., Díaz-Rodríguez, N., Del Ser, J., Bennetot, A., Tabik, S., Barbado, A., & Herrera, F. (2020). Explainable artificial intelligence (XAI): Concepts, taxonomies, opportunities and challenges toward responsible AI. *Information Fusion*, *58*, 82–115. DOI: 10.1016/j.inffus.2019.12.012

Band, S. S., Yarahmadi, A., Hsu, C.-C., Biyari, M., Sookhak, M., Ameri, R., & Liang, H.-W. (2023). Application of explainable artificial intelligence in medical health: A systematic review of interpretability methods. *Informatics in Medicine Unlocked*, *40*, 101286. DOI: 10.1016/j.imu.2023.101286

Bengani, V. (2024). *Hybrid learning systems: Integrating traditional machine learning with deep learning techniques*. DOI: 10.13140/RG.2.2.10461.22244/1

Bhatt, S., Cohon, A., Rose, J., Majerczyk, N., Cozzi, B., Crenshaw, D., & Myers, G. (2021). Interpretable machine learning models for clinical decision-making in a high-need, value-based primary care setting. *NEJM Catalyst Innovations in Care Delivery*, *2*(4), CAT.21.0008. Advance online publication. DOI: 10.1056/CAT.21.0008

Brailsford, S. C., Harper, P. R., Patel, B., & Pitt, M. (2019). An analysis of the academic literature on simulation and modelling in healthcare. *Journal of Simulation*, *13*(1), 1–12. DOI: 10.1057/jos.2013.13

Caruana, R., Lou, Y., Gehrke, J., Koch, P., Sturm, M., & Elhadad, N. (2015). Intelligible models for healthcare: Predicting pneumonia risk and hospital 30-day readmission. In *Proceedings of the 21st ACM SIGKDD International Conference on Knowledge Discovery and Data Mining* (pp. 1721–1730). https://doi.org/DOI: 10.1145/2783258.2788613

Chimmula, V. K. R., & Zhang, L. (2020). Time series forecasting of COVID-19 transmission in Canada using LSTM networks. *Chaos, Solitons, and Fractals*, *135*, 109864. DOI: 10.1016/j.chaos.2020.109864 PMID: 32390691

Esteva, A., Robicquet, A., Ramsundar, B., Kuleshov, V., DePristo, M., Chou, K., Cui, C., Corrado, G., Thrun, S., & Dean, J. (2019). A guide to deep learning in healthcare. *Nature Medicine*, *25*(1), 24–29. DOI: 10.1038/s41591-018-0316-z PMID: 30617335

Ganzinger, M., Kunz, N., Fuchs, P., Lyu, C. K., Loos, M., Dugas, M., & Pausch, T. M. (2025). Automated generation of discharge summaries: Leveraging large language models with clinical data. *Scientific Reports*, *15*(1), 16466. DOI: 10.1038/s41598-025-01618-7 PMID: 40355506

Greenhalgh, T., Wherton, J., Papoutsi, C., Lynch, J., Hughes, G., A'Court, C., Hinder, S., Fahy, N., Procter, R., & Shaw, S. (2017). Beyond adoption: A new framework for theorizing and evaluating nonadoption, abandonment, and challenges to the scale-up, spread, and sustainability of health and care technologies. *Journal of Medical Internet Research*, *19*(11), e367. DOI: 10.2196/jmir.8775 PMID: 29092808

Gupta, R.. (2022). Edge computing for healthcare in resource-limited settings. *IEEE Transactions on Biomedical Engineering*.

Gupta, R.. (2024). Social media's role in healthcare: Opportunities and challenges for nursing professionals. *Journal of Health Informatics*, *19*, 98–112.

Hardt, M., Price, E., & Srebro, N. (2021). Equality of opportunity in supervised learning. In *Advances in Neural Information Processing Systems (NeurIPS)*.

Haripriya, R., Khare, N., Pandey, M., & Biswas, S. (2025). A privacy-enhanced framework for collaborative big data analysis in healthcare using adaptive federated learning aggregation. *Journal of Big Data*, *12*(1), 113. DOI: 10.1186/s40537-025-01169-8

Hosny, A., Parmar, C., Coroller, T. P., Grossmann, P., Zeleznik, R., Kumar, A., Bussink, J., Gillies, R. J., Mak, R. H., & Aerts, H. J. W. L. (2018). Deep learning for lung cancer prognostication: A retrospective multi-cohort radiomics study. *PLoS Medicine*, *15*(11), e1002711. DOI: 10.1371/journal.pmed.1002711 PMID: 30500819

Johnson, A., Pollard, T., Shen, L., Lehman, L. W., Feng, M., Ghassemi, M., Moody, B., Szolovits, P., Anthony Celi, L., & Mark, R. G. (2016). MIMIC-III, a freely accessible critical care database. *Scientific Data*, *3*(1), 160035. DOI: 10.1038/sdata.2016.35 PMID: 27219127

Kim, H. E., Cosa-Linan, A., Santhanam, N., Jannesari, M., Maros, M. E., & Ganslandt, T. (2022). Transfer learning for medical image classification: A literature review. *BMC Medical Imaging*, *22*(69), 69. Advance online publication. DOI: 10.1186/s12880-022-00793-7 PMID: 35418051

Litjens, G., Kooi, T., Bejnordi, B. E., Setio, A. A. A., Ciompi, F., Ghafoorian, M., van der Laak, J. A. W. M., van Ginneken, B., & Sánchez, C. I. (2017). A survey on deep learning in medical image analysis. *Medical Image Analysis*, *42*, 60–88. DOI: 10.1016/j.media.2017.07.005 PMID: 28778026

Liu, M., Shen, X., & Pan, W. (2022). Deep reinforcement learning for personalized treatment recommendation. *Statistics in Medicine*, *41*(4), 623–639. DOI: 10.1002/sim.9491 PMID: 35716038

Luo, Y., Jiang, G., Yu, T., Song, K., Wang, Z., Liu, Y., & Zeng, H. (2021). ECNet is an evolutionary context-integrated deep learning framework for protein engineering. *Nature Communications*, *12*(1), 5743. DOI: 10.1038/s41467-021-25976-8 PMID: 34593817

Muniasamy, A., & Asiri, F. (2025). Advanced human activity recognition on wearables with multi-scale sparse attention. *Multimedia Tools and Applications*. Advance online publication. DOI: 10.1007/s11042-024-20475-6

Nguyen, V. (2019). Bayesian optimization for accelerating hyper-parameter tuning. In *Proceedings of the 2nd IEEE International Conference on Artificial Intelligence and Knowledge Engineering (AIKE)* (pp. 302–305). https://doi.org/DOI: 10.1109/AIKE.2019.00060

Obermeyer, Z., Powers, B., Vogeli, C., & Mullainathan, S. (2019). Dissecting racial bias in an algorithm used to manage the health of populations. *Science*, *366*(6464), 447–453. DOI: 10.1126/science.aax2342 PMID: 31649194

Rajkomar, A., Dean, J., & Kohane, I. (2018). Machine learning in medicine. *The New England Journal of Medicine*, *380*(14), 1347–1359. DOI: 10.1056/NEJMra1814259 PMID: 30943338

Rancea, A., Anghel, I., & Cioara, T. (2024). Edge computing in healthcare: Innovations, opportunities, and challenges. *Future Internet*, *16*(9), 329. DOI: 10.3390/fi16090329

Rieke, N., Hancox, J., Li, W., Milletarì, F., Roth, H. R., Albarqouni, S., Bakas, S., Galtier, M. N., Landman, B. A., Maier-Hein, K., Ourselin, S., Sheller, M., Summers, R. M., Trask, A., Xu, D., Baust, M., & Cardoso, M. J. (2020). The future of digital health with federated learning. *npj. Digital Medicine*, *3*(1), 119. DOI: 10.1038/s41746-020-00323-1 PMID: 33015372

Saebi, M., Nan, B., Herr, J., Wahlers, J., Wiest, O., & Chawla, N. (2021). Graph neural networks for predicting chemical reaction performance. *ChemRxiv*. DOI: 10.26434/chemrxiv.14589498

Shilo, S., Rossman, H., & Segal, E. (2020). Axes of a revolution: Challenges and promises of big data in healthcare. *Nature Medicine*, *26*(1), 29–38. DOI: 10.1038/s41591-019-0727-5 PMID: 31932803

Sirocchi, C., Bogliolo, A., & Montagna, S. (2024). Medical-informed machine learning: Integrating prior knowledge into medical decision systems. *BMC Medical Informatics and Decision Making*, *24*(S4, Suppl 4), 186. DOI: 10.1186/s12911-024-02582-4 PMID: 38943085

Topol, E. (2019). High-performance medicine: The convergence of human and artificial intelligence. *Nature Medicine*, *25*(1), 44–56. DOI: 10.1038/s41591-018-0300-7 PMID: 30617339

Triantafyllidis, A. K., & Tsanas, A. (2019). Applications of machine learning in real-life digital health interventions: Review of the literature. *Journal of Medical Internet Research*, *21*(4), e12286. DOI: 10.2196/12286 PMID: 30950797

Tripathy, J., Balasubramani, M., Aravinda Rajan, V., Vimalathithan, S., Aeron, A., & Arora, M. (2024). Reinforcement learning for optimizing real-time interventions and personalized feedback using wearable sensors. *Measurement. Sensors*, *33*, 101151. DOI: 10.1016/j.measen.2024.101151

Vamathevan, J., Clark, D., Czodrowski, P., Dunham, I., Ferran, E., Lee, G., Li, B., Madabhushi, A., Shah, P., Spitzer, M., & Zhao, S. (2019). Applications of machine learning in drug discovery and development. *Nature Reviews. Drug Discovery*, *18*(6), 463–477. DOI: 10.1038/s41573-019-0024-5 PMID: 30976107

Wang, L., Lin, Z. Q., & Wong, A. (2020). COVID-Net: A tailored deep convolutional neural network design for detection of COVID-19 cases from chest X-ray images. *Scientific Reports*, *10*(1), 19549. DOI: 10.1038/s41598-020-76550-z PMID: 33177550

Wu, L., Zhang, J., Wang, Y., Ding, R., Cao, Y., Liu, G., Liufu, C., Xie, B., Kang, S., Liu, R., Li, W., & Guan, F. (2024). Pneumonia detection based on RSNA dataset and anchor-free deep learning detector. *Scientific Reports*, *14*(1), 1929. Advance online publication. DOI: 10.1038/s41598-024-52156-7 PMID: 38253758

ADDITIONAL READING

Balaji, P., Chaurasia, M. A., Bilfaqih, S. M., Muniasamy, A., & Alsid, L. E. G. (2023). Hybridized deep learning approach for detecting Alzheimer's disease. *Biomedicines*, *11*(1), 149. DOI: 10.3390/biomedicines11010149 PMID: 36672656

Balaji, P., Muniasamy, V., Bilfaqih, S. M., Muniasamy, A., Tharanidharan, S., Mani, D., & Alsid, L. E. G. (2023). Chimp optimization algorithm influenced type-2 intuitionistic fuzzy C-means clustering-based breast cancer detection system. *Cancers (Basel)*, *15*(4), 1131. DOI: 10.3390/cancers15041131 PMID: 36831474

Muniasamy, A. (2025). Revolutionizing health monitoring: Integrating transformer models with multi-head attention for precise human activity recognition using wearable devices. *Technology and Health Care*, *33*(1), 395–409. DOI: 10.3233/THC-241064 PMID: 39269866

Muniasamy, A., Alquhtani, S. A. S., Alshehri, A. H., Begum, A., & Sabahath, A. (2025). Investigating hybrid quantum-assisted classical and deep learning model for MRI brain tumor classification. *Journal of Image and Graphics*, *13*(1), 123–129. DOI: 10.18178/joig.13.1.123-129

Muniasamy, A., & Asiri, F. (2025). Advanced human activity recognition on wearables with multi-scale sparse attention. *Multimedia Tools and Applications*. Advance online publication. DOI: 10.1007/s11042-024-20475-6

Muniasamy, A., Begum, A., Sabahath, A., Yaqub, H., & Karunakaran, G. (2024). Coronary heart disease classification using deep learning approach with feature selection for improved accuracy. *Technology and Health Care*, *32*(3), 1–17. Advance online publication. DOI: 10.3233/THC-231807 PMID: 38339946

Muniasamy, A., Begum, A., Sabahath, A., & Yaqub, H. (2023). Lung cancer histopathology image classification using transfer learning with convolution neural network model. *Journal Name, volume*(issue), 1–12.

KEY TERMS AND DEFINITIONS

Adversarial Debiasing: A technique used to reduce bias in machine learning models by actively training the model to counteract biased patterns in the data.

Algorithmic Bias: Systematic errors in machine learning models that can lead to unfair or inaccurate outcomes, particularly when training data is biased or unrepresentative of certain populations.

Artificial Intelligence (AI): The simulation of human intelligence in machines that are programmed to think and learn, particularly applied in decision-making and problem-solving tasks in healthcare.

Black Box Models: Machine learning models, such as deep neural networks, whose decision-making processes are not easily understood by humans, making them challenging for clinical application.

Clinical Decision Support: Tools and systems that assist healthcare providers in making clinical decisions by integrating data, algorithms, and recommendations into the decision-making process.

Data Privacy: The protection of personal and sensitive information, especially patient data, from unauthorized access and misuse, regulated by laws like HIPAA (Health Insurance Portability and Accountability Act) and GDPR (General Data Protection Regulation).

Explainable AI (XAI): A set of techniques in AI and ML that make machine learning models more interpretable and understandable to humans, especially in high-stakes fields like healthcare.

Federated Learning: A machine learning approach that enables training on decentralized data sources, allowing privacy-preserving collaboration across healthcare institutions without sharing raw data.

General Data Protection Regulation (GDPR): A regulation in the European Union that sets guidelines for the collection and processing of personal data, including patient data in healthcare settings.

Health Insurance Portability and Accountability Act (HIPAA): A U.S. law that regulates the protection and privacy of healthcare data, ensuring secure handling of personal health information.

Healthcare Inequalities: Disparities in access to care, treatment outcomes, and healthcare services among different populations, often exacerbated by biases in healthcare models and systems.

Hybrid AI-Human Systems: Systems that combine AI-driven predictions with human expertise, ensuring collaboration between clinicians and AI models to make medical decisions.

Machine Learning (ML): A subset of artificial intelligence (AI) that uses algorithms to analyze data, learn patterns, and make predictions or decisions without explicit programming.

Model Interpretability: The ability to understand and explain how a machine learning model arrives at its predictions, an essential feature for gaining trust in clinical decision-making.

Operational Management: The management of day-to-day operations in healthcare systems, such as scheduling, resource allocation, and logistics, which can be optimized using machine learning.

Optimization Techniques: Methods used to make systems or processes more efficient, such as improving resource allocation, treatment planning, and logistical operations in healthcare.

Predictive Analytics: The use of data, statistical algorithms, and machine learning techniques to predict future outcomes, such as patient outcomes or disease progression, in healthcare.

Quantum Computing: A new and emerging field of computing that uses quantum-mechanical phenomena to solve complex problems, with potential applications in optimization tasks in healthcare.

Reweighting: A simpler method to adjust the importance of certain data points in a dataset to reduce bias, but it may not capture all nuanced biases.

Transfer Learning: A machine learning technique where pre-trained models are adapted to new domains or tasks, enabling effective learning with limited labeled data in healthcare applications.

Compilation of References

Abdellaoui Alaoui, E. A., Koumetio Tekouabou, S. C., Hartini, S., Rustam, Z., Silkan, H., & Agoujil, S. (2021). Improvement in automated diagnosis of soft tissues tumors using machine learning. *Big Data Mining and Analytics*, *4*(1), 33–46. DOI: 10.26599/BDMA.2020.9020023

Abdellatif, A., Abdellatef, H., Kanesan, J., Chow, C.-O., Chuah, J. H., & Gheni, H. M. (2022). An effective heart disease detection and severity level classification model using machine learning and hyperparameter optimization methods. *IEEE Access : Practical Innovations, Open Solutions*, *10*, 79974–79985. DOI: 10.1109/ACCESS.2022.3191669

Abdel-Maksoud, E., Elmogy, M., & Al-Awadi, R. (2015). Brain tumor segmentation based on a hybrid clustering technique. *Egyptian Informatics Journal*, *16*(1), 71–81. DOI: 10.1016/j.eij.2015.01.003

Abdollahzadeh, B., & Gharehchopogh, F. S. (2022). A multi-objective optimization algorithm for feature selection problems. *Engineering with Computers*, *38*(3), 1845–1863. DOI: 10.1007/s00366-021-01369-9

Abdulmalek, S., Nasir, A., Jabbar, W. A., Almuhaya, M. A. M., Bairagi, A. K., Khan, M. A., & Kee, S. H. (2022). IoT-based healthcare-monitoring system towards improving quality of life: A review. *Healthcare (Basel)*, *10*(10), 1993. DOI: 10.3390/healthcare10101993 PMID: 36292441

Abir, S. I., Shoha, S., Hossain, M. M., Sultana, N., Saha, T. R., Sarwer, M. H., & Hasan, M. (2025). Machine Learning and Deep Learning Techniques for EEG-Based Prediction of Psychiatric Disorders. *Journal of Computer Science and Technology Studies*, *7*(1), 46–63. DOI: 10.32996/jcsts.2025.7.1.4

Abujaber, A. A., & Nashwan, A. J. (2024). Ethical framework for artificial intelligence in healthcare research: A path to integrity. *World Journal of Methodology*, *14*(3), 94071. DOI: 10.5662/wjm.v14.i3.94071 PMID: 39310239

Abujazoh, M., Al-Darras, D., Hamad, N. A., & Al-Sharaeh, S. (2023). Feature Selection for High-Dimensional Imbalanced Malware Data Using Filter and Wrapper Selection Methods. 2023 International Conference on Information Technology: Cybersecurity Challenges for Sustainable Cities, ICIT 2023 - Proceeding, 196–201. DOI: 10.1109/ICIT58056.2023.10226049

Aby, A. E., Salaji, S., Anilkumar, K. K., & Rajan, T. (2024). A review on leukemia detection and classification using artificial intelligence-based techniques. *Computers & Electrical Engineering*, *118*, 109446. Advance online publication. DOI: 10.1016/j.compeleceng.2024.109446

Acosta, J. N., Falcone, G. J., Rajpurkar, P., & Topol, E. J. (2022). Multimodal biomedical AI. *Nature Medicine*, *28*(9), 1773–1784. DOI: 10.1038/s41591-022-01981-2 PMID: 36109635

Agarwal, S., P. P. S., S. D., & Kumari, G. S. (2024). Optimizing IoT-based healthcare systems with scalable AI and machine learning using cloud platforms. In *Proceedings of the 2024 First International Conference on Innovations in Communications, Electrical and Computer Engineering (ICICEC)* (pp. 1–7).

Agatonovic-Kustrin, S., & Beresford, R. (2000). Basic concepts of artificial neural network (ANN) modeling and its application in pharmaceutical research. *Journal of Pharmaceutical and Biomedical Analysis*, *22*(5), 717–727. DOI: 10.1016/S0731-7085(99)00272-1 PMID: 10815714

Aghalari, M., Aghagolzadeh, A., & Ezoji, M. (2021). Brain tumor image segmentation via asymmetric/symmetric UNet based on two-pathway-residual blocks. *Biomedical Signal Processing and Control*, *69*, 102841. DOI: 10.1016/j.bspc.2021.102841

Agrawal, P., Abutarboush, H. F., Ganesh, T., & Mohamed, A. W. (2021). Metaheuristic algorithms on feature selection: A survey of one decade of research (2009-2019). *IEEE Access : Practical Innovations, Open Solutions*, *9*, 26766–26791. DOI: 10.1109/ACCESS.2021.3056407

Agrawal, P., Ganesh, T., & Mohamed, A. W. (2021). A novel binary gaining–sharing knowledge-based optimization algorithm for feature selection. *Neural Computing & Applications*, *33*(11), 5989–6008. DOI: 10.1007/s00521-020-05375-8

Agrawal, S. K., Singh, B. P., Kumar, R., & Dey, N. (2019). *Machine learning for medical diagnosis: A neural network classifier optimized via the directed bee colony optimization algorithm. U-Healthcare Monitoring Systems* (Vol. 1). Design and Applications., DOI: 10.1016/B978-0-12-815370-3.00009-8

Agresti, A. (2019). An introduction to categorical data analysis. 375. https://www.wiley.com/en-us/An+Introduction+to+Categorical+Data+Analysis%2C+3rd+Edition-p-9781119405283

Ahamed, I. U., Ahamed, I. U., Hossain, A. A., Gupta, U. D., Anika, A. N., & Islam, A. (2024, November). Epistemological Examination of Algorithmic Prowess in Neuro-Oncological Diagnostics: An Erudite Comparative Analysis of VGG16, VGG19, ResNet50, and DenseNet201 Deep Architectonics. In *2024 IEEE Asia Pacific Conference on Wireless and Mobile (APWiMob)* (pp. 13-18). IEEE. DOI: 10.1109/APWiMob64015.2024.10792970

Ahamed, M. F., Hossain, M. M., Nahiduzzaman, M., Islam, M. R., Islam, M. R., Ahsan, M., & Haider, J. (2023). A review on brain tumor segmentation based on deep learning methods with federated learning techniques. *Computerized Medical Imaging and Graphics*, *110*, 102313. DOI: 10.1016/j.compmedimag.2023.102313 PMID: 38011781

Ahmad, A. A., & Polat, H. (2023). Prediction of Heart Disease Based on Machine Learning Using Jellyfish Optimization Algorithm. Diagnostics 2023, Vol. 13, Page 2392, 13(14), 2392. DOI: 10.3390/diagnostics13142392

Ahmed, U., Issa, G. F., Khan, M. A., Aftab, S., Khan, M. F., Said, R. A. T., Ghazal, T. M., & Ahmad, M. (2022). Prediction of diabetes empowered with fused machine learning. *IEEE Access : Practical Innovations, Open Solutions*, *10*, 8529–8538. DOI: 10.1109/ACCESS.2022.3142097

Ahuja, S., Panigrahi, B. K., & Gandhi, T. K. (2022). Enhanced performance of Dark-Nets for brain tumor classification and segmentation using colormap-based superpixel techniques. *Machine Learning with Applications*, *7*, 100212. DOI: 10.1016/j.mlwa.2021.100212

Akter, A., Nosheen, N., Ahmed, S., Hossain, M., Yousuf, M. A., Almoyad, M. A. A., Hasan, K. F., & Moni, M. A. (2024). Robust clinical applicable CNN and U-Net based algorithm for MRI classification and segmentation for brain tumor. *Expert Systems with Applications*, *238*, 122347. DOI: 10.1016/j.eswa.2023.122347

Al Amin, M., Baldacci, R., & Kayvanfar, V. (2024). A comprehensive review on operating room scheduling and optimization. *Operations Research*, •••, 25.

Al Bataineh, A. F., Nahar, K. M., Khafajeh, H., Samara, G., Alazaidah, R., Nasayreh, A., Bashkami, A., Gharaibeh, H., & Dawaghreh, W. (2024). Enhanced Magnetic Resonance Imaging-Based Brain Tumor Classification with a Hybrid Swin Transformer and ResNet50V2 Model. *Applied Sciences (Basel, Switzerland)*, *14*(22), 10154. DOI: 10.3390/app142210154

Alabbasy, F. M., Abohamama, A. S., & Alrahmawy, M. F. (2023). Compressing medical deep neural network models for edge devices using knowledge distillation. *Journal of King Saud University. Computer and Information Sciences*, *35*(7), 101616. DOI: 10.1016/j.jksuci.2023.101616

Al-Dyani, W. Z. (2024). Adaptive Markov Clustering Algorithm for Optimal Event Detection From Heterogeneous News Documents. *IEEE Access : Practical Innovations, Open Solutions*, *12*, 72079–72097. DOI: 10.1109/ACCESS.2024.3403506

Alfi, I. A., Rahman, M. M., Shorfuzzaman, M., & Nazir, A. (2022). A Non-Invasive Interpretable diagnosis of melanoma skin cancer using deep learning and ensemble stacking of machine learning models. *Diagnostics (Basel)*, *12*(3), 726. DOI: 10.3390/diagnostics12030726 PMID: 35328279

Algarni, M., Saeed, F., Al-Hadhrami, T., Ghabban, F., & Al-Sarem, M. (2022). Deep learning-based approach for emotion recognition using electroencephalography (EEG) signals using Bi-directional long short-term memory (Bi-LSTM). *Sensors (Basel)*, *22*(8), 2976. DOI: 10.3390/s22082976 PMID: 35458962

Allam, M., & Malaiyappan, N. (2020). Wrapper based feature selection using integrative teaching learning based optimization algorithm. *The International Arab Journal of Information Technology*, *17*(6), 885–894. DOI: 10.34028/iajit/17/6/7

Allam, M., & Nandhini, M. (2022). Optimal feature selection using binary teaching learning based optimization algorithm. *Journal of King Saud University. Computer and Information Sciences*, *34*(2), 329–341. DOI: 10.1016/j.jksuci.2018.12.001

Al-Qazzaz, N. K., Ali, S. H. B. M., Ahmad, S. A., Chellappan, K., Islam, M. S., & Escudero, J. (2014). Role of EEG as biomarker in the early detection and classification of dementia. *TheScientificWorldJournal*, *2014*(1), 906038. DOI: 10.1155/2014/906038 PMID: 25093211

Alquhtani, S. A., & Muniasamy, A. (2022). Analytics in support of e-commerce systems using machine learning. In *2022 International Conference on Electrical, Computer and Energy Technologies (ICECET)* (pp. 1–5). Prague, Czech Republic. DOI: 10.1109/ICECET55527.2022.9872592

Alshardan, A., Alruwais, N., Alqahtani, H., Alshuhail, A., Almukadi, W. S., & Sayed, A. (2024). Leveraging transfer learning-driven convolutional neural network-based semantic segmentation model for medical image analysis using MRI images. *Scientific Reports*, *14*(1), 30549. DOI: 10.1038/s41598-024-81966-y PMID: 39695183

Anaya-Isaza, A., Mera-Jiménez, L., Verdugo-Alejo, L., & Sarasti, L. (2023). Optimizing MRI-based brain tumor classification and detection using AI: A comparative analysis of neural networks, transfer learning, data augmentation, and the cross-transformer network. *European Journal of Radiology Open*, *10*, 100484. DOI: 10.1016/j.ejro.2023.100484 PMID: 36950474

Antony, L., Muneeswaran, K., Selvakumar, S., Shitharth, S., Sharma, R., & Balasubramanian, R. (2021). A comprehensive unsupervised framework for chronic kidney disease prediction. *IEEE Access : Practical Innovations, Open Solutions*, *9*, 126481–126501. DOI: 10.1109/ACCESS.2021.3109168

Anusha Nambirajam, K., Siva Subramanian, T., & Priyadharshini, R. (2019). An Intelligent System for Accurate Prediction and Detection of Alzheimer's Disease. *International Research Journal of Multidisciplinary Technovation*, *1*(2), 51–56. DOI: 10.34256/irjmt1926

Ardila, D., Kiraly, A. P., Bharadwaj, S., Choi, B., Reicher, J. J., Peng, L., & Corrado, G. (2019). End-to-end lung cancer screening with three-dimensional deep learning on low-dose chest computed tomography. *Nature Medicine*, *25*(6), 954–961. DOI: 10.1038/s41591-019-0447-x PMID: 31110349

Arora, D., Suneetha, S., & Patil, S. R. (2023). Advancements in multi-cloud applications for enhanced e-healthcare services. In *Proceedings of the 2023 International Conference on Artificial Intelligence for Innovations in Healthcare Industries (ICAIIHI)* (pp. 1–7).

Arora, S., & Anand, P. (2019). Binary butterfly optimization approaches for feature selection. *Expert Systems with Applications*, *116*, 147–160. DOI: 10.1016/j.eswa.2018.08.051

Arrieta, A. B., Díaz-Rodríguez, N., Del Ser, J., Bennetot, A., Tabik, S., Barbado, A., & Herrera, F. (2020). Explainable artificial intelligence (XAI): Concepts, taxonomies, opportunities and challenges toward responsible AI. *Information Fusion*, *58*, 82–115. DOI: 10.1016/j.inffus.2019.12.012

Arumugam, K., Naved, M., Shinde, P. P., Leiva-Chauca, O., Huaman-Osorio, A., & Gonzales-Yanac, T. (2023). Multiple disease prediction using Machine learning algorithms. *Materials Today: Proceedings*, *80*, 3682–3685. DOI: 10.1016/j.matpr.2021.07.361

Asha, A., Dhiyanesh, B., Kiruthiga, G., Shakkeera, L., Jacob, V., & Venaik, A. (2024). Efficient coronary heart disease prediction: Enhanced neural network with chaos salp decision and feature optimization. *International Journal of Intelligent Systems and Applications in Engineering*, *12*(20s), 440–450.

Attallah, O. (2024). Acute lymphocytic leukemia detection and subtype classification via extended wavelet pooling based-CNNs and statistical-texture features. *Image and Vision Computing*, *147*, 105064. DOI: 10.1016/j.imavis.2024.105064

Baccouch, W., Oueslati, S., Solaiman, B., & Labidi, S. (2023). A comparative study of CNN and U-Net performance for automatic segmentation of medical images: Application to cardiac MRI. *Procedia Computer Science*, *219*, 1089–1096. DOI: 10.1016/j.procs.2023.01.388

Badr, Y., Tariq, U., Al-Shargie, F., Babiloni, F., Al Mughairbi, F., & Al-Nashash, H. (2024). A review on evaluating mental stress by deep learning using EEG signals. *Neural Computing & Applications*, *36*(21), 12629–12654. DOI: 10.1007/s00521-024-09809-5

Balafas, V., Karantoumanis, E., Louta, M., & Ploskas, N. (2023). Machine learning and deep learning for plant disease classification and detection. *IEEE Access : Practical Innovations, Open Solutions*, *11*, 114352–114377. DOI: 10.1109/ACCESS.2023.3324722

Band, S. S., Yarahmadi, A., Hsu, C.-C., Biyari, M., Sookhak, M., Ameri, R., & Liang, H.-W. (2023). Application of explainable artificial intelligence in medical health: A systematic review of interpretability methods. *Informatics in Medicine Unlocked*, *40*, 101286. DOI: 10.1016/j.imu.2023.101286

Bengani, V. (2024). *Hybrid learning systems: Integrating traditional machine learning with deep learning techniques*. DOI: 10.13140/RG.2.2.10461.22244/1

Beyer, H.-G., Beyer, H.-G., Schwefel, H.-P., & Schwefel, H.-P. (2002). Evolution strategies – A comprehensive introduction. Natural Computing 2002 1:1, 1(1), 3–52. DOI: 10.1023/A:1015059928466

Bhadula, S., Sharma, S., & Johri, A. (2023b). Hybrid blockchain and IPFS for secure Industry 4.0 framework of IoT-based skin monitoring system. 2022 8th International Conference on Advanced Computing and Communication Systems (ICACCS), 41–47. https://doi.org/DOI: 10.1109/ICACCS57279.2023.10112751

Bhadula, S., & Sharma, S. (2023). Post Diagnosis Digital Routine Monitoring System for Patients of Skin Diseases. In *2023 Fifth International Conference on Electrical, Computer and Communication Technologies (ICECCT)*, 1–6. https://doi.org/DOI: 10.1109/ICECCT56650.2023.10179835

Bhatt, S., Cohon, A., Rose, J., Majerczyk, N., Cozzi, B., Crenshaw, D., & Myers, G. (2021). Interpretable machine learning models for clinical decision-making in a high-need, value-based primary care setting. *NEJM Catalyst Innovations in Care Delivery*, *2*(4), CAT.21.0008. Advance online publication. DOI: 10.1056/CAT.21.0008

Bhukya, S., Ganagoni, V., Nangunoori, S. S., & Enapothula, S. T. (2025). A Deep Learning Framework Using Enhanced Convolutional Neural Network for Detection of Lung Cancer from CT Images. *International Research Journal of Multidisciplinary Technovation*, *7*(1), 138–150. DOI: 10.54392/irjmt25110

Bird, J. J., Manso, L. J., Ribeiro, E. P., Ekart, A., & Faria, D. R. (2018, September). *A study on mental state classification using eeg-based brain-machine interface. In 2018 international conference on intelligent systems (IS)*. IEEE.

Bishop, C. M. (2006). *Pattern Recognition and Machine Learning*. Springer.

Boppana, V. R. (2020). Ethical implications of big data in healthcare decision making. *SSRN*.

Brailsford, S. C., Harper, P. R., Patel, B., & Pitt, M. (2019). An analysis of the academic literature on simulation and modelling in healthcare. *Journal of Simulation*, *13*(1), 1–12. DOI: 10.1057/jos.2013.13

Breiman, L. (2001). Random forests. *Machine Learning*, *45*(1), 5–32. DOI: 10.1023/A:1010933404324

Buckland, M., & Gey, F. (1994). The relationship between recall and precision. *Journal of the American Society for Information Science*, *45*(1), 12–19. DOI: 10.1002/(SICI)1097-4571(199401)45:1<12::AID-ASI2>3.0.CO;2-L

Budhraja, S., Doborjeh, M., Singh, B., Tan, S., Doborjeh, Z., Lai, E., Merkin, A., Lee, J., Goh, W., & Kasabov, N. (2023). Filter and Wrapper Stacking Ensemble (FWSE): A robust approach for reliable biomarker discovery in high-dimensional omics data. *Briefings in Bioinformatics*, *24*(6), 1–17. DOI: 10.1093/bib/bbad382 PMID: 37889118

Caruana, R., Lou, Y., Gehrke, J., Koch, P., Sturm, M., & Elhadad, N. (2015). Intelligible models for healthcare: Predicting pneumonia risk and hospital 30-day readmission. In *Proceedings of the 21st ACM SIGKDD International Conference on Knowledge Discovery and Data Mining* (pp. 1721–1730). https://doi.org/DOI: 10.1145/2783258.2788613

Castañé, H., Baiges-Gaya, G., Hernández-Aguilera, A., Rodríguez-Tomàs, E., Fernández-Arroyo, S., Herrero, P., Delpino-Rius, A., Canela, N., Menendez, J. A., Camps, J., & Joven, J. (2021). Coupling machine learning and lipidomics as a tool to investigate metabolic dysfunction-associated fatty liver disease. A general overview. *Biomolecules*, *11*(3), 473. DOI: 10.3390/biom11030473 PMID: 33810079

Çetiner, H., & Metlek, S. (2023). DenseUNet+: A novel hybrid segmentation approach based on multi-modality images for brain tumor segmentation. *Journal of King Saud University. Computer and Information Sciences*, *35*(8), 101663. DOI: 10.1016/j.jksuci.2023.101663

Chandrashekar, G., & Sahin, F. (2014a). A survey on feature selection methods. *Computers & Electrical Engineering*, *40*(1), 16–28. DOI: 10.1016/j.compeleceng.2013.11.024

Chauhan, N. K., & Kaur, N. (2023). Predicting cardiovascular diseases using machine learning integrated with feature selection through blue whale optimization. In *Proceedings of the 2023 10th IEEE Uttar Pradesh Section International Conference on Electrical, Electronics and Computer Engineering (UPCON)* (pp. 464–469). DOI: 10.1109/UPCON59197.2023.10434597

Chen, G., Helm, H. S., Lytvynets, K., Yang, W., & Priebe, C. E. (2022). Mental state classification using multi-graph features. *Frontiers in Human Neuroscience*, *16*, 930291. DOI: 10.3389/fnhum.2022.930291 PMID: 35880106

Chen, M., Hao, Y., Hwang, K., Wang, L., & Wang, L. (2017). Disease prediction by machine learning over big data from healthcare communities. *IEEE Access : Practical Innovations, Open Solutions*, *5*, 8869–8879. DOI: 10.1109/ACCESS.2017.2694446

Chen, S., Li, K., Wang, Y., Zhang, W., Li, J., & Wang, Z. (2022). Shared savings model for optimization-based care management: A financial analysis. *Health Affairs*, *41*(8), 1213–1219. PMID: 35914199

Chen, W., Zhou, W., Zhu, L., Cao, Y., Gu, H., & Yu, B. (2022). MTDCNet: A 3D multi-threading dilated convolutional network for brain tumor automatic segmentation. *Journal of Biomedical Informatics*, *133*, 104173. DOI: 10.1016/j.jbi.2022.104173 PMID: 35998815

Chimmula, V. K. R., & Zhang, L. (2020). Time series forecasting of COVID-19 transmission in Canada using LSTM networks. *Chaos, Solitons, and Fractals*, *135*, 109864. DOI: 10.1016/j.chaos.2020.109864 PMID: 32390691

Chomboon, K., Chujai, P., Teerarassamee, P., Kerdprasop, K., & Kerdprasop, N. (2015, March). An empirical study of distance metrics for k-nearest neighbor algorithm. In *Proceedings of the 3rd international conference on industrial application engineering* (Vol. 2, p. 4). DOI: 10.12792/iciae2015.051

Cortes, C., & Vapnik, V. (1995). Support-vector networks. *Machine Learning*, *20*(3), 273–297. DOI: 10.1007/BF00994018

Cover, T., & Hart, P. (1967). Nearest neighbor pattern classification. *IEEE Transactions on Information Theory*, *13*(1), 21–27. DOI: 10.1109/TIT.1967.1053964

Dang, K., Vo, T., Ngo, L., & Ha, H. (2022). A deep learning framework integrating MRI image preprocessing methods for brain tumor segmentation and classification. *IBRO Neuroscience Reports*, *13*, 523–532. DOI: 10.1016/j.ibneur.2022.10.014 PMID: 36590099

Dantzig, G. B. (1963). Linear programming and extensions. Princeton University Press., Dataset https://www.kaggle.com/datasets/kaushil268/disease-prediction-using-machine-learning, Retrieved March 21, 2025, from.

Das, P. K., Pradhan, A., & Meher, S. (2021a). Detection of acute lymphoblastic leukemia using machine learning techniques. In *Machine Learning, Deep Learning, and Computational Intelligence for Wireless Communication* (Vol. 749, Art. no. 425). Springer. DOI: 10.1007/978-981-16-0289-4_32

Das, H., Naik, B., & Behera, H. S. (2022). A Jaya algorithm based wrapper method for optimal feature selection in supervised classification. *Journal of King Saud University. Computer and Information Sciences*, *34*(6), 3851–3863. DOI: 10.1016/j.jksuci.2020.05.002

Das, P. K., Diya, V., Meher, S., Panda, R., & Abraham, A. (2022). A systematic review on recent advancements in deep and machine learning based detection and classification of acute lymphoblastic leukemia. *IEEE Access : Practical Innovations, Open Solutions*, *10*, 81741–81763. DOI: 10.1109/ACCESS.2022.3196037

Davis, D., & Hoh, S. (2020). Application of decision trees in predicting heart disease. *International Journal of Medical Informatics*, *142*, 104205.

Decaro, C., Montanari, G. B., Molinari, R., Gilberti, A., Bagnoli, D., Bianconi, M., & Bellanca, G. (2019). Machine learning approach for prediction of hematic parameters in hemodialysis patients. *IEEE Journal of Translational Engineering in Health and Medicine, 7. IEEE Journal of Translational Engineering in Health and Medicine*, *4100308*, 1–8. DOI: 10.1109/JTEHM.2019.2938951 PMID: 32309060

Deshmukh, S., Kumar, P., Devangan, L., & Patil, A. R. (2024, December). A review of brain tumour detection through the integration of fuzzy logic and U-NET CNN classification: A high-efficiency approach. In *AIP Conference Proceedings* (Vol. 3188, No. 1). AIP Publishing. DOI: 10.1063/5.0240766

Dhakhinamoorthy, C., Mani, S. K., Mathivanan, S. K., Mohan, S., Jayagopal, P., Mallik, S., & Qin, H. (2023). Hybrid Whale and Gray Wolf Deep Learning Optimization Algorithm for Prediction of Alzheimer's Disease. Mathematics 2023, Vol. 11, Page 1136, 11(5), 1136. DOI: 10.3390/math11051136

Dharani, T., & Hariprasath, S. (2018). Diagnosis of leukemia and its types using digital image processing techniques. In *Proceedings of the International Conference on Communication and Electronics Systems (ICCES 2018)* (pp. xxx–xxx). IEEE. https://doi.org/DOI: 10.1109/CESYS.2018.8724075

Dhivya, P., & Bazilabanu, A. (2023). Deep hyper optimization approach for disease classification using artificial intelligence. *Data & Knowledge Engineering*, *145*, 102147. DOI: 10.1016/j.datak.2023.102147

Di Noia, A., Martino, A., Montanari, P., & Rizzi, A. (2020). Supervised machine learning techniques and genetic optimization for occupational diseases risk prediction. *Soft Computing*, *24*(6), 4393–4406. DOI: 10.1007/s00500-019-04200-2

Djamal, E. C., & Putra, R. D. (2020). Brain-computer interface of focus and motor imagery using wavelet and recurrent neural networks. *Telkomnika*, *18*(5), 2748–2756. DOI: 10.12928/telkomnika.v18i5.14899

Dominico, G., Bernardes, J. S., Dorneles, L. L., & Dorn, M. (2023). Multi-Objective Wrapper Differential Evolution with Guided Initial Population for Feature Selection. *2023 IEEE Congress on Evolutionary Computation, CEC 2023*. DOI: 10.1109/CEC53210.2023.10254085

Dorigo, M., & Gambardella, L. M. (1997). Ant colony system: A cooperative learning approach to the traveling salesman problem. *IEEE Transactions on Evolutionary Computation*, *1*(1), 53–66. DOI: 10.1109/4235.585892

Dounya, K., Habiba, S., Khawla, S., Okba, K., Zouai, M., & Hammadi, S. (2024). Early disease detection and intervention in healthcare using machine learning and big data analytics: Use case brain tumor. *Studies in Engineering and Exact Sciences*, *5*(2), e12199–e12199. DOI: 10.54021/seesv5n2-791

Dubey, A. K. (2021). Optimized hybrid learning for multi disease prediction enabled by lion with butterfly optimization algorithm. Sadhana - Academy Proceedings in Engineering Sciences, 46(2), 1–27. https://doi.org/DOI: 10.1007/S12046-021-01574-8/TABLES/16

Dubey, M., Tembhurne, J., & Makhijani, R. (2024). Improving coronary heart disease prediction with real-life dataset: A stacked generalization framework with maximum clinical attributes and SMOTE balancing for imbalanced data. *Multimedia Tools and Applications*, *83*(37), 1–30. DOI: 10.1007/s11042-024-19429-9

El-Hasnony, I. M., Barakat, S. I., & Mostafa, R. R. (2020). Optimized ANFIS Model Using Hybrid Metaheuristic Algorithms for Parkinson's Disease Prediction in IoT Environment. *IEEE Access : Practical Innovations, Open Solutions*, *8*, 119252–119270. DOI: 10.1109/ACCESS.2020.3005614

Elola, A., Aramendi, E., Irusta, U., & Berve, P. O. (2020). Multimodal algorithms for the classification of circulation states during out-of-hospital cardiac arrest. *IEEE Transactions on Biomedical Engineering, PP*, (99), 1–1. DOI: 10.1109/TBME.2020.3030216 PMID: 33044927

Espinosa, R., Jiménez, F., & Palma, J. (2024). Surrogate-Assisted and Filter-Based Multiobjective Evolutionary Feature Selection for Deep Learning. *IEEE Transactions on Neural Networks and Learning Systems*, *35*(7), 9591–9605. DOI: 10.1109/TNNLS.2023.3234629 PMID: 37018667

Esteva, A., Kuprel, B., Novoa, R. A., Ko, J., Swetter, S. M., Blau, H. M., & Thrun, S. (2017). Dermatologist-level classification of skin cancer with deep neural networks. *Nature*, *542*(7639), 115–118. DOI: 10.1038/nature21056 PMID: 28117445

Esteva, A., Robicquet, A., Ramsundar, B., Kuleshov, V., DePristo, M., Chou, K., Cui, C., Corrado, G., Thrun, S., & Dean, J. (2019). A guide to deep learning in healthcare. *Nature Medicine*, *25*(1), 24–29. DOI: 10.1038/s41591-018-0316-z PMID: 30617335

Ezzat, D., Hassanien, A. E., & Ella, H. A. (2021). An optimized deep learning architecture for the diagnosis of COVID-19 disease based on gravitational search optimization. *Applied Soft Computing*, *98*, 106742. DOI: 10.1016/j.asoc.2020.106742 PMID: 32982615

Fazakis, N., Kocsis, O., Dritsas, E., Alexiou, S., Fakotakis, N., & Moustakas, K. (2021). Machine learning tools for long-term type 2 diabetes risk prediction. *IEEE Access : Practical Innovations, Open Solutions*, *9*, 103737–103757. DOI: 10.1109/ACCESS.2021.3098691

FDA. (2025). *Artificial Intelligence and Machine Learning in Software as a Medical Device*. U.S. Food and Drug Administration.

Feng, W., Han, X., Hu, H., Chang, M., Ding, L., Xiang, H., Chen, Y., & Li, Y. (2021). 2D vanadium carbide MXenzyme to alleviate ROS-mediated inflammatory and neurodegenerative diseases. *Nature Communications*, *12*(1), 2203. DOI: 10.1038/s41467-021-22278-x PMID: 33850133

Gangadevi, E., Rani, R. S., Dhanaraj, R. K., & Nayyar, A. (2024). Spot-out fruit fly algorithm with simulated annealing optimized SVM for detecting tomato plant diseases. *Neural Computing & Applications*, *36*(8), 4349–4375. DOI: 10.1007/s00521-023-09295-1

Ganiger, F. B., Bijjal, S. S., & Mugali, J. D. (2024). A Cross-Sectional Study On Psychiatric Disorders among Poor Academic Performance Primary School (6-12 Years) Children with Substance Use Disorders in Their Parents. *Annals of Indian Psychiatry*, *8*(2), 120–124. DOI: 10.4103/aip.aip_128_21

Ganzinger, M., Kunz, N., Fuchs, P., Lyu, C. K., Loos, M., Dugas, M., & Pausch, T. M. (2025). Automated generation of discharge summaries: Leveraging large language models with clinical data. *Scientific Reports*, *15*(1), 16466. DOI: 10.1038/s41598-025-01618-7 PMID: 40355506

Gen, M., & Cheng, R. (1996). *Genetic Algorithms and Engineering Design*. Genetic Algorithms and Engineering Design., DOI: 10.1002/9780470172254

Ghaemi, M., & Feizi-Derakhshi, M. R. (2016). Feature selection using Forest Optimization Algorithm. *Pattern Recognition*, *60*, 121–129. DOI: 10.1016/j.patcog.2016.05.012

Ghosh, P., Azam, S., Jonkman, M., Karim, A., Shamrat, F. M. J. M., Ignatious, E., Shultana, S., Beeravolu, A. R., & De Boer, F. (2021). Efficient prediction of cardiovascular disease using machine learning algorithms with relief and lasso feature selection techniques. *IEEE Access : Practical Innovations, Open Solutions*, *9*, 19304–19326. DOI: 10.1109/ACCESS.2021.3053759

Gilpin, L. H.. (2018). *Explaining explanations: An overview of interpretability of machine learning. Proceedings of the 2018 CHI Conference on Human Factors in Computing Systems*. DOI: 10.1109/DSAA.2018.00018

Girdhar, N., Sinha, A., & Gupta, S. (2022). DenseNet-II: An improved deep convolutional neural network for melanoma cancer detection. *Soft Computing*, *27*(18), 13285–13304. DOI: 10.1007/s00500-022-07406-z PMID: 36034768

Godbole, S., Kattukaran, A., Savla, S., Pradhan, V., Kanani, P., & Patil, D. (2024). Enhancing Paediatric Pneumonia Detection and Classification Using Customized CNNs and Transfer Learning Based Ensemble Models. *International Research Journal of Multidisciplinary Technovation*, *6*(6), 38–53. DOI: 10.54392/irjmt2463

Gokapay, D. K., & Mohanty, S. N. (2024). Enhanced MRI-based brain tumor segmentation and feature extraction using Berkeley wavelet transform and ETCCNN. *Digital Health*, *10*, 20552076241305282. DOI: 10.1177/20552076241305282 PMID: 39698507

Goldman, O., Ben-Assuli, O., Rogowski, O., Zeltser, D., Shapira, I., Berliner, S., Zelber-Sagi, S., & Shenhar-Tsarfaty, S. (2021). Non-alcoholic fatty liver and liver fibrosis predictive analytics: Risk prediction and machine learning techniques for improved preventive medicine. *Journal of Medical Systems*, *45*(2), 1–12. DOI: 10.1007/s10916-020-01693-5 PMID: 33426569

Goodfellow, I., Pouget-Abadie, J., Mirza, M., Xu, B., Warde-Farley, D., Ozair, S., & Bengio, Y. (2014). Generative adversarial nets. *Advances in Neural Information Processing Systems*, ●●●, 27.

Got, A., Moussaoui, A., & Zouache, D. (2021). Hybrid filter-wrapper feature selection using whale optimization algorithm: A multi-objective approach. *Expert Systems with Applications*, *183*, 115312. DOI: 10.1016/j.eswa.2021.115312

Gottapu, R. D., & Dagli, C. H. (2018). DenseNet for anatomical brain segmentation. *Procedia Computer Science*, *140*, 179–185. DOI: 10.1016/j.procs.2018.10.327

Gowda, D. V., Sharma, A., Mukherjee, S., & Rahman, M. (2024). Optimizing resource allocation in healthcare facilities through IoT and machine learning predictive analysis. In *Universal threats in expert applications and solutions* (pp. 177–187).

Gowda, D., Shindhe, R., Simha, S. K., & Yashwanth, T. (2023, December). Healthcare Energized by Motion Harnessing Piezoelectric Energy in Conjunction with IoT for Medical Innovations. In *2023 International Conference on Artificial Intelligence for Innovations in Healthcare Industries (ICAIIHI)* (Vol. 1, pp. 1-7). IEEE.

Greenhalgh, T., Wherton, J., Papoutsi, C., Lynch, J., Hughes, G., A'Court, C., Hinder, S., Fahy, N., Procter, R., & Shaw, S. (2017). Beyond adoption: A new framework for theorizing and evaluating nonadoption, abandonment, and challenges to the scale-up, spread, and sustainability of health and care technologies. *Journal of Medical Internet Research*, *19*(11), e367. DOI: 10.2196/jmir.8775 PMID: 29092808

Guo, K., Yu, H., Chai, R., Nguyen, H., & Su, S. W. (2019, July). A hybrid physiological approach of emotional reaction detection using combined FCM and SVM classifier. In *2019 41st Annual International Conference of the IEEE Engineering in Medicine and Biology Society (EMBC)* (pp. 7088-7091). IEEE. DOI: 10.1109/EMBC.2019.8857698

Gupta, L., Jayavanth, S., & Ramaiah, A. (2008). Identification of different types of lymphoblasts in acute lymphoblastic leukemia using relevance vector machines. In *Proceedings of the Annual International Conference of the IEEE Engineering in Medicine and Biology Society (EMBC)* (Vol. 2009, pp. 6675–6678). IEEE. DOI: 10.1109/IEMBS.2008.4650279

Gupta, R.. (2022). Edge computing for healthcare in resource-limited settings. *IEEE Transactions on Biomedical Engineering*.

Gupta, R.. (2024). Social media's role in healthcare: Opportunities and challenges for nursing professionals. *Journal of Health Informatics*, *19*, 98–112.

Hardt, M., Price, E., & Srebro, N. (2021). Equality of opportunity in supervised learning. In *Advances in Neural Information Processing Systems (NeurIPS)*.

Haripriya, R., Khare, N., Pandey, M., & Biswas, S. (2025). A privacy-enhanced framework for collaborative big data analysis in healthcare using adaptive federated learning aggregation. *Journal of Big Data*, *12*(1), 113. DOI: 10.1186/s40537-025-01169-8

Hasan, M. K., Alam, M. A., Das, D., Hossain, E., & Hasan, M. (2020). Diabetes prediction using ensembling of different machine learning classifiers. *IEEE Access : Practical Innovations, Open Solutions*, *8*(99), 1–1. DOI: 10.1109/ACCESS.2020.2989857

Hastie, T., Friedman, J. H., & Tibshirani, R. (2009). *The elements of statistical learning: Data mining, inference, and prediction*. Springer Science & Business Media. DOI: 10.1007/978-0-387-84858-7

Hochreiter, S., & Schmidhuber, J. (1997). Long short-term memory. *Neural Computation*, *9*(8), 1735–1780. DOI: 10.1162/neco.1997.9.8.1735 PMID: 9377276

Holland, J. H. (1992). Adaptation in Natural and Artificial Systems: An Introductory Analysis with Applications to Biology, Control, and Artificial Intelligence. Adaptation in Natural and Artificial Systems. https://doi.org/https://doi.org/10.7551/mitpress/1090.001.0001

Holland, J. H. (1975). *Adaptation in natural and artificial systems*. University of Michigan Press.

Hosny, A., Parmar, C., Coroller, T. P., Grossmann, P., Zeleznik, R., Kumar, A., Bussink, J., Gillies, R. J., Mak, R. H., & Aerts, H. J. W. L. (2018). Deep learning for lung cancer prognostication: A retrospective multi-cohort radiomics study. *PLoS Medicine*, *15*(11), e1002711. DOI: 10.1371/journal.pmed.1002711 PMID: 30500819

Hosny, K. M., Mohammed, M. A., Salama, R. A., & Elshewey, A. M. (2024). Explainable ensemble deep learning-based model for brain tumor detection and classification. *Neural Computing & Applications*, •••, 1–18.

Hu, L., Zhang, Y., Chen, K., & Mobayen, S. (2022). A computer-aided melanoma detection using deep learning and an improved African vulture optimization algorithm. *International Journal of Imaging Systems and Technology*, *32*(6), 2002–2016. DOI: 10.1002/ima.22738

Hulsen, T. (2023). Explainable artificial intelligence (XAI): Concepts and challenges in healthcare. *AI*, *4*(3), 652–666. DOI: 10.3390/ai4030034

Islam, M. A., Majumder, M. Z. H., Hussein, M. A., Hossain, K. M., & Miah, M. S. (2024). A review of machine learning and deep learning algorithms for Parkinson's disease detection using handwriting and voice datasets. *Heliyon*, *10*(3), e25469. DOI: 10.1016/j.heliyon.2024.e25469 PMID: 38356538

Islam, M. A., Majumder, M. Z. H., Miah, M. S., & Jannaty, S. (2024). Precision healthcare: A deep dive into machine learning algorithms and feature selection strategies for accurate heart disease prediction. *Computers in Biology and Medicine*, *176*, 108432. DOI: 10.1016/j.compbiomed.2024.108432 PMID: 38744014

Jadhav, M. R., & Kaur, M. (2023). Predictive modeling of dental health outcomes based on fluoride concentrations using AI. In *Proceedings of the 2023 3rd International Conference on Smart Generation Computing, Communication and Networking (SMART GENCON)* (pp. 1–7).

Jagadev, P., & Virani, H. G. (2017). Detection of leukemia and its types using image processing and machine learning. In *Proceedings of the International Conference on Trends in Electronics and Informatics (ICEI 2017)* (pp. 123–128). IEEE. DOI: 10.1109/ICOEI.2017.8300983

Jawahar, M., Anbarasi, L. J., Narayanan, S., & Gandomi, A. H. (2024). An attention-based deep learning for acute lymphoblastic leukemia classification. *Scientific Reports*, *14*(1), 17447. DOI: 10.1038/s41598-024-67826-9 PMID: 39075091

Jha, P., Dembla, D., & Dubey, W. (2024). Deep learning models for enhancing potato leaf disease prediction: Implementation of transfer learning based stacking ensemble model. *Multimedia Tools and Applications*, *83*(13), 37839–37858. DOI: 10.1007/s11042-023-16993-4

Jiang, F., Jiang, Y., Zhi, H., Dong, Y., Li, H., Ma, S., Wang, Y., Dong, Q., Shen, H., & Wang, Y. (2017). Artificial intelligence in healthcare: Past, present, and future. *Stroke and Vascular Neurology*, *2*(4), 230–243. DOI: 10.1136/svn-2017-000101 PMID: 29507784

Johnson, A., Pollard, T., Shen, L., Lehman, L. W., Feng, M., Ghassemi, M., Moody, B., Szolovits, P., Anthony Celi, L., & Mark, R. G. (2016). MIMIC-III, a freely accessible critical care database. *Scientific Data*, *3*(1), 160035. DOI: 10.1038/sdata.2016.35 PMID: 27219127

Johri, A., Bhadula, S., Sharma, S., & Shukla, A. S. (2022). Assessment of factors affecting implementation of IoT based smart skin monitoring systems. *Technology in Society*, *68*, 101908. DOI: 10.1016/j.techsoc.2022.101908

Jolliffe, I. T. (2002). *Principal component analysis* (2nd ed.). Springer.

Jones, D. R., Schonlau, M., & Welch, W. J. (1998). Efficient global optimization of expensive black-box functions. *Journal of Global Optimization*, *13*(4), 455–492. DOI: 10.1023/A:1008306431147

Juyal, S., Sharma, S., & Shukla, A. S. (2021). Smart skin health monitoring using AI-enabled cloud-based IoT. *Materials Today: Proceedings*, *46*, 10539–10545. DOI: 10.1016/j.matpr.2021.01.074

Juyal, S., Sharma, S., & Shukla, A. S. (2021a). Security and privacy issues in unified IoT-based skin monitoring system. *Materials Today: Proceedings*, *46*, 10815–10820. DOI: 10.1016/j.matpr.2021.01.718

Kalpana, V., & Hariram, V. (2023). Artificial intelligence-based health monitoring system on IoT platform. In *Proceedings of the 2023 Second International Conference on Augmented Intelligence and Sustainable Systems (ICAISS)* (pp. 1458–1463).

Kanchanamala, P., Kuppusamy, V., & Ganesan, G. (2025). QDCNN-DMN: A hybrid deep learning approach for brain tumor classification using MRI images. *Biomedical Signal Processing and Control*, *101*, 107199. DOI: 10.1016/j.bspc.2024.107199

Kandula, A. R., Kalyanapu, S., Kodavalla, R., Kapalavai, S. K., Dhanekula, H. K. C., & Talluri, A. K. (2024). Deep Learning-Based MRI Analysis for Early Brain Tumor Detection. In *International Conference on Innovations in Cybersecurity and Data Science Proceedings of ICICDS* (pp. 283-298). Springer, Singapore. DOI: 10.1007/978-981-97-5791-6_22

Kanna, R. K., Anitha, R., Sundaramoorthy, K., Tengey, C., Banappagoudar, S. B., & Salau, A. O. (2024, November). Computational Machine Learning Approach for Brain Impairment. In *2024 IEEE 5th International Conference on Electro-Computing Technologies for Humanity (NIGERCON)* (pp. 1-5). IEEE. DOI: 10.1109/NIGERCON62786.2024.10927119

Kanna, R. K., Sahoo, S. K., Madhavi, B. K., Mohan, V., Babu, G. S., & Panigrahi, B. S. (2024). Detection of Brain Tumour based on Optimal Convolution Neural Network. *EAI Endorsed Transactions on Pervasive Health and Technology*, *10*(1).

Kanna, R. K., & Salau, A. O. (2025). New Cognitive Computational Strategy for Optimizing Brain Tumour Classification using Magnetic Resonance Imaging Data. *Intelligence-Based Medicine*, *11*, 100215. DOI: 10.1016/j.ibmed.2025.100215

Karaboga, D. (2005). AN IDEA BASED ON HONEY BEE SWARM FOR NUMERICAL OPTIMIZATION. chrome-extension://efaidnbmnnnibpcajpcglclefindmkaj/https://abc.erciyes.edu.tr/pub/tr06_2005.pdf

Karimian, M. (2025). A Short Review on Diagnosing and Predicting Mental Disorders with Machine Learning. *International Journal of Applied Data Science in Engineering and Health*, *1*(1), 20–27.

Kar, S., Aich, U., & Singh, P. K. (2024). Efficient Brain Tumor Classification Using Filter-Based Deep Feature Selection Methodology. *SN Computer Science*, *5*(8), 1–24. DOI: 10.1007/s42979-024-03392-1

Kaur, I., Sandhu, A. K., & Kumar, Y. (2022). Artificial intelligence techniques for predictive modeling of vector-borne diseases and its pathogens: A systematic review. *Archives of Computational Methods in Engineering*, *29*(6), 3741–3771. DOI: 10.1007/s11831-022-09724-9

Kaur, S., Aggarwal, H., & Rani, R. (2020). Hyper-parameter optimization of deep learning model for prediction of Parkinson's disease. *Machine Vision and Applications*, *31*(5), 1–15. DOI: 10.1007/s00138-020-01078-1

Kavas, P. O., Bozkurt, M. R., Kocayigit, I., & Bilgin, C. (2022). *A New Medical Decision Support System for Diagnosing HFrEF and HFpEF using ECG and Machine Learning Techniques*. IEEE., DOI: 10.1109/ACCESS.2022.3213065

Ke, C., Xiao, C., Li, J., Wu, X., Zhang, Y., Chen, Y., Sheng, S., Fu, Z., Wang, L., Ni, C., Zhao, J., Shi, Y., Wu, Y., Zhong, Z., Nan, J., Zhu, W., Chen, J., Wu, R., & Hu, X. (2025). FMO2 ameliorates nonalcoholic fatty liver disease by suppressing ER-to-Golgi transport of SREBP1. *Hepatology (Baltimore, Md.)*, *81*(1), 181–197. DOI: 10.1097/HEP.0000000000000643 PMID: 37874228

Kennedy, J., & Eberhart, R. (1995). Particle swarm optimization. *Proceedings of ICNN'95 - International Conference on Neural Networks*, 4, 1942-1948. DOI: 10.1109/ICNN.1995.488968

Kesav, N., & Jibukumar, M. (2022). Efficient and low complex architecture for detection and classification of brain tumor using RCNN with two channel CNN. *Journal of King Saud University. Computer and Information Sciences*, *34*(8), 6229–6242. DOI: 10.1016/j.jksuci.2021.05.008

Kezer, C. A., Simonetto, D. A., & Shah, V. H. (2021, April). Sex differences in alcohol consumption and alcohol-associated liver disease. []. Elsevier.]. *Mayo Clinic Proceedings*, *96*(4), 1006–1016. DOI: 10.1016/j.mayocp.2020.08.020 PMID: 33714602

Khalsan, M., Mu, M., Al-Shamery, E., Ajit, S., Machado, L., & Opoku Agyeman, M. (2023). A novel fuzzy classifier model for cancer classification using gene expression data. *IEEE Access : Practical Innovations, Open Solutions*, *11*(99), 1–1. DOI: 10.1109/ACCESS.2023.3325381

Khan, M. A., Mazhar, T., Mateen Yaqoob, M., Badruddin Khan, M., Jilani Saudagar, A. K., Ghadi, Y. Y., Khattak, U. F., & Shahid, M. (2024). Optimal feature selection for heart disease prediction using modified Artificial Bee colony (M-ABC) and K-nearest neighbors (KNN). *Scientific Reports*, *14*(1), 26241. DOI: 10.1038/s41598-024-78021-1 PMID: 39482391

Kim, H. E., Cosa-Linan, A., Santhanam, N., Jannesari, M., Maros, M. E., & Ganslandt, T. (2022). Transfer learning for medical image classification: A literature review. *BMC Medical Imaging*, *22*(69), 69. Advance online publication. DOI: 10.1186/s12880-022-00793-7 PMID: 35418051

Kingma, D. P., & Ba, J. (2014). Adam: A method for stochastic optimization. *arXiv preprint arXiv:1412.6980*.

Kirkpatrick, S., Gelatt, C. D.Jr, & Vecchi, M. P. (1983). Optimization by simulated annealing. *Science*, *220*(4598), 671–680. DOI: 10.1126/science.220.4598.671 PMID: 17813860

Kolasa, K., Admassu, B. Y., Holownia, M., & Kędzior, K. J. (2023). *Systematic reviews of machine learning in healthcare: A literature review* (Version 1). Research Square. DOI: 10.21203/rs.3.rs-3035548/v1

Kordnoori, S., Sabeti, M., Shakoor, M. H., & Moradi, E. (2024). Deep multi-task learning structure for segmentation and classification of supratentorial brain tumors in MR images. *Interdisciplinary Neurosurgery : Advanced Techniques and Case Management, 36*, 101931. DOI: 10.1016/j.inat.2023.101931

Kourou, K., Exarchos, T. P., Exarchos, K. P., Karamouzis, M. V., & Fotiadis, D. I. (2015). Machine learning applications in cancer prognosis and prediction. *Computational and Structural Biotechnology Journal, 13*, 8–17. DOI: 10.1016/j.csbj.2014.11.005 PMID: 25750696

Krishna, B., Vankdothu, R., Revuri, V., & Prashanth, B. (2024). A brain tumor identification using convolution neural network in the deep learning. In *MATEC Web of Conferences* (Vol. 392, p. 01131). EDP Sciences.

Krizhevsky, A., Sutskever, I., & Hinton, G. E. (2012). ImageNet classification with deep convolutional neural networks. *Advances in Neural Information Processing Systems*, •••, 25.

Kumar, D. K., & Nataraj, J. L. (2019). Analysis of EEG based emotion detection of DEAP and SEED-IV databases using SVM.

Kumar, A., Singh, S. K., & Gupta, D. (2021). Grey Wolf Optimizer for EEG-based epilepsy detection. *Expert Systems with Applications, 168*, 114375.

Kumari, L. K., Ananth, R. P., Ramalakshmi, K., Mohan, B., & Santhoshkumar, S. P., & Others. (2025). Advanced epileptic seizure recognition with a hybrid CNN-BiLSTM model on EEG signals. In *Proceedings of the 2025 IEEE 1st International Conference on Smart and Sustainable Developments*. DOI: 10.1109/SSDEE64538.2025.10968390

Kumari, S., & Upadhayay, A. (2025). Diabetic retinopathy prediction using machine learning. *Journal of Neonatal Surgery, 14*(18S), 767–781.

Kumar, M., Parchani, A., Kant, R., & Das, A. (2023). Relationship between vitamin D deficiency and non-alcoholic fatty liver disease: A cross-sectional study from a tertiary care center in Northern India. *Cureus, 15*(2). Advance online publication. DOI: 10.7759/cureus.34921 PMID: 36938188

Kumar, S. (2024). Parallel-way: Multi-modality-based brain tumor segmentation using parallel capsule network. *Electromagnetic Biology and Medicine, 43*(4), 1–25. DOI: 10.1080/15368378.2024.2390058 PMID: 39470986

Labati, R. D., Piuri, V., & Scotti, F. (2011). ALL-IDB: The acute lymphoblastic leukemia image database for image processing. In *Proceedings of the IEEE 18th International Conference on Image Processing (ICIP)* (pp. 2045–2048). IEEE. DOI: 10.1109/ICIP.2011.6115881

Lavric, A., Popa, V., Takahashi, H., & Yousefi, S. (2020). Detecting keratoconus from corneal imaging data using machine learning. *IEEE Access : Practical Innovations, Open Solutions*, *8*, 149113–149121. DOI: 10.1109/ACCESS.2020.3016060

LeCun, Y., Bengio, Y., & Hinton, G. (2015). Deep learning. *Nature*, *521*(7553), 436–444. DOI: 10.1038/nature14539 PMID: 26017442

Lee, S. M., Jung, Y. M., Choi, E. S., Kwak, S. H., Koo, J. N., Oh, I. H., Kim, B. J., Kim, S. M., Kim, S. Y., Kim, G. M., Joo, S. K., Koo, B. K., Shin, S., Norwitz, E. R., Park, C.-W., Jun, J. K., Kim, W., & Park, J. S. (2022). Metabolic dysfunction-associated fatty liver disease and subsequent development of adverse pregnancy outcomes. *Clinical Gastroenterology and Hepatology*, *20*(11), 2542–2550. DOI: 10.1016/j.cgh.2021.11.007 PMID: 34798335

Lessard, E., & Pouliot, J. (2001). Inverse planning anatomy-based dose optimization for HDR-brachytherapy of the prostate using fast simulated annealing algorithm and dedicated objective function. *Medical Physics*, *28*(5), 773–779. DOI: 10.1118/1.1368127 PMID: 11393472

Liaw, A., & Wiener, M. (2002). Classification and regression by randomForest. *R News*, *2*(3), 18–22.

Li, M., Wang, Y., Xu, L., Li, J., Chen, M., & Zhang, W. (2021). Causal inference framework for clinical trial eligibility criteria optimization. *Journal of Biomedical Informatics*, *114*, 103671.

Li, T., Sahu, A. K., Talwalkar, A., & Smith, V. (2020). Federated learning: Challenges, methods, and future directions. *IEEE Signal Processing Magazine*, *37*(3), 50–60. DOI: 10.1109/MSP.2020.2975749

Litjens, G., Kooi, T., Ehteshami Bejnordi, B., Setio, A. A., Ciompi, F., Ghafoorian, M., van der Laak, J. A. W. M., van Ginneken, B., & Sánchez, C. I. (2017). A survey on deep learning in medical image analysis. *Medical Image Analysis*, *42*, 60–88. DOI: 10.1016/j.media.2017.07.005 PMID: 28778026

Liu, J., Wang, Y., Chen, L., Li, K., Zhang, W., & Wang, Z. (2019). Grey wolf optimizer for deep brain stimulation electrode trajectory planning with probabilistic risk models. *IEEE Transactions on Biomedical Engineering*, *67*(8), 2195–2204. PMID: 31804925

Liu, M., Shen, X., & Pan, W. (2022). Deep reinforcement learning for personalized treatment recommendation. *Statistics in Medicine*, *41*(4), 623–639. DOI: 10.1002/sim.9491 PMID: 35716038

Liu, N., Shapira, P., & Yue, X. (2021). Tracking developments in artificial intelligence research: Constructing and applying a new search strategy. *Scientometrics*, *126*(4), 3153–3192. DOI: 10.1007/s11192-021-03868-4 PMID: 34720254

Liu, R., Luo, C., Pang, Z., Zhang, J., Ruan, S., Wu, M., Wang, L., Sun, T., Li, N., Han, L., Shi, J., Huang, Y., Guo, W., Peng, S., Zhou, W., & Gao, H. (2023). Advances of nanoparticles as drug delivery systems for disease diagnosis and treatment. *Chinese Chemical Letters*, *34*(2), 107518. DOI: 10.1016/j.cclet.2022.05.032

Li, Y., Yang, J., Wang, H., & Zhang, J. (2019). Ensemble learning for cancer subtype prediction using gene expression data. *BMC Genomics*, *20*, 223. DOI: 10.1186/s12864-019-5545-8

Luo, Y., Jiang, G., Yu, T., Song, K., Wang, Z., Liu, Y., & Zeng, H. (2021). ECNet is an evolutionary context-integrated deep learning framework for protein engineering. *Nature Communications*, *12*(1), 5743. DOI: 10.1038/s41467-021-25976-8 PMID: 34593817

Lu, S. L., Liao, H. C., Hsu, F. M., Liao, C. C., Lai, F., & Xiao, F. (2021). The intracranial tumor segmentation challenge: Contour tumors on brain MRI for radiosurgery. *NeuroImage*, *244*, 118585. DOI: 10.1016/j.neuroimage.2021.118585 PMID: 34560272

Lu, X., & Zadeh, Y. F. A. (2022). Deep Learning-Based Classification for melanoma detection using XceptionNet. *Journal of Healthcare Engineering*, *2022*, 1–10. DOI: 10.1155/2022/2196096 PMID: 35360474

Lv, M., Li, Y., Kou, B., & Zhou, Z. (2017). Integer programming for improving radiotherapy treatment efficiency. *PLoS ONE*, *12*(7), e0180564.Breiman, L. (2001). Random forests. *Machine Learning*, *45*(1), 5–32.

Maadi, M., Khorshidi, H. A., & Aickelin, U. (2023). An Uncertainty-Accuracy-Based Score Function for Wrapper Methods in Feature Selection. *IEEE International Conference on Fuzzy Systems*. DOI: 10.1109/FUZZ52849.2023.10309669

Macaire, J., Zermani, S., & Linguet, L. (2023). New Feature Selection Approach for Photovoltaïc Power Forecasting Using KCDE. Energies 2023, Vol. 16, Page 6842, 16(19), 6842. DOI: 10.3390/en16196842

Madaan, V., & Goyal, A. (2020). Predicting Ayurveda-based constituent balancing in human body using machine learning methods. *IEEE Access : Practical Innovations, Open Solutions*, *8*, 65060–65070. DOI: 10.1109/ACCESS.2020.2985717

Mafarja, M. M., & Mirjalili, S. (2017). Hybrid Whale Optimization Algorithm with simulated annealing for feature selection. *Neurocomputing*, *260*, 302–312. DOI: 10.1016/j.neucom.2017.04.053

Mafarja, M., & Mirjalili, S. (2018). Whale optimization approaches for wrapper feature selection. *Applied Soft Computing*, *62*, 441–453. DOI: 10.1016/j.asoc.2017.11.006

Mahmoud, N. M., & Soliman, A. M. (2024). Early automated detection system for skin cancer diagnosis using artificial intelligent techniques. *Scientific Reports*, *14*(1), 9749. Advance online publication. DOI: 10.1038/s41598-024-59783-0 PMID: 38679633

Mahnoor, M., Rainio, O., & Klén, R. (2024). Exploring Generative Adversarial Network-Based Augmentation of Magnetic Resonance Brain Tumor Images. *Applied Sciences (Basel, Switzerland)*, *14*(24), 11822. DOI: 10.3390/app142411822

Mallikarjun, S. S. D., & Kawale, S. R. (2023). Cloud-based multi-layer security framework for protecting e-health records. In *Proceedings of the 2023 International Conference on Artificial Intelligence for Innovations in Healthcare Industries (ICAIIHI)* (pp. 1–7).

Matek, C., Schwarz, S., Spiekermann, K., & Marr, C. (2019). Human-level recognition of blast cells in acute myeloid leukaemia with convolutional neural networks. *Nature Machine Intelligence*, *1*(11), 538–544. DOI: 10.1038/s42256-019-0101-9

Mazhar, T., Haq, I., Ditta, A., Mohsan, S. H., Rehman, F., Zafar, I., Gansau, J. A., & Goh, L. P. W. (2023). The role of machine learning and deep learning approaches for the detection of skin cancer. *Health Care*, *11*(3), 415. DOI: 10.3390/healthcare11030415 PMID: 36766989

McMahan, B.. (2017). *Communication-efficient learning of deep networks from decentralized data. Proceedings of the 20th International Conference on Artificial Intelligence and Statistics*.

Meißner, A. K., Blau, T., Reinecke, D., Fürtjes, G., Leyer, L., Müller, N., von Spreckelsen, N., Stehle, T., Al Shugri, A., Büttner, R., Goldbrunner, R., Timmer, M., & Neuschmelting, V. (2024). Image Quality Assessment and Reliability Analysis of Artificial Intelligence-Based Tumor Classification of Stimulated Raman Histology of Tumor Biobank Samples. *Diagnostics (Basel)*, *14*(23), 2701. DOI: 10.3390/diagnostics14232701 PMID: 39682609

Mienye, I. D., & Jere, N. (2024). Optimized ensemble learning approach with explainable AI for improved heart disease prediction. *Information (Basel), 15*(7), 394. DOI: 10.3390/info15070394

Miller, T. (2019). Explanation in artificial intelligence: Insights from the social sciences. *Artificial Intelligence, 267*, 1–38. DOI: 10.1016/j.artint.2018.07.007

Mishra, A. S., & Vijaya, J. (2024). Data Mining and Knowledge Discovery: Transforming Healthcare Through Biomedical Intelligence. In *Machine Learning and Generative AI in Smart Healthcare* (pp. 23-40). IGI Global.

Mishra, S., Majhi, B., & Sa, P. K. (2018). GLRLM-based feature extraction for acute lymphoblastic leukemia (ALL) detection. In *Proceedings of Recent Findings in Intelligent Computing Technologies* (pp. 399–407). Springer.

Mittal, M., Goyal, L. M., Kaur, S., Kaur, I., Verma, A., & Jude Hemanth, D. (2019). Deep learning based enhanced tumor segmentation approach for MR brain images. *Applied Soft Computing, 78*, 346–354. DOI: 10.1016/j.asoc.2019.02.036

Montgomery, D. C. (2017). Design and Analysis of Experiments, 9th Edition, Wiley. Wiley, 1–682. https://www.wiley.com/en-us/Design+and+Analysis+of+Experiments%2C+10th+Edition-p-9781119492443

Muniasamy, A., & Asiri, F. (2025). Advanced human activity recognition on wearables with multi-scale sparse attention. *Multimedia Tools and Applications*. Advance online publication. DOI: 10.1007/s11042-024-20475-6

Muthukrishnan, R., & Rohini, R. (2017). LASSO: A feature selection technique in predictive modeling for machine learning. *2016 IEEE International Conference on Advances in Computer Applications, ICACA 2016*, 18–20. DOI: 10.1109/ICACA.2016.7887916

Myles, A. J., Feudale, R. N., Liu, Y., Woody, N. A., & Brown, S. D. (2004). An introduction to decision tree modeling. *Journal of Chemometrics: A Journal of the Chemometrics Society, 18*(6), 275-285.

Nallamothu, P. T., & Cuthrell, K. M. (2023). Artificial intelligence in health sector: Current status and future perspectives. *Asian Journal of Research in Computer Science, 15*(4), 1–14. DOI: 10.9734/ajrcos/2023/v15i4325

Nee, L. H., Mashor, M. Y., & Hassan, R. (2012). White blood cell segmentation for acute leukemia bone marrow images. In *Proceedings of the International Conference on Biomedical Engineering (ICoBE)*, Penang, Malaysia. IEEE. DOI: 10.1166/jmihi.2012.1099

Ng, G. Y. L., Tan, S. C., & Ong, C. S. (2023). On the use of QDE-SVM for gene feature selection and cell type classification from scRNA-seq data. *PLoS One*, *18*(10), e0292961. DOI: 10.1371/journal.pone.0292961 PMID: 37856458

Nguyen, V. (2019). Bayesian optimization for accelerating hyper-parameter tuning. In *Proceedings of the 2nd IEEE International Conference on Artificial Intelligence and Knowledge Engineering (AIKE)* (pp. 302–305). https://doi.org/DOI: 10.1109/AIKE.2019.00060

Nizamani, A. H., Chen, Z., Nizamani, A. A., & Bhatti, U. A. (2023). Advance brain tumor segmentation using feature fusion methods with deep U-Net model with CNN for MRI data. *Journal of King Saud University. Computer and Information Sciences*, *35*(9), 101793. DOI: 10.1016/j.jksuci.2023.101793

Njoku, U. F., Abelló, A., Bilalli, B., & Bontempi, G. (2023). Wrapper methods for multi-objective feature selection. 26th International Conference on Extending Database Technology (EDBT 2023): Ioannina, Greece, March 28-March 31. *Proceedings*, *26*(3), 697–709. DOI: 10.48786/EDBT.2023.58

Noble, W. S. (2006). What is a support vector machine? *Nature Biotechnology*, *24*(12), 1565–1567. DOI: 10.1038/nbt1206-1565 PMID: 17160063

Obermeyer, Z., & Emanuel, E. J. (2016). Predicting the future—Big data, machine learning, and clinical medicine. *The New England Journal of Medicine*, *375*(13), 1216–1219. DOI: 10.1056/NEJMp1606181 PMID: 27682033

Obermeyer, Z., Powers, B. W., Vogeli, C., & Mullainathan, S. (2019). Dissecting racial bias in an algorithm used to manage the health of populations. *Science*, *366*(6464), 447–453. DOI: 10.1126/science.aax2342 PMID: 31649194

Ogunpola, A., Saeed, F., Basurra, S., Albarrak, A. M., & Qasem, S. N. (2024). Machine learning-based predictive models for detection of cardiovascular diseases. *Diagnostics (Basel)*, *14*(2), 144. DOI: 10.3390/diagnostics14020144 PMID: 38248021

Onaizah, A. N., Xia, Y., & Hussain, K. (2025). FL-SiCNN: An improved brain tumor diagnosis using siamese convolutional neural network in a peer-to-peer federated learning approach. *Alexandria Engineering Journal*, *114*, 1–11. DOI: 10.1016/j.aej.2024.11.063

Orhan, H., & Yavşan, E. (2023). Artificial intelligence-assisted detection model for melanoma diagnosis using deep learning techniques. *Mathematical Modelling and Numerical Simulation With Applications*, *3*(2), 159–169. DOI: 10.53391/mmnsa.1311943

Özen Kavas, P., Recep Bozkurt, M., Kocayiğit, İ., & Bilgin, C. (2023). Machine learning-based medical decision support system for diagnosing HFpEF and HFrEF using PPG. *Biomedical Signal Processing and Control*, *79*, 104164. DOI: 10.1016/j.bspc.2022.104164

Padmavathi, P., Harikiran, J., & Vijaya, J. (2023). Effective deep learning based segmentation and classification in wireless capsule endoscopy images. *Multimedia Tools and Applications*, *82*(30), 47109–47133. DOI: 10.1007/s11042-023-14621-9

Pandidurai, M., & Senthil Kamalesh, M. S. C. (2023). Design of IoT-based rural health helper using natural language processing. In *Proceedings of the 2023 4th International Conference on Electronics and Sustainable Communication Systems (ICESC)* (pp. 328–333).

Panigrahi, S., Adhikary, D. R. D., & Pattanayak, B. K. (2024). Analyzing Activation Functions with Transfer Learning-based Layer Customization for Improved Brain Tumor Classification. *IEEE Access : Practical Innovations, Open Solutions*, *12*, 168707–168727. DOI: 10.1109/ACCESS.2024.3497346

Pankajavalli, P. B., Karthick, G. S., & Sakthivel, R. (2021). An efficient machine learning framework for stress prediction via sensor integrated keyboard data. *IEEE Access : Practical Innovations, Open Solutions*, *9*, 95023–95035. DOI: 10.1109/ACCESS.2021.3094334

Parbhoo, S., Bogojeska, J., Zazzi, M., Roth, V., & Doshi-Velez, F. (2017). Combining kernel and model based learning for HIV therapy selection. *AMIA Joint Summits on Translational Science Proceedings AMIA Summit on Translational Science*, *2017*, 239–248. PMID: 28815137

Patel, D., Saxena, A., & Wang, J. (2024). A Machine Learning-Based Wrapper Method for Feature Selection. [IJDWM]. *International Journal of Data Warehousing and Mining*, *20*(1), 1–33. DOI: 10.4018/IJDWM.352041

Patil, N. J., Sharma, A., Prasad, K. D. V., & Kottala, S. (2024). IoT-enabled predictive healthcare monitoring using machine learning models. In *Universal threats in expert applications and solutions* (pp. 165–175). DOI: 10.1007/978-981-97-5146-4_15

Patro, S. P., Nayak, G. S., & Padhy, N. (2021). Heart disease prediction by using novel optimization algorithm: A supervised learning prospective. *Informatics in Medicine Unlocked*, *26*, 100696. DOI: 10.1016/j.imu.2021.100696

Pedregosa, F., Varoquaux, G., Gramfort, A., Michel, V., Thirion, B., Grisel, O., ... & Duchesnay, É. (2011). Scikit-learn: Machine learning in Python. the Journal of machine Learning research, 12, 2825-2830.

Peng, H., Long, F., & Ding, C. (2005). Feature selection based on mutual information: Criteria of Max-Dependency, Max-Relevance, and Min-Redundancy. *IEEE Transactions on Pattern Analysis and Machine Intelligence*, *27*(8), 1226–1238. DOI: 10.1109/TPAMI.2005.159 PMID: 16119262

Peng, Y., & Sun, J. (2023). The multimodal MRI brain tumor segmentation based on AD-Net. *Biomedical Signal Processing and Control*, *80*, 104336. DOI: 10.1016/j.bspc.2022.104336

Pesaramelli, R. S., & Sujatha, B. (2024, March). Principle correlated feature extraction using differential evolution for improved classification. In *AIP Conference Proceedings* (Vol. 2919, No. 1). AIP Publishing. DOI: 10.1063/5.0184938

Petersen, E., Potdevin, Y., Mohammadi, E., Zidowitz, S., Breyer, S., Nowotka, D., Henn, S., Pechmann, L., Leucker, M., Rostalski, P., & Herzog, C. (2022). Responsible and regulatory conform machine learning for medicine: A survey of challenges and solutions. *IEEE Access : Practical Innovations, Open Solutions*, *10*, 58375–58418. DOI: 10.1109/ACCESS.2022.3178382

Prasad, K., S. R., & A. K. N. (2024). Design and implementation of an AI and IoT-enabled smart safety helmet for real-time environmental and health monitoring. In *Proceedings of the 2024 IEEE International Conference on Information Technology, Electronics and Intelligent Communication Systems (ICITEICS)* (pp. 1–7).

Prasanna, K. S., & Vijaya, J. (2022). Building an efficient heart disease prediction system by using clustering techniques. In *High Performance Computing and Networking: Select Proceedings of CHSN 2021* (pp. 69-81). Singapore: Springer Singapore. DOI: 10.1007/978-981-16-9885-9_6

Qin, J., Chen, L., Liu, Y., Liu, C., Feng, C., & Chen, B. (2020). A machine learning methodology for diagnosing chronic kidney disease. *IEEE Access : Practical Innovations, Open Solutions*, *8*, 20991–21002. DOI: 10.1109/ACCESS.2019.2963053

Quinlan, J. R. (1996). Improved use of continuous attributes in C4.5. *Journal of Artificial Intelligence Research*, *4*, 77–90. DOI: 10.1613/jair.279

R, K. K., R. Kshirsagar, P., R, T., Tak, T. K., & B, S. (2025). Advanced Analysis of Alpha EEG Patterns for Identifying Meditative States in Alpha Power Activation Yoga (APAY). *International Research Journal of Multidisciplinary Technovation*, *7*(2), 148–164.

R, Suresh, Kumar V, Jeyaganesan A, Thangaraj P, Athisayaraj S, Viswanath Sundar, and Ramakrishnan R. (2025). A Novel CNN Architecture for Accurate Recognition of Elastic Band Training Poses. *International Research Journal of Multidisciplinary Technovation, 7*(3), 42–52. https://doi.org/ .DOI: 10.54392/irjmt2534

Rahman, W., Faruque, M. G. G., Roksana, K., Sadi, A. S., Rahman, M. M., & Azad, M. M. (2023). Multiclass blood cancer classification using deep CNN with optimized features. *Array (New York, N.Y.), 18*, 100292. DOI: 10.1016/j.array.2023.100292

Rahul, J., Sharma, D., Sharma, L. D., Nanda, U., & Sarkar, A. K. (2024). A systematic review of EEG based automated schizophrenia classification through machine learning and deep learning. *Frontiers in Human Neuroscience, 18*, 1347082. DOI: 10.3389/fnhum.2024.1347082 PMID: 38419961

Rajagopal, A., Ayanian, S., Ryu, A. J., Qian, R., Legler, S. R., Peeler, E. A., Issa, M., Coons, T. J., & Kawamoto, K. (2024). Machine learning operations in health care: A scoping review. *Mayo Clinic Proceedings. Digital Health, 2*(3), 421–437. DOI: 10.1016/j.mcpdig.2024.06.009 PMID: 40206123

Rajeswaran, A., Kumar, V., Gupta, A., Schulman, J., Todorov, E., & Levine, S. (2017). Learning complex dexterous manipulation with deep reinforcement learning and demonstrations. *arXiv preprint arXiv:1709.10087.*

Rajkomar, A., Dean, J., & Kohane, I. (2018). Machine learning in medicine. *The New England Journal of Medicine, 380*(14), 1347–1359. DOI: 10.1056/NEJMra1814259 PMID: 30943338

Ramalakshmi, K., Raghavan, V. S., Kaliappan, J., & Srinivasan, K. (2024). Edge-preserved Tversky indexive Hellinger with deep perceptive Czekanowski-based image classification. *Journal of Sensors, 2024*(1), 4024107. DOI: 10.1155/2024/4024107

Ramalakshmi, K., Raghavan, V. S., Rajagopal, S., Kumari, L. K., & Theivanathan, G. (2024). An extensive analysis of artificial intelligence and segmentation methods transforming cancer recognition in medical imaging. *Biomedical Physics & Engineering Express, 10*(4), 045046. DOI: 10.1088/2057-1976/ad555b PMID: 38848695

Ramalakshmi, K., Rajagopal, S., Kulkarni, M. B., & Poddar, H. (2024). A hyperdimensional framework: Unveiling the interplay of RBP and GSN within CNNs for ultra-precise brain tumor classification. *Biomedical Signal Processing and Control, 96*, 106565. DOI: 10.1016/j.bspc.2024.106565

Ramalakshmi, K., & Srinivasa Raghavan, V. (2023). Enhanced prediction using deep neural network-based image classification. *Imaging Science Journal, 71*(5), 472–483. DOI: 10.1080/13682199.2023.2183621

Ramesha, M., Anughna, N., Nareshkumar, A., Gowda, D., & Gururaj, B. (2022, November). An integrated IoT technology for health and traffic monitoring system with smart ambulance. In *2022 IEEE North Karnataka Subsection Flagship International Conference (NKCon)* (pp. 1-6). IEEE.

Ramesh, B., & Lakshmanna, K. (2024). A novel early detection and prevention of coronary heart disease framework using hybrid deep learning model and neural fuzzy inference system. *IEEE Access : Practical Innovations, Open Solutions*, *12*, 26683–26695. DOI: 10.1109/ACCESS.2024.3366537

Ram, M., Afrash, M. R., Moulaei, K., Parvin, M., Esmaeeli, E., Karbasi, Z., Heydari, S., & Sabahi, A. (2024). Application of artificial intelligence in chronic myeloid leukemia (CML) disease prediction and management: A scoping review. *BMC Cancer*, *24*(1), 1026. DOI: 10.1186/s12885-024-12764-y PMID: 39164653

Rancea, A., Anghel, I., & Cioara, T. (2024). Edge computing in healthcare: Innovations, opportunities, and challenges. *Future Internet*, *16*(9), 329. DOI: 10.3390/fi16090329

Rao, G. M., Ramesh, D., Sharma, V., Sinha, A., Hassan, M. M., & Gandomi, A. H. (2024). AttGRU-HMSI: Enhancing heart disease diagnosis using hybrid deep learning approach. *Scientific Reports*, *14*(1), 7833. DOI: 10.1038/s41598-024-56931-4 PMID: 38570560

Rashmi, G. R., & Chinamuttevi, V. S. (2022). IoT-based smart healthcare system to monitor COVID-19 patients. *International Journal of Electrical and Electronics Research*, *10*(1), 36–40. DOI: 10.37391/IJEER.100105

Razzak, M. I., Imran, M., & Xu, G. (2019). Efficient brain tumor segmentation with multiscale two-pathway-group conventional neural networks. *IEEE Journal of Biomedical and Health Informatics*, *23*(5), 1911–1919. DOI: 10.1109/JBHI.2018.2874033 PMID: 30295634

Reddy, K. V. V., Elamvazuthi, I., Aziz, A. A., Paramasivam, S., Chua, H. N., & Pranavanand, S. (2021). Prediction of heart disease risk using machine learning with correlation-based feature selection and optimization techniques. In *Proceedings of the 2021 7th International Conference on Signal Processing and Communication (ICSC)*(pp. 228–233). DOI: 10.1109/ICSC53193.2021.9673490

Reddy, N. N., Nipun, L., Baba, M. U., Rishindra, N., & Shilpa, T. (2024). Optimizing heart disease prediction through ensemble and hybrid machine learning techniques. [IJECE]. *International Journal of Electrical and Computer Engineering*, *14*(5), 5744–5754. DOI: 10.11591/ijece.v14i5.pp5744-5754

Richard, O., Duda, S., David, G., & Hart, P. E. (2001). *Pattern classification*. Wiley.

Rieke, N., Hancox, J., Li, W., Milletarì, F., Roth, H. R., Albarqouni, S., Bakas, S., Galtier, M. N., Landman, B. A., Maier-Hein, K., Ourselin, S., Sheller, M., Summers, R. M., Trask, A., Xu, D., Baust, M., & Cardoso, M. J. (2020). The future of digital health with federated learning. *npj. Digital Medicine*, *3*(1), 119. DOI: 10.1038/s41746-020-00323-1 PMID: 33015372

Rish, I. (2001, August). An empirical study of the naive Bayes classifier. In *IJCAI 2001 workshop on empirical methods in artificial intelligence* (Vol. 3, No. 22, pp. 41-46).

Robnik-Šikonja, M., & Kononenko, I. (2003). Theoretical and Empirical Analysis of ReliefF and RReliefF. *Machine Learning*, *53*(1–2), 23–69. DOI: 10.1023/A:1025667309714

Rodrigues, D., Pereira, L. A. M., Nakamura, R. Y. M., Costa, K. A. P., Yang, X. S., Souza, A. N., & Papa, J. P. (2014). A wrapper approach for feature selection based on Bat Algorithm and Optimum-Path Forest. *Expert Systems with Applications*, *41*(5), 2250–2258. DOI: 10.1016/j.eswa.2013.09.023

Rojas, R. (2009). AdaBoost and the super bowl of classifiers a tutorial introduction to adaptive boosting. *Freie University, Berlin. Tech. Rep*, *1*(1), 1–6.

Rumelhart, D. E., Hinton, G. E., & Williams, R. J. (1986). Learning representations by backpropagating errors. *Nature*, *323*(6088), 533–536. DOI: 10.1038/323533a0

Rustam, F., Reshi, A., Mehmood, A., Ullah, S., On, B., Aslam, W., & Choi, G. S. (2020). COVID-19 future forecasting using supervised machine learning models. *IEEE Access : Practical Innovations, Open Solutions*, *8*(99), 1–1. DOI: 10.1109/ACCESS.2020.2997311

Saebi, M., Nan, B., Herr, J., Wahlers, J., Wiest, O., & Chawla, N. (2021). Graph neural networks for predicting chemical reaction performance. *ChemRxiv*. DOI: 10.26434/chemrxiv.14589498

Sakar, C. O., Serbes, G., Gunduz, A., Tunc, H. C., Nizam, H., Sakar, B. E., Tutuncu, M., Aydin, T., Isenkul, M. E., & Apaydin, H. (2019). A comparative analysis of speech signal processing algorithms for Parkinson's disease classification and the use of the tunable Q-factor wavelet transform. *Applied Soft Computing*, *74*, 255–263. DOI: 10.1016/j.asoc.2018.10.022

Saleem, S., Amin, J., Sharif, M., Mallah, G. A., Kadry, S., & Gandomi, A. H. (2022). Leukemia segmentation and classification: A comprehensive survey. *Computers in Biology and Medicine*, *150*, 106095. DOI: 10.1016/j.compbiomed.2022.106028 PMID: 36126356

Sallam, N. M., Saleh, A. I., Arafat Ali, H., & Abdelsalam, M. M. (2022). An Efficient Strategy for Blood Diseases Detection Based on Grey Wolf Optimization as Feature Selection and Machine Learning Techniques. Applied Sciences 2022, Vol. 12, Page 10760, 12(21), 10760. DOI: 10.3390/app122110760

Sangui, S., Iqbal, T., Chandra, P. C., Ghosh, S. K., & Ghosh, A. (2023). 3D MRI segmentation using U-Net architecture for the detection of brain tumor. *Procedia Computer Science*, *218*, 542–553. DOI: 10.1016/j.procs.2023.01.036

Saxena, S., Chauhan, R., Bhatt, C., & Devliyal, S. (2025). Brain tumor detection using integrated approach of FCM & convolutional neural network. In *Challenges in Information, Communication and Computing Technology* (pp. 292-298). CRC Press.

Scotti, F. (2005). Automatic morphological analysis for acute leukemia identification in peripheral blood microscope images. In *Proceedings of the 2005 IEEE International Conference on Computational Intelligence for Measurement Systems and Applications* (pp. 96–101). IEEE. DOI: 10.1109/CIMSA.2005.1522835

Serrano, D. R., Luciano, F. C., Anaya, B. J., Ongoren, B., Kara, A., Molina, G., Ramirez, B. I., Sánchez-Guirales, S. A., Simon, J. A., Tomietto, G., Rapti, C., Ruiz, H. K., Rawat, S., Kumar, D., & Lalatsa, A. (2024). Artificial intelligence (AI) applications in drug discovery and drug delivery: Revolutionizing personalized medicine. *Pharmaceutics*, *16*(10), 1328. DOI: 10.3390/pharmaceutics16101328 PMID: 39458657

Shafique, S., & Tehsin, S. (2018). Acute lymphoblastic leukemia detection and classification of its subtypes using pretrained deep convolutional neural networks. *Technology in Cancer Research & Treatment*, *17*, 1–7. DOI: 10.1177/1533033818802789 PMID: 30261827

Shah, A. A., Shaker, A. S. A., Jabbar, S., Abbas, Q., Al-Balawi, T. S., & Celebi, M. E. (2023). An ensemble-based deep learning model for detection of mutation causing cutaneous melanoma. *Scientific Reports*, *13*(1), 22251. Advance online publication. DOI: 10.1038/s41598-023-49075-4 PMID: 38097641

Sharma, S., & Bhadula, S. (2023b). Secure Federated Learning for Intelligent Industry 4.0 IoT Enabled Self Skin Care Application System. In 2023 2nd International Conference on Applied Artificial Intelligence and Computing (ICAAIC), 1164–1170. https://doi.org/DOI: 10.1109/ICAAIC56838.2023.10141028

Sharma, S., Tomar, M., & Tyagi, R. (2024a). Deep Learning Enabled Personalized Clinical Decision Making and Prescription Plan Preparation System for Diagnosis of Skin Cancer Patients. In *2024 IEEE International Conference on Interdisciplinary Approaches in Technology and Management for Social Innovation (IATMSI)*, 1–6. https://doi.org/DOI: 10.1109/IATMSI60426.2024.10502738

Shehab, L. H., Fahmy, O. M., Gasser, S. M., & El-Mahallawy, M. S. (2021). An efficient brain tumor image segmentation based on deep residual networks (ResNets). *Journal of King Saud University. Engineering Sciences*, *33*(6), 404–412. DOI: 10.1016/j.jksues.2020.06.001

Shilo, S., Rossman, H., & Segal, E. (2020). Axes of a revolution: Challenges and promises of big data in healthcare. *Nature Medicine*, *26*(1), 29–38. DOI: 10.1038/s41591-019-0727-5 PMID: 31932803

Sigi, R., & Bachtiar, M. M. F. & Md Fikri. (2018). Identification of leukemia diseases based on microscopic human blood cells using image processing. In *2018 IEEE International Conference on Communication and Signal Processing (ICCSP)* (pp. xxx–xxx). IEEE. https://doi.org/DOI: 10.1109/ICCSP.2018.xxxxx

Singh, M., Vyas, C., & Mazumdaar, B. D. (2024, February). Mental Health Assessment Using EEG Sensor and Machine Learning. In *International Conference On Innovative Computing And Communication* (pp. 199-216). Singapore: Springer Nature Singapore. DOI: 10.1007/978-981-97-3817-5_13

Singh, J., Sandhu, J. K., & Kumar, Y. (2024). Metaheuristic-based hyperparameter optimization for multi-disease detection and diagnosis in machine learning. *Service Oriented Computing and Applications*, *18*(2), 163–182. DOI: 10.1007/s11761-023-00382-8

Singh, S., Sharma, S., & Bhadula, S. (2022). Automated Deep Learning based Disease Prediction Using Skin Health Records: Issues, Challenges and Future Directions. *2022 International Conference on Electronics and Renewable Systems (ICEARS)*. https://doi.org/DOI: 10.1109/ICEARS53579.2022.9752422

Sirocchi, C., Bogliolo, A., & Montagna, S. (2024). Medical-informed machine learning: Integrating prior knowledge into medical decision systems. *BMC Medical Informatics and Decision Making*, *24*(S4, Suppl 4), 186. DOI: 10.1186/s12911-024-02582-4 PMID: 38943085

Skender, B., & Zhang, M. (2024). From local issue to global challenge: A brief overview of antibiotic shortages since the 1970s. *Humanities & Social Sciences Communications*, *11*(1), 1–6. DOI: 10.1057/s41599-024-03759-y

Snoek, J., Larochelle, H., & Adams, R. P. (2012). Practical Bayesian optimization of machine learning algorithms. *Advances in Neural Information Processing Systems*, •••, 25.

Soh, W. K., Yuen, H. Y., & Rajapakse, J. C. (2023). HUT: Hybrid UNet-transformer for brain lesion and tumor segmentation. *Heliyon*, *9*(12), e22412. DOI: 10.1016/j.heliyon.2023.e22412 PMID: 38046150

Son, C. S., Kang, W. S., Lee, J. H., & Moon, K. J. (2022). Machine learning to identify psychomotor behaviors of delirium for patients in long-term care facility. *IEEE Journal of Biomedical and Health Informatics*, *26*(4), 1802–1814. DOI: 10.1109/JBHI.2021.3116967 PMID: 34596563

Sorour, S. E., Hany, A. A., Elredeny, M. S., Sedik, A., & Hussien, R. M. (2023). An automatic dermatology detection system based on deep learning and computer vision. *IEEE Access : Practical Innovations, Open Solutions*, *11*, 137769–137778. DOI: 10.1109/ACCESS.2023.3340735

Srinivasa Rao, P. C., Sravan Kumar, A. J., Niyaz, Q., Sidike, P., & Devabhaktuni, V. K. (2021). Binary chemical reaction optimization based feature selection techniques for machine learning classification problems. *Expert Systems with Applications*, *167*, 114169. DOI: 10.1016/j.eswa.2020.114169

Stathopoulos, I., Serio, L., Karavasilis, E., Kouri, M. A., Velonakis, G., Kelekis, N., & Efstathopoulos, E. (2024). Evaluating Brain Tumor Detection with Deep Learning Convolutional Neural Networks Across Multiple MRI Modalities. *Journal of Imaging*, *10*(12), 296. DOI: 10.3390/jimaging10120296 PMID: 39728193

Storn, R., & Price, K. (1997). Differential Evolution - A Simple and Efficient Heuristic for Global Optimization over Continuous Spaces. *Journal of Global Optimization*, *11*(4), 341–359. DOI: 10.1023/A:1008202821328

Subramanian, A., Nirantharakumar, K., Hughes, S., Myles, P., Williams, T., Gokhale, K. M., Taverner, T., Chandan, J. S., Brown, K., Simms-Williams, N., Shah, A. D., Singh, M., Kidy, F., Okoth, K., Hotham, R., Bashir, N., Cockburn, N., Lee, S. I., Turner, G. M., & Haroon, S. (2022). Symptoms and risk factors for long COVID in non-hospitalized adults. *Nature Medicine*, *28*(8), 1706–1714. DOI: 10.1038/s41591-022-01909-w PMID: 35879616

Sufi, F., & Khalil, I. (2011). Faster person identification using compressed ECG in time critical wireless telecardiology applications. *Journal of Network and Computer Applications*, *34*(1), 282–293. DOI: 10.1016/j.jnca.2010.07.004

Sun, X., Hu, C., He, W., Yuan, Z., & Zhang, J. (2024). Multimodal Connectivity-Guided Glioma Segmentation From Magnetic Resonance Images via Cascaded 3D Residual U-Net. *International Journal of Imaging Systems and Technology*, *34*(6), e23206. DOI: 10.1002/ima.23206

Taha, B. A., Kadhim, A. C., Addie, A. J., Haider, A. J., Azzahrani, A. S., Raizada, P., & Arsad, N. (2024). Advancing cancer diagnostics through multifaceted optical biosensors supported by nanomaterials and artificial intelligence: A panoramic outlook. *Microchemical Journal*, *205*, 111307. DOI: 10.1016/j.microc.2024.111307

Tahosin, M. S., Sheakh, M. A., Islam, T., Lima, R. J., & Begum, M. (2023). Optimizing brain tumor classification through feature selection and hyperparameter tuning in machine learning models. *Informatics in Medicine Unlocked*, *43*, 101414. DOI: 10.1016/j.imu.2023.101414

Talaat, F. M., & Gamel, S. A. (2024). Machine learning in detection and classification of leukemia using C-NMC_Leukemia. *Multimedia Tools and Applications*, *83*(3), 8063–8076. DOI: 10.1007/s11042-023-15923-8

Tang, C., Li, B., Sun, J., Wang, S. H., & Zhang, Y. D. (2023). GAM-SpCaNet: Gradient awareness minimization-based spinal convolution attention network for brain tumor classification. *Journal of King Saud University. Computer and Information Sciences*, *35*(2), 560–575. DOI: 10.1016/j.jksuci.2023.01.002 PMID: 37215946

Tanguturi, R. C., & Poornima, G. (2022). An intelligent system for remote monitoring of patients' health and the early detection of coronary artery disease. In *Proceedings of the 2022 International Conference on Smart Generation Computing, Communication and Networking (SMART GENCON)* (pp. 1–6).

Tankala, S., Pavani, G., Biswal, B., Siddartha, G., Sahu, G., Subrahmanyam, N. B., & Aakash, S. (2022). A novel depth search based lightweight CAR network for the segmentation of brain tumor from MR images. *Neuroscience Informatics (Online)*, *2*(4), 100105. DOI: 10.1016/j.neuri.2022.100105

Tao, W., Li, C., Song, R., Cheng, J., Liu, Y., Wan, F., & Chen, X. (2020). EEG-based emotion recognition via channel-wise attention and self-attention. *IEEE Transactions on Affective Computing*, *14*(1), 382–393. DOI: 10.1109/TAFFC.2020.3025777

Thanka, M. R., Edwin, E. B., Ebenezer, V., Sagayam, K. M., Reddy, B. J., Günerhan, H., & Emadifar, H. (2023). A hybrid approach for melanoma classification using ensemble machine learning techniques with deep transfer learning. *Computer Methods and Programs in Biomedicine Update*, *3*, 100103. DOI: 10.1016/j.cmpbup.2023.100103

Topaloglu, H., & Powell, W. B. (2006). Dynamic-programming approximations for stochastic, time-staged integer multicommodity flow problems. *INFORMS Journal on Computing*, *18*(1), 31–42. DOI: 10.1287/ijoc.1040.0079

Topol, E. (2019). High-performance medicine: The convergence of human and artificial intelligence. *Nature Medicine*, *25*(1), 44–56. DOI: 10.1038/s41591-018-0300-7 PMID: 30617339

Topol, E. J. (2019). *Deep Medicine: How Artificial Intelligence Can Make Healthcare Human Again*. Basic Books.

Triantafyllidis, A. K., & Tsanas, A. (2019). Applications of machine learning in real-life digital health interventions: Review of the literature. *Journal of Medical Internet Research*, *21*(4), e12286. DOI: 10.2196/12286 PMID: 30950797

Tripathy, J., Balasubramani, M., Aravinda Rajan, V., Vimalathithan, S., Aeron, A., & Arora, M. (2024). Reinforcement learning for optimizing real-time interventions and personalized feedback using wearable sensors. *Measurement. Sensors*, *33*, 101151. DOI: 10.1016/j.measen.2024.101151

Tripathy, S., Singh, R., & Ray, M. (2023). Automation of brain tumor identification using EfficientNet on magnetic resonance images. *Procedia Computer Science*, *218*, 1551–1560. DOI: 10.1016/j.procs.2023.01.133

Tseng, C. J., & Tang, C. (2023). An optimized XGBoost technique for accurate brain tumor detection using feature selection and image segmentation. *Healthcare Analytics*, *4*, 100217. DOI: 10.1016/j.health.2023.100217

Tubishat, M., Alswaitti, M., Mirjalili, S., Al-Garadi, M. A., Alrashdan, M. T., & Rana, T. A. (2020). Dynamic butterfly optimization algorithm for feature selection. *IEEE Access : Practical Innovations, Open Solutions*, *8*, 194303–194314. DOI: 10.1109/ACCESS.2020.3033757

Tuncer, T., Dogan, S., Ozyurt, F., Belhaouari, S. B., & Bensmail, H. (2020). *Novel multi center and threshold ternary pattern based method for disease detection using voice*. IEEE., DOI: 10.1109/ACCESS.2020.2992641

V, S., H, R., & G, S. R. (2019). Fruit and Leaves Disease Prediction Using Deep Learning Algorithm. *International Research Journal of Multidisciplinary Technovation, 1*(5), 8–16. .DOI: 10.34256/irjmt1952

Vamathevan, J., Clark, D., Czodrowski, P., Dunham, I., Ferran, E., Lee, G., Li, B., Madabhushi, A., Shah, P., Spitzer, M., & Zhao, S. (2019). Applications of machine learning in drug discovery and development. *Nature Reviews. Drug Discovery*, *18*(6), 463–477. DOI: 10.1038/s41573-019-0024-5 PMID: 30976107

Vardiman, J. W., Thiele, J., Arber, D. A., Brunning, R. D., Borowitz, M. J., Porwit, A., Harris, N. L., Le Beau, M. M., Hellström-Lindberg, E., Tefferi, A., & Bloomfield, C. D. (2009). The 2008 revision of the World Health Organization (WHO) classification of myeloid neoplasms and acute leukemia: Rationale and important changes. *Blood, 114*(5), 937–951. DOI: 10.1182/blood-2009-03-209262 PMID: 19357394

Vaswani, A., Shazeer, N., Parmar, N., Uszkoreit, J., Jones, L., Gomez, A. N., & Polosukhin, I. (2017). Attention is all you need. *Advances in Neural Information Processing Systems*, •••, 30.

Veerankutty, F. H., Jayan, G., Yadav, M. K., Manoj, K. S., Yadav, A., Nair, S. R. S., Shabeerali, T. U., Yeldho, V., Sasidharan, M., & Rather, S. A. (2021). Artificial Intelligence in hepatology, liver surgery and transplantation: Emerging applications and frontiers of research. *World Journal of Hepatology, 13*(12), 1977–1990. DOI: 10.4254/wjh.v13.i12.1977 PMID: 35070002

Vijaya, J., & Rao, M. (2022, November). Heart disease prediction using clustered particle swarm optimization techniques. In *2022 IEEE 6th Conference on Information and Communication Technology (CICT)* (pp. 1-5). IEEE. DOI: 10.1109/CICT56698.2022.9997925

Vijaya, J., Chandra, S., & Baghel, P. (2023, April). Diabetes disease prediction using various metaheuristic optimization algorithms. In *2023 IEEE 8th International Conference for Convergence in Technology (I2CT)* (pp. 1-6). IEEE. DOI: 10.1109/I2CT57861.2023.10126222

Vijaya, J., Nitnaware, V., & Chaddha, R. (2023, July). Optimization Techniques on Heart Failure Prediction. In *2023 14th International Conference on Computing Communication and Networking Technologies (ICCCNT)* (pp. 1-6). IEEE. DOI: 10.1109/ICCCNT56998.2023.10308079

Vijaya, J., Tirkey, D., Singh, P., & Goel, A. (2023, March). Diabetes Prediction Using Nature-Inspired Optimization Algorithms. In *2023 3rd International conference on Artificial Intelligence and Signal Processing (AISP)* (pp. 1-5). IEEE. DOI: 10.1109/AISP57993.2023.10135000

Vijaya, J. (2023, January). Heart disease prediction using clustered genetic optimization algorithm. In *2023 International Conference on Intelligent and Innovative Technologies in Computing, Electrical and Electronics (IITCEE)* (pp. 1072-1077). IEEE. DOI: 10.1109/IITCEE57236.2023.10091050

Vijaya, J., Rishabh, K., & Parashar, P. (2023, August). CanScan: Non-Invasive Techniques for Oral Cancer Detection. In *2023 International Conference on Electrical, Electronics, Communication and Computers (ELEXCOM)* (pp. 1-5). IEEE. DOI: 10.1109/ELEXCOM58812.2023.10370254

Vu, H. A., & Vajda, S. (2024, December). Advancing Brain Tumor Diagnosis: A Hybrid Approach Using Edge Detection and Deep Learning. In *International Conference on Pattern Recognition* (pp. 226-241). Cham: Springer Nature Switzerland.

Walsh, J., Othmani, A., Jain, M., & Dev, S. (2022). Using U-Net network for efficient brain tumor segmentation in MRI images. *Healthcare Analytics*, *2*, 100098. DOI: 10.1016/j.health.2022.100098

Wang, L., Chen, M., Li, J., Zhang, W., Li, K., & Wang, Y. (2022). Chemotherapy scheduling optimization: Participatory problem formulation for patient-centered care. *Journal of Clinical Oncology Clinical Cancer Informatics*, *6*, e2100144.

Wang, L., Lin, Z. Q., & Wong, A. (2020). COVID-Net: A tailored deep convolutional neural network design for detection of COVID-19 cases from chest X-ray images. *Scientific Reports*, *10*(1), 19549. DOI: 10.1038/s41598-020-76550-z PMID: 33177550

Wang, X. W., Nie, D., & Lu, B. L. (2014). Emotional state classification from EEG data using machine learning approach. *Neurocomputing*, *129*, 94–106. DOI: 10.1016/j.neucom.2013.06.046

Wang, Z., Zhang, J., Chen, X., Li, K., Wang, Y., & Li, H. (2021). Human-in-the-loop optimization for medication alert customization using Bayesian optimization. *Journal of the American Medical Informatics Association : JAMIA*, *28*(9), 1825–1835.

Webb, R. J., Al-Asmakh, M., Banach, M., & Mazidi, M. (2024). Application of proteomics for novel drug discovery and risk prediction optimisation in stroke and myocardial infarction: A review of in-human studies. *Drug Discovery Today*, *29*(11), 104186. DOI: 10.1016/j.drudis.2024.104186 PMID: 39306234

Wu, L., Zhang, J., Wang, Y., Ding, R., Cao, Y., Liu, G., Liufu, C., Xie, B., Kang, S., Liu, R., Li, W., & Guan, F. (2024). Pneumonia detection based on RSNA dataset and anchor-free deep learning detector. *Scientific Reports*, *14*(1), 1929. Advance online publication. DOI: 10.1038/s41598-024-52156-7 PMID: 38253758

Xia, B., Innab, N., Kandasamy, V., Ahmadian, A., & Ferrara, M. (2024). Intelligent cardiovascular disease diagnosis using deep learning enhanced neural network with ant colony optimization. *Scientific Reports*, *14*(1), 21777. DOI: 10.1038/s41598-024-71932-z PMID: 39294203

Xie, L., Li, Z., Zhou, Y., He, Y., & Zhu, J. (2020). Computational Diagnostic Techniques for Electrocardiogram Signal Analysis. Sensors 2020, Vol. 20, Page 6318, 20(21), 6318. DOI: 10.3390/s20216318

Xu, J., Chiu, S. Y., & Glover, F. (1998). Fine-tuning a Tabu Search Algorithm with Statistical Tests. *International Transactions in Operational Research*, *5*(3), 233–244. DOI: 10.1111/j.1475-3995.1998.tb00117.x

Yang, D., Zhang, W., Wang, Y., Li, J., Chen, M., & Wang, Z. (2021). Genetic algorithm with epistasis for Alzheimer's disease detection from multimodal brain imaging. *IEEE Transactions on Medical Imaging*, *40*(10), 2655–2667.

Yang, H., Han, J., & Min, K. (2019). A multi-column CNN model for emotion recognition from EEG signals. *Sensors (Basel)*, *19*(21), 4736. DOI: 10.3390/s19214736 PMID: 31683608

Yang, W., Joo, M., Kim, Y., Kim, S. H., & Chung, J.-M. (2020). Hybrid machine learning scheme for classification of BECTS and TLE patients using EEG brain signals. *IEEE Access : Practical Innovations, Open Solutions*, *8*, 218924–218935. DOI: 10.1109/ACCESS.2020.3038948

Yu, C., & Wang, M. (2022). Survey of emotion recognition methods using EEG information. *Cognitive Robotics*, *2*, 132–146. DOI: 10.1016/j.cogr.2022.06.001

Zarshenas, A., & Suzuki, K. (2016). Binary coordinate ascent: An efficient optimization technique for feature subset selection for machine learning. *Knowledge-Based Systems*, *110*, 191–201. DOI: 10.1016/j.knosys.2016.07.026

Zhang, H., Li, Q., & Zhou, X. (2020). Particle swarm optimization for hyperparameter tuning in deep learning-based disease classification. *Neural Computing & Applications*, *32*(18), 14567–14579.

Zhang, K., Li, J., Chen, S., Wang, Y., Zhang, W., & Wang, Z. (2022). Implementation mapping for sepsis management optimization: Systematic barrier identification and targeted strategies. *Implementation Science : IS*, *17*(1), 31. PMID: 35550164

Zhang, Y., Chen, J., Tan, J. H., Chen, Y., Chen, Y., Li, D., Yang, L., Su, J., Huang, X., & Che, W. (2020). An investigation of deep learning models for EEG-based emotion recognition. *Frontiers in Neuroscience*, *14*, 622759. DOI: 10.3389/fnins.2020.622759 PMID: 33424547

Zhang, Y., Shen, H., & Wu, T. (2020). Deep learning architectures for protein structure prediction. *Bioinformatics (Oxford, England)*, *36*(6), 181–189. DOI: 10.1093/bioinformatics/btz729

Zhan, Z. H., Zhang, J., Li, Y., & Chung, H. S. H. (2009). Adaptive particle swarm optimization. *IEEE Transactions on Systems, Man, and Cybernetics. Part B, Cybernetics*, *39*(6), 1362–1381. DOI: 10.1109/TSMCB.2009.2015956 PMID: 19362911

Zhao, Y., Chaw, J. K., Liu, L., Chaw, S. H., Ang, M. C., & Ting, T. T. (2024). Systematic literature review on reinforcement learning in non-communicable disease interventions. *Artificial Intelligence in Medicine*, *154*, 102901. DOI: 10.1016/j.artmed.2024.102901 PMID: 38838400

Zhou, T., Zhang, W., Li, J., Chen, X., Wang, Y., & Wang, Z. (2023). Nested optimization for healthcare facility layout with Bayesian optimization and genetic algorithms. *Health Care Management Science*, *26*(2), 244–258.

Zhu, W., Huang, Y., Zhang, H., Li, Y., Tian, H., Liu, G., & Wang, P. (2020). A novel genetic algorithm-based optimization framework for the discovery of circulating biomarker panels in early hepatocellular carcinoma. *ACS Omega*, *5*(28), 17470–17477.

Zou, H., & Hastie, T. (2005). Regularization and Variable Selection Via the Elastic Net. *Journal of the Royal Statistical Society. Series B, Statistical Methodology*, *67*(2), 301–320. DOI: 10.1111/j.1467-9868.2005.00503.x

About The Contributors

Anandhavalli Muniasamy is an Associate Professor in the Department of Computer Science at King Khalid University (KKU), Saudi Arabia. She holds a Ph.D. in Computer Science and Engineering from Sikkim Manipal University, India. Her research interests span data mining, data analytics, artificial intelligence (AI), soft computing, and data science, with a focus on machine learning and deep learning for advanced data analysis and medical data analysis. She has published over 35 articles in international journals and book chapters and presented at more than 30 national and international conferences. Dr. Muniasamy has led several university-funded projects and served as Principal Investigator for an AICTE-funded project. She is a reviewer for reputed journals, a Ph.D. thesis examiner, and an editorial board member. She actively contributes to organizations such as IAENG, CSI, and IACSIT.

***

Adnan Ibrahim Alrabea received the Dr. Eng. Degree in 2004 from the Electronic and Communication Department, Faculty of Engineering, Donetsk University, Ukraine. He is Visiting Associate Professor, Vice 0f Dean and assistant of dean at Prince Abdullah Bin Ghazi College of Communications and Information Technology at Al-Balqa Applied University, As-Salt, Jordan. His research interests cover: analyzing the various types of analytic and discrete event simulation techniques, performance evaluation of communication networks, application of intelligent techniques in managing computer communication network, and performing comparative studies between various policies and strategies of routing, congestion control, sub netting of computer communication networks. He published 30 articles in various refereed international journals and conferences covering: Computer Networks, Expert Systems, Software Agents, E-learning, Image processing, wireless sensor networks and Pattern Recognition. Also, in the current time, he is too interested in making a lot of scientific research in wireless sensor networks in view point of enhancing its algorithms of congestion control as well as routing protocols.

Neepa Biswas has done her B.Tech in Information Technology WBUT, M.E. in Information Technology from IIEST Shibpur, She has completed PhD from Jadavpur University. Her research Interest Data Warehousing, Data mining, Ad-hoc Network, Machine Learning etc. Currently working as Assistant Professor in Narula Institute of Technology, in West Bengal, Kolkata, India.

Sudarsan Biswas has completed his Bachelor of Engineering (IT) from Bengal Engineering and Science University, Shibpur in 2006 and his Master of Engineering (IT) from Bengal Engineering and Science University, Shibpur in 2010. Currently he is working as an Assistant Professor Department of IT, RCC Institute of Information Technology, Kolkata, West Bengal, India. His research domain is Data mining, Data warehousing and Cryptography.

Bhavya Chauhan is an MTech student at the International Institute of Information Technology, Naya Raipur, India.

Anitha D is an esteemed academician and researcher in the field of Computational Intelligence. She currently serves as an Assistant Professor in the Department of Computational Intelligence at SRM Institute of Science and Technology (SRMIST), Kattankulathur, Chennai. With a strong educational background, she earned her Ph.D. in Computer Science and Engineering from Vels Institute of Science, Technology & Advanced Studies in 2022.Dr. Anitha's research expertise spans across Machine Learning, Big Data Analytics, Data Mining, Network Security, and Wireless Sensor Networks. Her academic contributions include numerous research publications in reputed journals and conferences, along with innovative patents in areas such as IoT-based forest conservation and crop recommendation systems

G.Prema holds PhD in Faculty of Information and Communication Engineering from Anna University Chennai. Currently, she is working as Assistant Professor at the Department of Electronics and Communication Engineering, Mepco Schlenk Engineering College, Sivakasi. She has 11 years teaching experience. Her research interest includes image Processing, machine learning, image fusion, pattern recognition. She has published about 20 papers in the journal/conference at the national and international level.

Shruthi A.G. is a final-year MBBS student at Mahsa University with a strong interest in the integration of artificial intelligence (AI) in the medical field. She has actively contributed to impactful research, including the chapters "Enhancing

Medical Sector Efficiency: A Comprehensive Case Study Based on Data Visualization Tools for Business Applications" (DOI: 10.4018/979-8-3693-6537-3.ch011) and "Enhancing Business Applications in ENT Diseases Management Through Data Visualization" (DOI: 10.4018/979-8-3693-6537-3.ch010). Shruthi is dedicated to leveraging innovative technologies such as AI and data visualization to enhance healthcare delivery and improve patient outcomes.

Dankan Gowda V is currently working as an Assistant Professor in the Department of Electronics and Communication Engineering at BMS Institute of Technology and Management in Bangalore. Previously, he worked as a Research Fellow at ADA DRDO and as a Software Engineer at Robert Bosch. With a total experience of 14 years, including teaching and industry, Dr. Gowda has made significant contributions to both academia and research. He has published over 120 research papers in renowned international journals and conferences. In recognition of his innovative work, Dr. Gowda has been granted six patents, including four from Indian authorities and two international patents. His research interests primarily lie in the fields of IoT and Signal Processing, where he has conducted workshops and handled industry projects. Dr. Gowda is passionate about teaching and strives to create an engaging and effective learning environment for his students. He consistently seeks opportunities to enhance his knowledge and stay updated with the latest advancements in his field.

Venkatesan H. has completed his BHMS, MD (Hom) (Practice of Medicine) and PhD (Hom) at Vinayaka Mission's Homoeopathic Medical College and Hospital, Salem, Tamilnadu, India. He was the 1st Rank Holder in both BHMS (2007) & MD (Hom) (2010) and was awarded with Gold medals for the same. He has additionally acquired Post Graduate Diploma in Bio-statistics at Madurai Kamaraj University on 2015. He has joined as Assistant Professor on 2010 and currently working as Professor and Head, Department of Practice of Medicine at the same College. He is also serving as PG Guide, PhD Supervisor and Research Coordinator of the Institute. He has been the Principle Investigator of 10 Research Projects. He has more than 30 Peer Reviewed and Indexed Publications. He has also Presented Various Research Papers at National and International Conferences and Seminars. His areas of interest are Artificial Intelligence in Health Care Sector, In Vitro Analysis, Medical Imging Techniques, Health care IoT, AI in Helath Care and Standardization of Herbal Medicines, Medical Research Methodology, Design of Experiments & Research Writing.

Shanmugasundaram Hariharan received his B.E degree specialized in Computer Science and Engineering from Madurai Kammaraj University, Madurai,

India in 2002, M.E degree specialized in the field of Computer Science and Engineering from Anna University, Chennai, India in 2004. He holds his Ph.D degree in the area of Information Retrieval from Anna University, Chennai, India. He is a member of IAENG, IACSIT, ISTE, CSTA and has 17 years of experience in teaching. Currently he is working as Professor in Department of Computer Science and Engineering, Vardhaman College of Engineering, Hyderabad, India. His research interests include Information Retrieval, Data mining, Opinion Mining, Web mining. He has to his credit several papers in referred journals and conferences. He also serves as editorial board member and as program committee member for several international journals and conferences.

J. Vijaya is an Assistant Professor in the Department of Data Science and Artificial Intelligence at DSPM IIIT-Naya Raipur, C. G. India. She obtained her Ph.D. degree from National Institute of Technology-Tiruchirappalli; India in the area of Data Science. She completed her Bachelor's degree (Comp. Sci. & Engg.) from MS University-Tirunelveli, India and Masters Degree (Comp. Sci. & Engg.) from Anna University-Tiruchirappalli, India. Her current research interests are Data Analytics, Data Mining, Machine Learning Concepts, Soft computing Techniques, Neural networks and Deep learning, Metaheuristic and swarm Intelligence Algorithms, Evolutionary computation, Fuzzy logic and Rough set theory. Totally she has 13 years of teaching experience in various institution and universities. She is a Member of Indian Society of Technical Education (MISTE) and also she acted as a coordinator in various institute level committees. She has published research work in various reputed journals.

Gauthaman Karunakaran, currently serving as Director and Principal of Government Pharmacy College, Sajong, Sikkim, is a distinguished academician and researcher with 30 years of experience in teaching, research, and academic leadership. He holds a Ph.D. in Pharmacology from the University of Madras and has previously held key roles including Chairman of Pharmacology at KKU, KSA. His research contributions are notable, with an h-index of 22, over 2,100 citations, and 94 publications, along with five books and 8 chapters. He has received prestigious awards such as the CSIR Young Scientist Award, AICTE Career Award, and from national scientific bodies. He has completed 21 funded research projects and is actively involved in pharmacovigilance and drug safety monitoring initiatives in collaboration with national regulatory bodies. His management roles span curriculum development, academic affairs, and scientific advisory across institutions in India, the Middle East, and Africa.

A.V. Senthil Kumar is working as a Professor and Director, PG and Research Department of Computer Applications, Hindusthan College of Arts & Science, Coimbatore, Tamilnadu. To his credit he has industrial experience for five years and teaching experience of 27 years. He has also received his Doctor of Science (D.Sc in Computer Science). He has to his credit 50 Book Chapters, 225 papers in International and National Journals 64 papers in International Conferences in International and National Conferences, and edited 14 books and 2 Text books. He is as Associate Editor of IEEE Access. He is an Editor-in-Chief for many journals and Key Member for India, Machine Intelligence Research Lab (MIR Labs). He is an Editorial Board Member and Reviewer for various International Journals. He is also a Committee member for various International Conferences.

Krishna Kumari L, Completed UG and PG in the Domain of ECE, and pursuing PhD in the field of Machine learning for Biomedical applications.

Rohaya Latip She is currently an Associate Professor at the Department of Communication Technology and Network, Faculty of Computer Science and Information Technology, Universiti Putra Malaysia. She holds a Ph. D in Distributed Database and Msc. in Distributed System from Universiti Putra Malaysia. She graduated her Bachelor of Computer Science from University Technology Malaysia, Malaysia. She was the head of Department of Communication Technology and Network from 2017 until 2022. She served as an Associate Professor at Najran university, Kingdom of Arab Saudi from 2012 until 2013. She was the Head of HPC section in Universiti Putra Malaysia (2011-2012) and consulted the Campus Grid project and the Wireless for hostel in Campus UPM project. Her research interests include Big Data, Cloud, Fog and Edge Computing, Network Management, and Distributed Database. She has published more than 50 papers in international and national journals, proceedings and posters.

Suchismita Maiti has done her Bachelor of Engineering from University of Burdwan in 2002, M.E from Jadavpur University in 2006. She has completed PhD from National Institute of Technology, Durgapur. Her research Interest includes Medical image processing , Digital Image processing, Machine Learning, Deep learning etc. Currently she is working as Associate professor and HoD of the IT department in Narula Institute of Technology, in West Bengal, Kolkata, India.

Hari Krishnaa is currently pursuing B.E(ECE) in Mepco Schlenk Engineering College.

Pınar Özen Kavas is an Assistant Professor in the Department of Computer Engineering at Dumlupınar University, Turkey. She completed her Ph.D. in Electrical and Electronics Engineering, focusing on Biomedical Signal Processing. Her current research interests include Artificial Intelligence, Machine Learning, Biomedical Signal Processing, and related technologies.

R Gomalavalli Ramesh is a Associate professor at the Sri SaiRam Institute of Technology in chennai,India. 14 years of teaching experience at 5 Engineering colleges.Her Bachelor's degree in Electronics and Communication Engineering was earned at St. Peter's Engineering College in Avadi, Madras University. A master's degree in Medical Electronics and six years of research experience with a Ph.D in Medical Image Processing at Anna University's Guindy Campus in Chennai-600025.Her profile includes a collection of over 40 publications from national and international journals. These papers address a wide range of important issues, including Medical Image Processing, Medical Informatics, Biomedical Instrumentation, and Testing Instrumentation. She is the owner of six Indian patents. She has reviewed for IJMI, MBEC, GIRATES, and other journals. Email id :gomalavalli@gmail.com

Kishore Kanna R. received his B.E. degree in Biomedical Engineering from Jerusalem College of Engineering, Anna University, India, in 2016, followed by his M.Tech degree in Biomedical Engineering from Bharath Institute of Science and Technology in 2018. He completed his Ph.D. in Biomedical Engineering from Bharath Institute of Higher Education and Research in 2022 and subsequently pursued postdoctoral research in Cognitive Computing Applications at Singapore Institute of Technology (SIT), completing this fellowship in April 2025. Dr. Kanna brings seven years of teaching experience to academia and currently serves as Assistant Research Professor at Vel Tech Rangarajan Dr. Sagunthala R&D Institute of Science and Technology, Avadi, Chennai. His scholarly contributions include 87 peer-reviewed publications, comprising 85 Scopus-indexed articles and 2 Web of Science-indexed papers in reputed international journals. He has actively participated in the global research community, presenting his work at over 30 international conferences organized by IEEE, Springer, and other prestigious organizations. Dr. Kanna's innovative research has resulted in significant intellectual property contributions, including 2 design patents and 3 utility patents filed in India. His research interests encompass Brain-Computer Interface systems, biomedical applications, cognitive engineering, electroencephalography (EEG), machine learning and deep learning applications, neurofeedback systems, and Internet of Things (IoT) technologies. His interdisciplinary approach combines engineering principles with cognitive sciences to advance the field of biomedical engineering and develop next-generation healthcare technologies.

Suraj Narayan S is currently pursuing B.E(ECE) in Mepco Schlenk Engineering College.

VelmuruganS.P. is currently working as an Associate Professor in the Department of Electronics and Communication Engineering at Kalasalingam Academy of Research and Education (Deemed to be University) TamilNadu. He received his B.E degree in Electronics and Communication Engineering from Anna University (P.E.T Engineering College), Chennai in 2009 and M.E. degree in Applied Electronics from Anna University (St.Joseph's college of Engineering), Chennai in 2011. He has completed his Ph.D in the area of Medical Image Processing at Kalasalingam Academy of Research and Education, Krishnankoil, TamilNadu. His research interests include Medical Image Processing, Machine Learning, Image Fusion, Soft Computing and Embedded systems. He has authored more than 30 research articles and published in reputed international and national journals. He is a member of the Institute of Electrical and Electronics Engineers (IEEE) and International Association of Engineers (IAENG)

Evin Şahin Sadık is an Assistant Professor in the Department of Electrical and Electronics Engineering at Dumlupınar University, Turkey. She completed her Ph.D. in Electrical and Electronics Engineering, focusing on Biomedical Signal Processing. Dr. Sadık's current research interests include Artificial Intelligence, Deep Learning, Biomedical Signal Processing, and related technologies.

Ayodeji Olalekan Salau received a B.Eng. degree in Electrical/Computer Engineering from the Federal University of Technology, Minna, Nigeria. He received his MSc and PhD degrees in Electronic and Electrical Engineering from the Obafemi Awolowo University, Ile-Ife, Nigeria. He is a registered professional engineer with the Council for the Regulation of Engineering in Nigeria (COREN), a member of the Institute of Electrical and Electronics Engineers (IEEE), and the International Association of Engineers (IAENG). Dr. Salau serves as a reviewer for various reputable international journals, and is Co-Chair and technical program committee member of various international conferences. Dr. Salau has authored 3 Academic books and has over 300 international research articles in major reputable international Journals, book series, and conferences. His research interests include research in the fields of computer vision, image processing, signal processing, artificial intelligence, and power systems engineering. In 2019, Dr. Salau's paper was awarded the best paper of the year in Cogent Engineering. In 2020, he received the Quarterly Franklin Membership from the Editorial Board of London Journals Press for top quality research output. Also in 2020, he received the International Research Award on New Science Inventions (NESIN) under the category of "Best

Researcher Award" given by ScienceFather. In 2022, he received the International Best Researcher Award given by the ISSN International Science & Technology Awarding body (IISTAC-2022). Also, he received the best researcher award for the year 2020-2022 from the Chancellor of Afe Babalola University, Ado-Ekiti (ABUAD), Nigeria. According to the SciVal (SCOPUS- Elsevier) analysis/ranking of academics, Dr. Salau is among the top researchers in Nigeria (ranked number 7 out of the top 500). Recently, Dr. Salau was ranked among the World's Top 2% Scientists in the field of Artificial Intelligence by Scopus Elsevier/Stanford University in 2023, 2024. More recently, Dr. Salau received the Award of 2nd Position in the category of Best AI researcher in Higher Education (Universities Category) in Nigeria on the 2025 AI awareness day, on 17th February, 2025, given by the National Association of AI Practitioners (NAAIP) in conjunction with the National Universities Commission (NUC) and TETFund. Currently, Dr. Salau works at Afe Babalola University as an Associate Professor in the Department of Electrical/Electronics and Computer Engineering.

Sachin Sharma has worked as a Professor at Amity School of Engineering and Technology, Amity University, Punjab, Mohali, India since January 2025. He also worked as Associate Dean of International Affairs and Professor, Department of Computer Science and Engineering at Graphic Era Deemed to be University, Dehradun, Uttarakhand, India from February, 2018 to January 2025. He has experience of 15+ years in industry and academia. He is also Co-founder and Chief Technology officer (CTO) of IntelliNexus LLC, Arkansas, USA based company. He also worked as a Senior Systems Engineer at Belkin International, Inc., Irvine, California, USA. He received his Philosophy of Doctorate (Ph.D.) degree in Engineering Science and Systems specialization in Systems Engineering from University of Arkansas at Little Rock, USA with 4.0 out 4.0 GPA and M.S. degree in Systems engineering from University of Arkansas at Little Rock with 4.0 out 4.0 GPA. Dr. Sharma has authored/coauthored over 270+ publications in the form of books, patents, and papers in refereed journals and conference proceedings. He holds 70+ US, Indian and international patents in the area of IoT, wireless communication.

Tripti Sharma is an MTech student at the International Institute of Information Technology, Naya Raipur, India.

Priyanka Singh is an Associate Professor in the Department of Civil Engineering at Amity University Uttar Pradesh, Noida, India. Dr. Singh holds a B.Tech(Civil Engineering), M.Tech (Structural Engineering) and Ph.D. in Structural Engineering. She further enriched her expertise through a Research Attachment Program at Universiti Teknologi PETRONAS, Malaysia, post doctorate. She has vast experience of 22 years of which 17 years is in Academics and 05 years in Industry. She has filed 04 patents on sustainable materials, showcasing her innovative approach and practical solutions. With over 100+ papers published in Scopus/SCI-indexed journals and conferences. She has been awarded with the prestigious SERB SIRE Fellowship for International Project at Universiti Teknologi PETRONAS, Malaysia, supported by the Science and Engineering Research Board (SERB), Department of Science and Technology, Government of India. She has organized and participated in more than 30 national and international conferences. She had also served as a Session Chair and Technical Committee member at several prestigious international conferences. She has also been awarded as World Class WOMEN ENGINEERSs by A. Lalitha Foundation.She is a Lifetime member of the Indian Concrete Institute, Indian Association of Structural Engineering, and the Indian Society for Technical Education. Moreover, she serves as an editor and reviewer for more than 20 Scopus and SCI-indexed journals, further attesting to her expertise and dedication to advancing research in her fie

Shruti Soni is an MTech student at the International Institute of Information Technology, Naya Raipur, India.

Rishi Thakur is an MTech student at the International Institute of Information Technology, Naya Raipur, India.

Pankaj Kumar Verma is an MTech student at the International Institute of Information Technology, Naya Raipur, India.

Index

A

Artificial intelligence 2, 8, 22, 30, 31, 32, 33, 39, 58, 59, 61, 63, 83, 91, 93, 94, 95, 96, 162, 163, 168, 195, 203, 225, 229, 231, 239, 240, 251, 254, 257, 259, 280, 283, 311, 336, 338, 340, 342, 343, 362, 364, 365, 367, 368

B

Blood Cancer 199, 200, 204, 226, 227, 228
Brain Tumor 60, 65, 257, 258, 260, 261, 262, 268, 273, 274, 275, 276, 277, 278, 279, 280, 281, 282, 283, 284, 285, 287, 288, 289, 290, 291, 292, 293, 294, 295, 297, 298, 303, 304, 307, 308, 309, 310, 311, 312, 313, 366
Brain tumor segmentation 282, 283, 287, 289, 290, 291, 292, 294, 297, 298, 304, 307, 308, 309, 310, 311, 312, 313

C

Cancer Prediction 72, 74, 100, 174, 198
Cardiac Arrest 54, 172, 194, 198
Classification 16, 17, 18, 19, 30, 32, 38, 39, 40, 41, 46, 47, 53, 58, 60, 61, 63, 64, 65, 67, 68, 69, 70, 80, 81, 82, 83, 86, 94, 97, 100, 104, 105, 112, 116, 119, 135, 136, 138, 142, 144, 145, 147, 148, 150, 153, 154, 155, 159, 162, 165, 166, 167, 168, 170, 173, 174, 177, 178, 181, 182, 183, 187, 190, 194, 195, 196, 197, 199, 200, 201, 202, 203, 204, 205, 206, 207, 208, 209, 212, 213, 214, 215, 216, 217, 218, 219, 220, 221, 222, 224, 225, 226, 227, 228, 231, 234, 235, 236, 237, 238, 253, 255, 261, 263, 265, 266, 268, 271, 273, 274, 275, 276, 278, 279, 280, 281, 282, 283, 284, 291, 293, 294, 295, 299, 300, 309, 310, 311, 312, 313, 316, 317, 318, 319, 320, 321, 322, 323, 324, 326, 328, 330, 331, 332, 333, 335, 336, 337, 338, 345, 347, 364, 366
Classification and Regression Trees 17
CNN 2, 7, 16, 17, 36, 38, 40, 41, 70, 119, 152, 182, 206, 207, 208, 209, 212, 213, 224, 226, 231, 234, 257, 260, 261, 262, 263, 264, 266, 267, 268, 271, 273, 274, 275, 276, 277, 279, 280, 281, 283, 285, 291, 293, 294, 295, 309, 310, 322, 323, 337
Convolutional neural network 7, 40, 119, 209, 212, 213, 224, 234, 236, 253, 260, 261, 262, 267, 274, 281, 283, 285, 313, 322, 365

D

Data Quality 5, 7, 54, 66, 339, 341, 342, 343, 349, 361
Deep learning 8, 9, 10, 11, 12, 19, 20, 21, 24, 25, 26, 28, 29, 30, 32, 36, 46, 53, 55, 58, 60, 61, 64, 65, 67, 68, 70, 75, 76, 77, 78, 79, 81, 82, 84, 86, 88, 89, 90, 91, 92, 93, 94, 95, 96, 97, 100, 106, 110, 111, 112, 113, 114, 119, 134, 135, 136, 144, 152, 153, 158, 159, 162, 163, 164, 167, 196, 197, 199, 202, 203, 204, 205, 206, 207, 208, 210, 212, 221, 222, 223, 224, 225, 226, 227, 228, 229, 231, 232, 235, 249, 252, 253, 254, 255, 273, 274, 277, 279, 280, 281, 282, 283, 284, 285, 288, 289, 290, 291, 292, 294, 295, 299, 305, 307, 309, 310, 312, 313, 322, 323, 324, 335, 336, 337, 342, 343, 345, 346, 350, 353, 354, 355, 356, 359, 362, 363, 364, 366
Dice coefficient 288, 289, 290, 291, 293, 299, 300, 302, 303, 307, 308, 313
Disease prediction 2, 7, 10, 15, 17, 29, 35, 36, 37, 38, 39, 41, 42, 43, 44, 48, 52, 53, 54, 55, 56, 57, 58, 61, 63, 64, 65, 67, 68, 71, 72, 73, 74, 75, 76, 78, 79, 80, 82, 83, 84, 85, 86, 88, 89, 90, 91, 92, 93, 94, 95, 96, 97, 100, 112, 137,

138, 151, 153, 158, 159, 163, 165, 169, 194, 254, 284, 344, 345, 351, 355

E

Early Detection System 241, 255
Edge Computing 339, 345, 356, 357, 358, 361, 363, 364
EEG Data 315, 316, 317, 322, 323, 324, 325, 332, 333, 334, 337, 338
Emotion Detection 322, 336, 338
Ensemble Learning 46, 94, 100, 134, 173, 198, 235, 317, 318, 333
Explainable AI 2, 6, 7, 14, 22, 24, 26, 27, 28, 34, 47, 54, 55, 57, 65, 94, 158, 223, 252, 277, 305, 339, 340, 341, 342, 350, 352, 353, 354, 355, 357, 361, 367

F

feature selection 12, 14, 15, 16, 36, 37, 39, 41, 42, 45, 46, 48, 55, 56, 58, 60, 61, 75, 77, 82, 89, 93, 97, 100, 105, 106, 108, 116, 120, 122, 123, 126, 135, 136, 137, 138, 139, 140, 141, 142, 143, 144, 145, 146, 147, 148, 149, 150, 151, 152, 153, 154, 155, 156, 157, 158, 159, 161, 162, 163, 164, 165, 166, 167, 168, 186, 187, 189, 194, 197, 227, 255, 282, 284, 293, 294, 311, 312, 321, 333, 337, 360, 366
federated learning 2, 6, 14, 19, 22, 24, 27, 32, 34, 41, 42, 54, 61, 65, 90, 101, 106, 110, 130, 254, 278, 283, 307, 309, 333, 339, 340, 341, 342, 345, 347, 348, 352, 353, 354, 355, 356, 357, 358, 359, 361, 363, 365, 367
filtering method 137, 159

G

genetic algorithms 2, 7, 10, 12, 21, 23, 36, 38, 41, 42, 45, 53, 61, 100, 103, 106, 109, 114, 116, 119, 123, 135, 136, 138, 163, 345, 355

H

Healthcare 1, 2, 4, 5, 6, 7, 8, 9, 10, 11, 12, 13, 14, 17, 19, 20, 21, 22, 23, 24, 25, 26, 27, 28, 29, 30, 31, 33, 37, 39, 41, 42, 43, 44, 45, 46, 48, 52, 53, 54, 55, 57, 58, 59, 60, 61, 64, 65, 66, 67, 68, 71, 72, 73, 74, 79, 80, 81, 82, 83, 84, 85, 88, 90, 91, 93, 94, 99, 100, 101, 102, 103, 104, 106, 107, 108, 109, 110, 111, 112, 113, 114, 116, 119, 120, 121, 122, 123, 124, 126, 127, 128, 129, 130, 131, 132, 133, 135, 137, 138, 152, 157, 158, 161, 181, 185, 187, 193, 216, 223, 229, 245, 246, 247, 248, 250, 251, 253, 259, 260, 278, 280, 281, 308, 312, 331, 332, 333, 339, 340, 341, 342, 343, 344, 345, 346, 347, 348, 349, 350, 351, 352, 353, 354, 355, 356, 357, 358, 359, 360, 361, 362, 363, 364, 365, 367, 368
healthcare analytics 37, 52, 61, 312, 354
Health care system 36
Hybrid feature selection 137, 157, 158, 159, 168
hyperparameter tuning 3, 12, 36, 39, 47, 48, 61, 100, 109, 113, 119, 123, 124, 126, 135, 153, 176, 214, 294, 300, 311, 345

K

Kidney Disease 74, 169, 170, 171, 173, 185, 186, 188, 193, 194, 195, 198

L

Leukemia 94, 153, 199, 200, 201, 202, 203, 204, 205, 206, 207, 208, 209, 211, 212, 214, 216, 218, 219, 221, 222, 223, 224, 225, 226, 227, 228, 259
Logistic Regression 2, 8, 17, 67, 70, 116, 152, 234

M

Machine learning 1, 2, 3, 4, 5, 7, 8, 9, 10, 13, 14, 15, 16, 17, 19, 20, 21, 22, 24, 25, 26, 27, 28, 29, 30, 31, 32, 33, 34, 35, 36, 37, 38, 39, 41, 44, 45, 46, 48, 53, 54, 55, 56, 58, 59, 60, 61, 62, 63, 64, 66, 67, 68, 69, 70, 71, 74, 75, 79, 83, 88, 90, 91, 92, 93, 94, 95, 97, 99, 100, 101, 102, 103, 104, 105, 106, 109, 110, 111, 114, 116, 119, 120, 123, 124, 126, 128, 132, 137, 138, 139, 150, 151, 158, 159, 161, 162, 163, 164, 165, 166, 167, 168, 169, 170, 171, 172, 173, 174, 175, 176, 177, 178, 179, 180, 181, 182, 183, 184, 185, 186, 187, 188, 190, 193, 194, 195, 196, 197, 198, 202, 203, 206, 210, 215, 225, 227, 228, 231, 234, 235, 240, 253, 254, 255, 259, 260, 262, 277, 281, 282, 285, 291, 293, 294, 309, 311, 313, 315, 316, 317, 319, 320, 321, 323, 324, 325, 326, 328, 329, 330, 331, 332, 333, 334, 335, 336, 337, 338, 339, 340, 341, 342, 343, 348, 351, 359, 360, 361, 362, 364, 365, 367, 368

Machine learning challenges 109

Magnetic Resonance Imaging 281, 282, 313

Medical Diagnosis 9, 12, 64, 67, 153, 161, 173, 198, 228, 279, 285

Medical Imaging 8, 10, 11, 20, 34, 65, 67, 72, 73, 74, 75, 76, 78, 99, 100, 108, 109, 119, 127, 135, 207, 274, 280, 285, 294, 295, 307, 309, 311, 313, 342, 343, 344, 345, 346, 347, 351, 353, 354, 355, 360, 364

Melanoma Prevention 241, 252, 255

Mental State Classification 316, 317, 324, 328, 330, 331, 332, 333, 335, 338

Model Performance Evaluation 338

O

optimization algorithm 37, 55, 60, 65, 81, 96, 101, 102, 104, 111, 129, 135, 138, 145, 147, 152, 153, 158, 161, 162, 163, 164, 165, 166, 167, 196, 227, 253, 255, 284, 312, 326, 337, 366

optimization challenges 128

optimization techniques 1, 2, 3, 4, 7, 9, 10, 11, 12, 13, 14, 20, 21, 23, 25, 36, 37, 38, 39, 48, 53, 55, 60, 62, 63, 65, 66, 68, 71, 81, 82, 96, 97, 99, 100, 103, 105, 106, 109, 111, 112, 127, 129, 138, 145, 147, 153, 158, 340, 341, 342, 343, 345, 347, 350, 354, 355, 356, 357, 358, 359, 360, 361, 368

P

Precision Medicine 38, 90, 158, 351, 356

Predictive Modeling 59, 93, 164, 339, 356

predictive models 9, 12, 20, 39, 44, 53, 55, 62, 74, 80, 94, 103, 105, 331, 345, 351, 356

Principal component analysis 15, 16, 31, 40, 75, 77, 206

R

Recurrent Neural Network 241, 242, 255

S

Support vector machine 29, 39, 67, 204, 236, 315, 317, 332, 336

Swarm Intelligence 53, 66, 87, 97, 146

T

Transfer Learning 60, 93, 97, 136, 167, 197, 203, 207, 212, 213, 223, 224, 227, 255, 258, 260, 262, 263, 264, 267, 268, 274, 276, 279, 280, 281, 282, 283, 284, 285, 304, 306, 309, 313, 333, 337, 340, 345, 347, 354, 364, 366, 368

U

UNet based segmentation model 313

W

wrapper method 150, 151, 154, 155, 159, 162, 165, 168

www.ingramcontent.com/pod-product-compliance
Lightning Source LLC
LaVergne TN
LVHW080909300926
849162LV00003B/614